Prader-Willi Syndrome:

Quality of Life

Prader-Willi Syndrome:
Quality of Life

Terrance N. James, PhD

Poplar Publishing
Courtenay, BC, Canada

First published in 2011 by
Poplar Publishing
2766 O'Brien Road
Courtenay, BC V9N 9H9
Tel/Fax: (250) 338-0597

For more information on Canadian publications on Prader-Willi syndrome please visit: www.prader-willi.ca

Library and Archives Canada Cataloguing in Publication

James, Terrance N. (Terrance Norman), 1944-
    Prader-Willi syndrome : quality of life / Terrance N. James.

Includes bibliographical references and index.
ISBN 978-0-9685838-2-1

1. Prader-Willi syndrome. 2. Prader-Willi syndrome--Patients--Biography.
3. Prader-Willi syndrome--Patients--Care. I. Title.

RJ520.P7J27 2010   618.92'85884   C2010-902226-2

Credits:
    Cover photograph: Seal Bay, Vancouver Island, by Charity Munro;
    Photograph p. 262 used with permission of Alumni Support,
    Calgary, Alberta.

Printed and bound in Canada by
Printorium Bookworks
Victoria, BC

Contents

List of Tables

List of Figures

Acknowledgements

This book is based on data collected from Canadian families with a member with PWS, over a period of 25 years. Families generously contributed intimate details of their lives in the interest of research, with the hope that others would be able to benefit from their experiences. They permitted agencies and service providers to share their perspectives in order that the whole story might be told. They contributed photographs which add "thousands of words" to the impact of this manuscript. They demonstrated a PWS reality, that there is a strength of character and common bond that exists within the PWS community. Their hospitality, sometimes into late evening hours, made the time spent most enjoyable. I am thankful for all of the families that I have met. Without their interest and support this project would not have been possible.

Thanks are extended to the agency staff and other service providers who also shared their experiences. Their insights helped to better understand policy issues and best practices. To those who perhaps do not get many thanks on a day-to-day basis, your contributions are acknowledged with appreciation.

To the parents who provided feedback on chapter drafts, and all of those who encouraged me in this project, I extend my gratitude.

To my wife and family who supported me in this undertaking, I thank you for your patience and understanding.

Preface

In 1985-86 I had the privilege of gathering information and stories from 51 families in western Canada with a child or adult with Prader-Willi syndrome. The fieldwork was a rich experience as I travelled through four provinces, visiting homes, schools and agencies. I met and observed people with Prader-Willi syndrome as they went about their daily lives. My dissertation, completed for the University of Calgary in 1987, was titled *Social and Psychological Aspects of Prader-Willi Syndrome*. This was followed a few years later by *Prader-Willi Syndrome: Home, School and Community* (1992), co-authored with Roy Brown. Wearing the hat of a part-time rehabilitation consultant working with this syndrome, I met and assisted individuals and families throughout western Canada for more than twenty-five years. Retiring from my position as Director of Student Services for a public school system, I wanted to re-visit the original 51 families and others that I had met over the years. I wanted to know what had happened to them in the intervening time span.

Locating families after 22 years, in an expanse of 4,000 kilometers, was not easy. I started with Canada 411, using the last known address and telephone number. Then I networked through contacts within existing parent groups. The possibility that some of the original group had passed away lead me to research obituaries from community newspapers. Contact with family members confirmed deaths of individuals with PWS and their parents. They also provided current contact information, and personal stories. I was struck by how easy it was to pick up from where I had left off with families so many years earlier. I was greeted in a warm and hospitable fashion everywhere I travelled.

I was able to account for 43 out of the original 51 participants (84%). I am still eager to find out about the rest. As I began to gather information about these older individuals and families I decided to make some comparisons with the experiences of younger families. Through contact with parent associations, another 25 families volunteered to meet with me. Interviews were held with all parents, and siblings, extended family members, care workers and agency staff when available. Stories from my case files on another 40 families were incorporated in the writing, along with stories of Canadian families obtained from newspaper and magazine articles. The experiences of more than 125 Canadian families were considered in preparing this manuscript.

This book was written primarily for parents, although it is hoped that professionals will benefit from its content as well. It contains a snapshot of current best management practices in Canada. Quality of life provides a logical framework as it addresses the essence of what parents wanted to talk about: the quality of life for their child and themselves. In this book parents will find a balance of stories about the joys and the heartaches of parenting a child with special needs. Ample photographs illustrate the normalcy of life activities

It is hoped that this book will provide encouragement to families. Perhaps parents will enjoy a new understanding, see new possibilities, locate new resources, experience a new thankfulness, or have a greater appreciation for the efforts of those who were the pioneers. Maybe professionals will see the need for changes to social policies and for meaningful applied research. Hopefully, together they will forge a new partnership to advocate for the needs of children and adults with PWS.

Terrance James
December 2010

1

Quality of life

When asked about their hopes and ambitions for their child with PWS parents will often reply with "a reasonable quality of life." It is interesting that the word "reasonable" is used. It reflects the parental awareness that "optimal" quality of life may be hard to attain. It suggests that perhaps yet unknown forces will have a role to play in determining the quality of life of their child. While most parents desire a "better" quality of life for their off-spring, there is perhaps the underlying recognition that this might never be possible.

"Reasonable" is a subjective word. It may mean something different to each one. To parents of a child with PWS it often means long-term economic security, stable residential accommodation, meaningful social activities, regular occupational activity, and rigid weight management. Indeed, a reasonable quality of life embraces all of these things, and more.

Parents commonly project quality of life expectations for their children. These reflect their hopes and dreams. They also have quality of life expectations for themselves. These are often more pragmatic, such as peace and harmony in the home, evenings out, and annual vacations. Quality of life is something we all have, albeit with a different focus or in differing degrees.

There is a general acknowledgement by professionals who have been associated with PWS over the long term that quality of life has improved over the last few decades. People with PWS have benefited from the changes in societal attitudes toward individuals with disabilities, which in Canada were enshrined in the federal Charter of Rights and Freedoms in 1984. The Charter, along with provincial and federal human rights legislation, protects against discriminatory practices and envisages a future with a better quality of life for people with disabilities.

In the same time period, the concepts of deinstitutionalization, normalization, least restrictive environment, and inclusionary practice have impacted educational, residential, social, and vocational services. They have created greater acceptance and increased opportunities for people with disabilities. Individuals with PWS now live in community and not in institutions, as in the past. Surely this means a better quality of life.

While the protection of individual rights has been applauded for most, it has created a moral–ethical debate among some parents, caregivers, and service providers. For example, should adults with PWS be denied access to food if they want it? Do individuals have the right to place their health at risk? At what point does the duty to care trump personal rights and freedoms? The answers to such questions are not simple.

What is quality of life?

Concerns for the quality of daily living have emerged from many disciplines over the last couple of decades. Quality of life provides a useful philosophical framework for considering a cradle to grave discussion of PWS. Much of what is understood about quality of life for individuals with disabilities has come from the study of intellectual disability, and as such should be of interest for families with a member with PWS.

Children begin to think about quality of life at a young age. As they compare their own situation to those of their friends they are intuitively assessing their own quality of life. As they beg, share, or manipulate to achieve the same benefits as their friends they are attempting to improve their own quality of life. As they outgrow the self-centredness of childhood they begin to engage in longer-term thinking and planning about quality of life. The choices made in secondary school regarding application to studies, participation in extra curricular activities, or socializing with friends are made to enhance quality of life. The longer-term considerations of post-secondary education, choosing a mate, or relocating for employment are based on a maturing understanding of quality of life.

Children and teens are seldom satisfied with their quality of life. Parents often hear "that's not fair," "why can't I...?" or "everyone else is doing it." As adults they may be concerned with "keeping up with the Joneses," "upward mobility," and "living beyond one's means." All of these clichés reflect quality of life considerations. To want to be the same as, or to want more or better, is part of North American culture. Everyone seems to want a better quality of life.

A consideration of quality of life must focus on what is important to the individual. To this end, personal stories have been included in this book from individuals with PWS, their parents and caregivers to illustrate quality of life in various domains. These domains are reflected in chapter headings.

A framework for understanding

The work of Brown and Brown (2003) presents a comprehensive framework for understanding key ideas and principles involved in a quality of life approach to working with individuals with disabilities. The guiding principle is that all humans are entitled to enjoy quality lives. They identify five key ideas as central to this approach:

- quality of life addresses aspects of life that all humans share
- quality of life also addresses aspects of life that are unique to individuals
- individuals can indicate what quality means for them and how they wish to achieve it
- all parts of our lives and environments are interconnected
- quality of life is ever-changing (p. 108).

There are common characteristics which contribute to everyone's quality of life; at the same time, there are unique individual needs and behaviours. In order for self-actualization to occur, individuals must be given the opportunity to define the quality of their own lifestyle across all environments. Given the dynamic nature of human life, quality of life will need to be constantly revisited as it changes with individual growth and circumstances.

Drawing from these key ideas, Brown and Brown (2003) formulate eight application principles. They assert that a quality of life approach:

- focuses most on what is important to the individual
- supports action that increases personal satisfaction and decreases dissatisfaction

- stresses that opportunities to improve must be within the individual's grasp
- insists that personal choice should be exercised, when ever possible, in selecting opportunities
- improves the person's self-image
- increases levels of personal empowerment
- considers life span implications; and
- recognizes inter- and intra-individual variability (p. 108).

These principles emphasize personal meaning, value, enjoyment, and happiness of life. They recognize that opportunities to grow are lifelong and dependent on the environment. They affirm the importance of the expression of personal will and the empowerment of the individual to make choices. They underscore the importance of a positive view of self and recognize the uniqueness of all individuals.

A quality of life approach is progressive, focusing first on "attaining the basic necessities of life," then progressing to "experiencing satisfaction with aspects of life that are important to the person," and ultimately to "achieving high levels of personal enjoyment and fulfillment" (Brown & Brown, 2003, p. 109). The goals of this quality of life approach are easily understood, by both practitioners and parents:

- personal needs met
- enjoyment/satisfaction
- personal meaning
- positive self-image
- social inclusion
- improved well-being (p. 109).

Parents and practitioners generally agree on the importance of these goals for the child or the client. In reading this book parents should also consider these goals as they apply to their own quality of life.

In short, quality of life has to do with an individual's enjoyment of, or satisfaction with, personal life circumstances. In the past, questionnaires have been used to glean information about quality of life, requiring respondents to choose or rate items from a range of possibilities thought to be important to a quality lifestyle. At best, they have provided a snapshot of what researchers interpret the subjects' quality of life to be. While such an approach can lead to quantification and inferential statistics it does little to describe the range of possibilities or illustrate the realities of daily living. In contrast, the present document places a high value on interviews and observations over time, and the corroboration of significant others who know the individuals well. The longitudinal approach reflects the changes that have occurred in individual lives and family circumstances, for better and for worse.

Dilemma #1: Whose quality of life?

As just indicated, a quality of life approach should focus on what is important to the individual. However, what is important to the person with PWS is not likely to be the same as what is important to the parents. Indeed, what is important to one parent, may not be important to the other. So a dilemma often occurs when considering the question of quality of life: Whose quality of life are we talking about?

Before the age of majority, a child is generally under the care of a parent, or parents. Thereafter, if an adult with PWS remains under the care of the parent(s) the underlying principle that "all" are entitled to enjoy a quality of life gives rise to a second question: Whose quality of life takes priority, that of the adult with PWS or of the parent(s)? While "all" are entitled to enjoy quality lives, the application of this fundamental principle is not easy. There may be confusion and conflict as a result. The dilemma is more complex when the household includes siblings, grandparents or other extended family members. How does the life of the child with PWS augment or diminish their quality of life?

There is a natural tendency to think of one's own quality of life first. Parents of adults with PWS often report improvements in their own quality of life as a result of an out-of-home placement of their son or daughter. The quality of life dilemma may persist, however, for the individual with PWS in the new context. House mates are entitled to quality in their lives too. Sometimes, when the actions of a person with PWS become too intrusive, whether in the parents' home or that of a caregiver, it may be necessary to change the placement.

There are many decisions that are made for or about children and adults with PWS that they are not happy about. These decisions, while considered necessary or important from a parent, staff, or professional point of view, may impinge on the quality of life of the individual.

Dilemma #2: Longevity of life versus quality of life

To individuals with PWS, quality of life may be more important than longevity of life. In other words, they may prefer to be happy, making their own choices and defining their own lifestyle, even though they may be placing their health at risk and shortening their life expectancy.

Without choices they argue that there can be no quality to life. For adults, parents, and professionals with a responsibility to care, this usually creates a dilemma - to what extent to impose controls, contrary to the individual's wishes, in order to protect health and longevity of life.

Quality of life for the person with PWS

Parents are often polarized on the issue of independence. Most say to value longevity of life necessarily requires restrictions and controls; others say to value independence and self-determination necessarily means acceptance of choices and risks. Neither position is inherently 'right.' Parents do, and always will, have an interest and a role to play in the life of their child. However, decisions made on behalf of their child may, or may not, be based on quality of life considerations. Often there are more important cultural, familial, religious, or community perspectives which influence decisions about the life of an individual with PWS.

Parents should be encouraged to think about quality of life while their child is young. This means reading about quality of life, wrestling with its theory, arguing its merits, and preparing a framework for personal decisions. Quality of life offers a holistic approach from which to operate.

Normalcy of expectations

Higher functioning teens with PWS often express normal expecta-tions – to graduate, get a job, move away from home, get married, and have a family. They see this pattern modelled by older siblings or extended family members. They also see it in television programs and in movies. The integration experience of most school systems often sets them up to have the same expectations. The practice of inclusion in high school opens equal access to courses, clubs, and activities with few restrictions. Parents, on the other hand, espouse a broad range of responses to inclusionary practices, from the idealists who want their child to have equal access to every opportunity in their quest for normalcy, to the realists who recognize a need for more pragmatic preparation for the future.

Parents play a critical role in helping to shape the lifestyle expectations of their PWS teen. They know their child best. They, and not the school system, are the experts on PWS. Teachers will not want to burst the bubble of expectations for a child. Few counsellors will have enough knowledge of PWS to be able to realistically talk about the possibilities of marriage, future employment, or residential options.. Rather, it is the parents who must be proactive in helping to support realistic expectations and redefine unrealistic ones.

Wants

In 1992, James and Brown included a chapter on quality of life which discussed the lives of twelve Canadian adults with PWS. The views of the individuals with PWS were corroborated by commentary from parents and caregivers. Their questionnaire results indicated that people with PWS wanted:

- emotional support
- greater range of leisure experiences
- help with practical aspects of home management
- greater independence
- ownership of personal belongings
- private living area.

Adults with PWS also expressed concern about their own temper tantrums. Most were optimistic, seeing their lives improving in the future, although this view was not necessarily shared by their parents. The authors cautioned that people with PWS in most cases are very different from one another and that each case should be treated on an individual basis within the context of family.

The desire for greater independence is still one of the most universal themes expressed by individuals with PWS. They are tired of close supervision all of the time. Like their non-handicapped peers, they want their own space and the opportunity to make their own decisions. This is, of course, a major quality of life concern.

Needs

PWS needs are usually understood from a parent perspective. For example, parent literature talks about the need for supervision, food access controls, and behaviour management strategies. While these interventions may be needed to help manage the syndrome according to the parents, they probably would not be viewed as needs from the PWS perspective. Similarly, doctors may explain that there is a need for medication, physiotherapists may say that specific exercises are needed, and dietitians may define the number of calories that are needed. While meeting such needs may improve the physical quality of life of a person with PWS, there may also be a negative impact on stress levels, behaviours, and relationships.

In the current study there were examples of individuals needing emotional support to deal with significant life event issues such as the death of a parent, a broken relationship, or issues of abuse. While it may be obvious that such specific events create needs which require support, there may be more subtle situations which generate needs that are overlooked. For example, the on-going lack of opportunity to be meaningfully involved in family discussions, continual treatment as a perennial child, or conflicts with siblings may drain the emotions of a teen or adult with PWS on a regular basis. Parents may not recognize the emotional needs and the individual may not be able to articulate the needs. To whom do they turn to get support to confront such issues?

Values

Not surprisingly, the questionnaire by James and Brown (1992) indicated that those with PWS value things in common with most adults:
- personal belongings
- private living area
- the ability to make choices and decisions over what one wants.

Social services policies support the normalcy of such expectations. Most importantly, however, do parents recognize and accept these same values for their child?

Sometimes quality of life becomes such a huge issue that the only resolution is to change residence and start over again. When new caregivers respect those things that people with PWS value, that is to say space for privacy, the accommodation of personal belongings, and the opportunity to make choices, then quality of life will improve for the new resident. Simultaneously, quality of life will improve in the family home. Most individuals with PWS in this book have experienced multiple residential placements in their adult years.

Choices

Teens and adults with PWS want to exercise personal decision making. They want to have choices in their lives. At age 40, John wrote:

> I want to have the CHOICE to decide what I want in my life. I want to have an apartment with my own support workers to help me keep myself and my apartment clean, to monitor my food intake and keep me safe. I know that I need someone to keep the cupboards locked, and I need someone to keep me active to control my weight. I want to have some fun in my life.

> I have the right to have the same CHOICES in life that you do. Without choices my right to freedom is being denied. Your child has the right to choose the quality of their life. (James, 2010, p. 93).

John had a clear understanding of the supports that he required and how he wanted those supports to be provided. He understood what would improve his quality of life. John was more articulate than many with PWS and he became an advocate in order to defend the rights of others with special needs to express their choices.

Growth and learning

Choices are also important for personal growth and learning. Those who are able to hold a full or part-time job, engage in entrepreneurial activities, or volunteer in the community are placed in situations where they must acquire additional skills and knowledge. When appropriate job tasks are assigned, and training provided, there are few complaints related to job performance. As will become apparent later in this book, it is the lack of opportunity for employment during tight economic times and the need for supervision which contribute to the vocational disappointments.

Learning doesn't stop when high school or college ends; most people with PWS are capable of continued learning into the adult years. By choice, some individuals have registered for academic upgrading, worker preparation programs, vocational skills training, or community recreation and leisure learning opportunities. They have earned certificates, diplomas, bursaries, and recognition awards. A lack of personal growth and learning is often a symptom of a lack of opportunity in the environment.

Independence versus inter-dependence

Public education teaches a strong ethic of independence; most teens are programmed toward independence before high school graduation. Families encourage this notion as they support camp, travel and exchange opportunities for their children. They maintain independence as the norm as they encourage leaving home after graduation, in order to pursue employment or post-secondary education.

Children with special needs are largely raised in the same culture of independence, yet they need to learn more about inter-dependence. They will need to depend on the support of family and friends, programs and services of community living, employment, and recreation agencies throughout their lifetime. Knowing how to appreciate, accept, and optimize the resources within a more inter-dependent model will contribute importantly to quality of life considerations.

Parents must wrestle with the inter-dependence versus independence positions. In doing so it is important to have a knowledge of what happens to adults with PWS, the social services available to support them, and a realistic view of the future family team.

♋

In order to know what individuals with PWS feel about their quality of life it is necessary to listen to them. Parents should neither project their own quality of life biases nor assume that they understand the quality of life concerns of their child. Entering into the dialogue, however, may be difficult.

The following chapters are organized according to widely recognized "domains" of life. They incorporate descriptive data, observations, and personal testimonies from Canadian families with a PWS member. Families have shared intimately in the interest of helping others. They have been quite clear about things that add to individual and corporate quality of life. Best practice can be inferred from their experiences.

2

Family

Today it is a given that children with special needs will live at home with their families. This was not always so. Some of today's seniors with PWS spent years in institutional settings removed from family life.

The presence of a family member with PWS affects families differently. While there may be some merit to talking about a behavioural phenotype, that is to say a common set of behavioural descriptors for PWS, it is more difficult to describe the impact of such behaviours on families. Each family circumstance is unique.

Not all families look the same. Families may be biological, adoptive or foster. In fact, they can be any group of people who consider themselves to be part of the family. "Uncle" or "auntie" may not be related by blood or marriage, but have been granted the status because of frequency and quality of involvement with the family. Others may function with a similar degree of intimacy without the honourary title.

Family quality of life is a composite of each individual's quality of life and the interaction effects that all the individuals bring. For example, work contributes in a large way to the quality of life of parents, and school to the quality of life of siblings. The experiences of a parent at work or a child in school contributes to their individual quality of life, but will also be a factor in the corporate family life. A mother or father who is under stress on the job will likely bring some of the tension into the home. Similarly, a child who has an unresolved major meltdown at the end of the school day may bring upheaval into the home, affecting siblings and parents. The recurrent nature of such episodes can be ongoing sources of stress and act as an emotional drain on family members.

With the birth of the first child, and each ensuing sibling, the dynamics of the family are altered. It is not unusual for family life to be centred on the needs of the member with PWS. The demands on everyone detracts from time, energy and resources available for preferred activities that would otherwise contribute to a higher quality of life for parents and siblings.

The level of care required to support a child with PWS in the family home may be beyond that encountered by families of children with other developmental disabilities. While life's course for many categories of special needs is well documented and professionals understand the nature of supports that are necessary to provide a high level of well-being, this is not necessarily the case with PWS.

Over the long haul, terms such as "chronic burden," "extended burden of care," and "lifelong responsibility" can be heard. This is particularly evidenced with parents who continue as caregivers for adults with PWS. The demands of caregiving also detract from the time and energy available for a spouse and other children. Siblings variously describe the impact of PWS on their own upbringing – some with good memories, some not so good.

Many families display a surprising resiliency to constant stressors. Some choose to make it on their own, and do not seek much help, while others take full advantage of all resources available. Family stories indicate differences in the availability of resources across provinces and communities.

Quality of life should have both short-term and long-term goals. Parents who sacrifice their own quality of life in the short term, without the benefits of long-term planning, shortchange themselves and place family quality of life at risk. To not take advantage of available respite, for example, might contribute to early parental burnout or breakdown in spousal or parent-child relations.

Parents

Today in Canada, people with mental handicaps live their childhood in a normalized fashion with their parents within the community, rather than in institutions. However, since the responsibility for social care programs is a provincial one there may be variations in care and support options across provinces. Teens and adults with PWS have acknowledged, and expressed appreciation for, the support of their families. Families fulfill two primary functions, those of caregivers and advocates.

Parents as caregivers

Parenting a child with PWS is a complex task involving all aspects of life. With the transition to adulthood, the same comprehensive approach to care is required, whether provided by the parents or others who are hired to do the task.

Many parents, seeing few residential options for their children with PWS, choose to keep their young adult at home. Parents often view a basement suite option as very desirable, affording a limited degree of independence and optimal degree of supervision. Such planning seems reasonable to parents as their child leaves the public education system and enters the adult world. Unfortunately, this long-term solution may lead to two significant difficulties:

- strained relations between child and parent, and
- dependency and helplessness upon death of the parent(s).

Whether the adult with PWS lives in the basement suite in their parents' home or upstairs with the family, the parents will always be in a parenting role. This usually leads to strained child and parent relations at some point in time. The parent, in providing supervision over food access and other aspects of the adult's life, may be resented. The adult with PWS may rebel against the eternal child role. Contrast this situation of parents as primary caregivers with a situation where the adult lives with another family or in the basement suite of another family's home. In this scenario, the parents are no longer the heavies enforcing the rules, as there is a third party in this role. The PWS adult enjoys a greater degree of independence and more normalized relations with the parents, even though the supervision level is still the same.

Perhaps the most tragic consequence of parental caregiving occurs when a parent dies or becomes incapacitated in their later years and the remaining spouse can no longer carry on with the required caregiving. Suddenly, the government system must find accommodation for a 40 or 50-year-old dependent adult, who has lived a very sheltered life. Having been denied the opportunity for greater independence, the individual is now more handicapped than many peers and faced with the trauma associated with the loss of a parent, disruption to home life, and adjustment to a new type of dependence or semi-independence.

But times are changing. Certainly government ministries want to prevent the previous scenario from occurring. Today social services policies empower individual choice and support more independent lifestyles. Younger parents are aware of this reality. In a recent Alberta study, parents of school-aged children expressed fear that socio-cultural norms and the desire for independence would no longer permit them to play such a protective role in the lives of their children in the future (Kinash, 2007c).

Parents as advocates

Parents play an important role as advocates for their children. For pioneer parents advocacy was important in seeking a diagnosis. James and Brown (1992) reported that patients saw an average of six physicians, including GPs and specialists before getting a diagnosis. Ten percent of couples saw more than 10 physicians. The highest number of medical practitioners seen was 30, for a woman who was not diagnosed until age 32. Thankfully, such persistence and advocacy is no longer required as most diagnoses now occur within the first year. The major areas of advocacy with the medical system are now the fight to establish eligibility for growth hormone treatment and appropriate medical care during emergencies.

Special education supports did not exist for the oldest individuals with PWS in the current study. Secondary special education may have denied the child the opportunity for twelve years of schooling, and educational assistants didn't exist in most jurisdictions prior to the 1980s. Older parents battled against social views that placed individuals with special needs in institutions or in segregated schools. They advocated for integrated settings and inclusionary practices. Today education continues to be one of the major areas of advocacy. Parents relate having to fight with school jurisdictions for educational assistant time, meaningful individualized programs, and food-free activities and environments.

Early advocacy was also needed with the social services system. The two main issues from the past, eligibility and funding, are still present today. Parents relate battling with the system in order to establish eligibility for services. Often they are frustrated because they assume that the diagnostic label of Prader-Willi syndrome will mean automatic services. While this may appear to happen in infancy, it does not occur in child and adult services. Parents have to be proactive and prove need in order to get services. And once services are in place there is the perennial concern about wait lists and reductions in service due to economic cut-backs.

In addition to advocacy aimed at government services, parents have always needed to be advocates for behavioural understanding and social inclusion with family, friends, and neighbours.

Parental conflicts

The presence of a child with special needs creates extra stresses in marriages. Some spouses will handle the pressures well, others will falter. Conflict may result. Some parents become closer as they fight the common enemy of PWS; others drift apart, and still others find their marriage disintegrating under the pressures. The quality of married life is affected by how couples handle the typical parental conflicts which follow.

Different values in child rearing. It is important for parents to "be on the same page" when it comes to child rearing. Often, however, there are different perceptions or philosophies on how to raise a child with special needs. This is understandable given that there are few courses on parenting and that most parents depend on the recollections of their own childhood experiences.

As the primary caregiver, often at home alone with the child, the mother may feel resentment, frustration, or anger toward her spouse for being absent, being "too soft," or not adhering to similar behavioural controls. For his part, the father wants to be able to enjoy some positive one-on-one time with his child and has a very limited window of opportunity between suppertime and bedtime in which to do so. He may place a higher value at this point on enjoyable positive interaction than on enforcing behavioural consequences for events which occurred earlier in the day.

Alternatively, mothers may be frustrated by a spouse's lack of understanding and tolerance, for example the father who returns from work with a "short fuse" and steps immediately into a disciplinary role. In this situation mother may be overly protective, believing that the child deserves better treatment.

Children clue into the differences in treatment from parents. It is not unusual for them to play one parent against the other. They learn who will give in to their demands first, who to avoid, and who will accept a fib or a lie. Parents need to be together philosophically in their approach to behaviour management and consistent in the application of child management principles.

Dealing differentially with siblings. While most parents expect to treat each of their children in a fair and equal manner, the presence of a child with special needs challenges their understanding of these concepts. Because of limitations in cognitive level and the lack of satiety, children with PWS require "different" treatment than their siblings. They usually function better with routines and schedules. Mealtimes, for example, require punctuality. Having second helpings or special treats may be out of the question. Flexibility to respond to needs of other siblings, or spontaneity to take advantage of an opportunity, may be curtailed. Sibling privileges may need to be hidden or disguised, and not shared. The child with PWS requires individualized treatment in the home as is the case elsewhere. Fair treatment of siblings means to recognize their individual differences and needs as well. "Fair" doesn't necessarily mean "equal" in all circumstances.

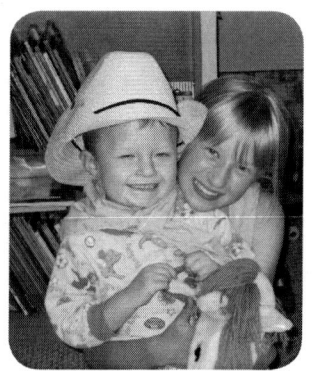

Cody and his sister enjoy play time together

All children need their share of parental attention. From infancy, children with PWS require or demand a disproportionate amount of parental, particularly maternal, time. When this occurs siblings may complain, act out, or withdraw. Planned, uninterrupted, one-on-one time may be needed as a preventive measure. This is good use of respite according to mothers of PWS children dealing with sibling issues.

Fair treatment is a particularly difficult concept to apply in blended families, where a parent will have a strong, protective bond with a natural child and a commitment to be fair to all new siblings. The common good can be in direct conflict with the individual needs of a special child. For example, to apply a rule of "no junk food" is a cornerstone of PWS dietary management, yet will be viewed as unfair and punitive by many siblings unless parents devise some differentiated strategies.

Changes to food routines. Over the years, the primary food concerns of fathers have been the limitation on junk food and the increased volume of vegetables (especially salads). Men who have been used to a diet centred on meat and potatoes may have considerable difficulty with the changes required to food routines. Along with new food items they must also learn the basics of new concepts such as: calorie counting, food exchanges, and nutritional management.

Family eating habits and routines must necessarily adjust to accommodate the food issues associated with PWS. "House rules" become more stringent and limiting for other family members. Table 1 illustrates some adjustments that families have recommended. Most report that meal schedules become more rigorous. Grocery shopping, food storage, meal preparation, clean-up, and garbage disposal all become highly routinized. And yet there are some families who seem to be able to get by with less controls. They emphasize a proactive approach to teaching good nutrition, choice making and self-regulation. But these don't work for all situations.

Table 1
Some adjustments to home food routines
• ensure regular schedule of meals
• be punctual with snacks and meals
• eat only in dining area
• serve single portions only (no seconds)
• restrict serving of desserts
• eat more vegetables, salads
• count calories, use food exchange system or other dietary plan
• adjust food preparation (e.g., no frying or use of sauces)
• clear table and clean up immediately after meals
• restrict access to kitchen during food preparation
• provide only low-calorie snack items
• avoid junk food
• limit dining out

Limitations to social activities.   The inability to maintain an active social life is also problematic for some parents. It can be a form of alienation. Mothers are particularly vulnerable, especially if they are stay-at-home moms with little opportunity for social contacts.

One mother explained that she was tired of always having to explain about her daughter. It was simply easier to stay at home than have to face social situations. While avoidance may be an effective stress reduction technique it is not socially fulfilling.

Another set of parents were able to maintain a weekly commitment to a social-recreational activity because of the respite support of relatives. Regular attendance for such activities is only possible when parents have confidence in those providing respite. Several parents who said that they do not go out, explained that they had negative experiences with baby-sitters who were not able to manage behaviours or maintain food controls.

One family that received house guests as part of the father's employment role, created PWS literature to share with guests which explained routines in their home. In this case the social activity was not limited, but rather enhanced with a proactive message.

Parent stress

People handle stress in different ways. Some internalize, others externalize. Some become overwhelmed and show signs of anxiety or depression; others rise to the challenge and fight to overcome. How do parents of children with PWS handle stress?

Finding time for each other. There are often differences in spousal acceptance of adjustments that are necessary in home routines with the presence of a child with PWS. Mothers are generally quicker to accept changes to lifestyle; for fathers the changes are often more difficult. For mothers the care and nurturing of a child is the primary responsibility. With the arrival of the first child, a father must begin to adjust his expectations. Spousal time and spontaneous activities now require scheduling and arrangements. With each successive child, and particularly a child with special needs, the father receives less spousal attention. If the mother is carrying too much of the responsibility she may not have much energy left at the end of the day. It may be difficult to find time for each other.

Younger parents seem to have a greater commitment to, or are more creative at, finding time for each other. Perhaps it is one of the benefits of early diagnosis and parent education. The presence and support of extended family is a big help. Having trusted family to provide respite to allow for a date night, or just to be able to run errands together, supports the marital relationship.

Marital challenges. Decreased time, when combined with tensions over child rearing and behaviour management practices, may contribute to serious marital problems. In *The Way Life Is* (Johnson, 2004), Rick shares intimately the marital pressures that he and Pat endured in their early marriage:

> The honeymoon was definitely over. Sara's arrival had brought us depression, anxiety, financial difficulty, more depression, more worry, and, of course, a loss of intimacy in our relationship. In the face of it all, it was probably inevitable we would, sooner or later, envision better prospects for happiness apart....
>
> I had been pretty selfish and unrealistic, pretty much addicted to my work, and would have preferred Patty support me in my career, be there for me physically and emotionally,

keep herself fit and happy and, of course, look after Sara without complaint or demands on me.

The Way Life Is is the inspirational true story of the Johnson family. It is about "love and faith and standing fast against adversity." It is an honest account of marital stress, the type of stress often hidden from others. Many parents will identify with their story.

Of course, not all marriages end in crisis. Heinemann (2003), penned an article with an interrogative title – *Does a child with disabilities = A disabled marriage?* She concluded that the answer is "no - as long as you put the same effort into "yourself, your relationship and your other children as you do your child with a disability" (p. 10). She offers the following survival strategies:

- absolve yourself of guilt
  "if we don't nurture ourselves as individuals and
  as a couple, we cannot joyfully give to our children."
- take a good look at your stress factors
  "it helps to know where the enemy lies rather than
  have a vague feeling of being bombarded on all sides."
- share the parenting role
  "it is important that mothers allow the dads the opportunity to play and bond with their children."
- savour the good times
  "we often worry about what will happen next week,
  next month or next year - and don't really appreciate
  today."
- don't take your relationship for granted
  "a good relationship won't stay good without a lot
  of time and effort put into it."

Separation and/or divorce. The Johnson family story has a happy ending. However, for others excessive marital problems can lead to permanent separation or divorce. In 1992 James and Brown reported that 28% of children with PWS in western Canada were living with parents who were separated, divorced, remarried or cohabiting. By comparison, there was only one case of separation and one of remarriage in the new group of 25 parents interviewed in 2007-08. It is likely that earlier identification, increased supports and greater syndrome knowledge contribute to marital stability.

Stress and coping. James and Brown (1992) found similar high levels of stress for mothers and fathers of PWS children who completed the SCL90-R (Derogatis, 1983), a self-measure of psychopathological aspects of stress. Maternal stress levels were comparable to those of mothers of children with Down syndrome and more than twice those of mothers of non-handicapped children. Paternal stress, on the other hand, was approximately twice that experienced by fathers of children with Down syndrome and four times that of fathers of non-handicapped children. For mothers, traditionally the primary parent in child-rearing, the stresses associated with caring for a child with special needs were similar regardless of the type of syndrome. It was speculated that adjustments in family eating patterns and the need for paternal involvement in child management may have contributed to the higher stress levels for PWS fathers.

According to Dykens and Hodapp (1995), investigators moved from examining families as "pathological" to considering them to be under more stress, but often times coping very well. Research shifted to examining how and why families are stressed and to identify particular social supports that best help families to function effectively. They identified the three major findings from this work:

- families were most worried and concerned about the func-tioning level and future care of the PWS member, and the degree to which family members had to "compromise, sacri-fice, and do without" because of the demands of PWS.
- most of the stress factors occurred during the adult and not the childhood years. As families provided care into the adult years, caretaking demands became more stressful. "Families of individuals who were more obese felt more stress."
- support from friends and neighbours seemed most important in lessening stress levels, particularly in the adult years.

Hodapp, Dykens and Masino (1997) found that PWS families have relatively high levels of support (average of 7.5 supporters per family); only 8% of support came from professionals. Parent-family problems and pessimism were identified as the most stressful areas. "Almost all parents expressed concern about their child's future, were bothered by characteristics of their child, and expressed sadness, disappointment and concern about their families" (p. 21). Interestingly, in this study there was no relationship between the child's degree of obesity or IQ and the stress level of parents. Families experienced greater stress when a child showed more maladaptive behaviours.

Families respond to stress in different ways. Given an unbearable family stress load, the Johnson family, like others, made arrangements for Sara to move into another living situation. As a result the atmos-phere of stress was reduced. Pat wrote:

Family stress is now greatly reduced. The relationship between Sara and her siblings has vastly improved. Also the relationship with us, her parents, and especially me, her mother, is 100% better now than when she was home. We look forward to her visits home every two weeks and are much better advocates for her care because we have more energy for her now.

Many parents have testified to the improvement in relationships once the young adult with PWS moves out of the family home. This move is often easier for the young adult than it is for the parents.

Quality of life for parents with a child with PWS

While parents with PWS children share similar responsibilities for child-rearing, their experiences vary widely. Quality of life is dependent on a host of individual circumstances. Even the quality of life of two adults living within the same home can vary widely.

Impact of a child with special needs. Unfortunately, the presence of a child with special needs has been a factor in some broken marriages. The impact on quality of life for the husband and wife can range from seemingly imperceptible to traumatic. For example, how one handles the demands of supervision, the chronic nature of caring, dietary restrictions and social limitations will have a bearing on one's satisfaction with life. In an attempt to enhance the quality of life for a child with PWS, parents may sacrifice important aspects of their own quality of life. Devotion to, or preoccupation with, a child with PWS may interfere with important considerations such as marital harmony, extended family relations, social opportunities and employment options. On the other hand, it may provide new opportunities for growth, service and meaning. For example, the experience of parenting a child with special needs has been the impetus for several mothers to seek employment in school systems as teacher assistants supporting other children with special needs. Satisfaction gained from this area of employment service enhances their quality of life.

The old adage, "once a parent always a parent," is certainly a truism for PWS parents. What is experienced by some as a prolonged burden of caring, however, might be viewed by others as a lifelong blessing. Again, quality of life is a uniquely personal assessment of circumstances. Cindy, the mother of a 16-year-old with PWS, reflected:

How my life changed the day he was born ... I have been able to find my 'passion' in life - my involvement in the world of special needs has been so rewarding and energizing.

Projecting child quality of life. All parents have hopes and aspirations for their children. Most learn by trial and error, however, that they cannot force their expectations on children as they emerge into adulthood, including children with special needs. As much as parents might want to determine the quality of life for their child, they may not have the right to do so. Parents will project their own values and priorities when making decisions for a child. While some may be aware of their biases, others are not.

Some parents naively argue that it is their right to make decisions for their child who has attained the age of majority. Unfortunately, they may be acting contrary to law. Ignorance in this area may perpetuate over-protective and controlling attitudes. Parents' rights change dramatically when the child reaches the age of majority. In reality, however, many parents do continue to make decisions for their adult child with PWS, without experiencing negative repercussions. On the one hand, they may not understand the matter of rights; on the other, they may well understand but place a higher value on the necessity of making decisions for them.

Often parent protective actions are driven by fear - fear of harm, fear of the future, fear of the unknown. Such fears can be terribly inhibiting. They can limit a child's social opportunities, emotional development, and growth toward greater independence. The desire to protect can perpetuate eternal childhood in the parents' home. Despite the best of intentions to ensure a quality life for their adult with PWS, a parent's actions, however, may be counterproductive when upon their death the adult goes into care without advocacy.

After years of advocacy, an activity which has given them a mission, meaning and self-worth, it is hard for some parents to give up control over their adult child's life. Retaining control gives them purpose and allows them to minimize factors which might negatively impact their own quality of life.

Parent quality of life concerns. There are two important junctures when parents are most likely to raise quality of life concerns:
- at the transition from teen to adult, generally coinciding with graduation from secondary school, and
- at the time of planning for transfer of guardianship, in anticipation of their own inability to continue to provide care and/or advocacy.

Graduation, or leaving secondary school, roughly coincides with the recognition of adult status. Parents usually experience anxiety as they anticipate changes from child to adult social services, and a change of focus from education to vocational activity. Uncertainties regarding the future lead logically to questions central to quality of life, for example: What work will my child be able to do? Where will my child live? What community supports will be available?

Similarly, as parents approach their senior years, there is commonly a concern for the future care of their adult with PWS. Recognizing their own inability to continue to provide the level of support necessary, they raise questions central to the future quality of life of their adult child, for example: Who will provide economically for my child when I am gone? Who will monitor/supervise the life of my child? Who will advocate for my child's needs?

As far as they are able, most parents undertake planning for the future quality of life of their child. The inclusion of topics related to wills and estate planning at PWS conferences attest to parent interest in this topic. In some cases, there are siblings or other family members who are able to step into the caregiver or advocate roles; in other cases the government must assume these roles. Most parents, however, fear a reduced quality of life for their child if placed under the care of the Public Trustee.

Parents are quick to talk about quality of life for their child, but more hesitant to talk much about their own quality of life. Older parents are perhaps more philosophical in their reflection, recognizing ways in which a child with special needs enriched their family experiences. Some, however, harbour hurts and resentments and complain about the stresses caused by individual doctors, social workers, teachers, and program workers. They criticize government policies and agency practices. Others, are more personal, admitting to difficulties with siblings and grandparents or the mistakes they made in not using respite or looking after themselves. The quality of life of parents is inextricably intertwined with that of their PWS child, as will be seen throughout this book. Parents are encouraged to read between the lines and imagine how similar experiences might affect their own quality of life.

Siblings

Parents express concern about the imbalance in family life created by the presence of a child with PWS. They are concerned about how to be "fair" or how to treat siblings "equally." They recognize that the demands of one child's special needs will detract from time and energy available for the other children.

Number and birth order of children

The roles of siblings are affected by the number of children and the birth order of the child with PWS. When considered by age groupings, those over age 40 with PWS (to be referred to as the "over-40 group"; i.e., born prior to 1970) all had siblings; this was not necessarily the case for those under age 40. No one in the over-40 group came from a single child family. Statistically, families of the over-40 group had 3.5 children. Families with a PWS child born in the 1970s had 2.55 children, those born in the 1980s had 2.58 children, and those born in the 1990s had only 1.5 suggesting a trend to smaller families.

When the first child has PWS there are likely to be fewer children in the family. In some instances, there are no others. When the child with PWS is the youngest child, older siblings are required to assume extra responsibilities. In play, older children are usually role models and teachers. In the words of an eight-year-old sister, "I play with him. I teach him his numbers."

Younger siblings often become playmates. Parents and teachers have commented that children with PWS are more comfortable around younger children. Likely the slower pace and less complex play activities of younger children are less stressful and more enjoyable.

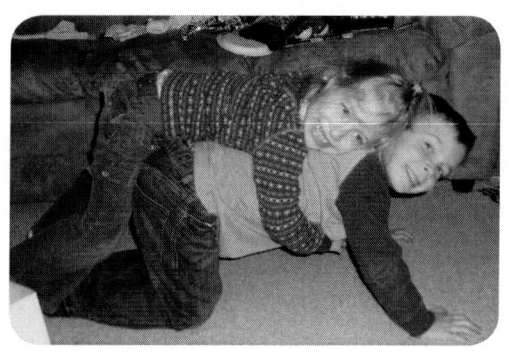

Isabelle and Maxim - playful siblings

Unmet needs

Throughout childhood there is a parent concern for the unmet needs of the other siblings (James & Brown, 1992). Parents always wrestle with the extraordinary time requirements for supervision and appointments for their PWS child, which take time away from other family members.

Given that children with special needs require a disproportionate amount of parent time some siblings, particularly by the teen years, have become resentful, even to the point of withdrawing, acting out, or escaping from the situation. Siblings have indicated that the responsibility to babysit, chaperone, or supervise activities interfered with their preferred activities and that the limitations imposed on diet and junk food in the house created resentment.

Adult siblings, reflecting on their personal experiences of growing up, have urged parents to better understand the impact of a sibling with special needs on the other children, particularly younger ones, reminding them that all children need a share of their parents' time, energy, and love.

In extreme cases, it has been necessary to seek an out-of-home placement for a child with PWS in order to address the unmet needs of other family members. Rick and Pat, describing the out-of-home placement for their daughter, explained:

> Our hopes and prayers were that, with separation, we would eventually have more patience for her, and save the other two from the unhealthy environment that had become our home - give them some experience of a more normal childhood (Johnson, 2004, p. 145).

Self-image

A teen's image of self and quality of life may be negatively affected when there is a sibling with PWS. Tantrums and locks in the kitchen may cause embarrassment when having friends home. Hence, there may be a desire to be out of the house more often. When in the same school, a sibling may be very protective. or may try to avoid being seen together. At home, there may be resistance to participating in family activities and one-to-one involvement with the sibling with PWS. One eleven-year-old sometimes just wished that her brother would go away - not in a permanent sense, but in order to allow her space to be herself, to be her own person. A boy of about the same age said he was embarrassed by his sister's tantrums and didn't like the fact that adults expected him to be a problem solver.

Another sibling described how her sister with PWS got all of the attention as a child. She remembered being dragged to activities to support her sister, yet felt little support for herself. She lamented that she never had the opportunity to meet others in a similar situation. She had nobody with whom she could identify or who could understand her. As a teen she resented her sister and her home situation. Such experiences contributed to her rebelliousness and loneliness.

How a sibling reacts to the presence of a sister or brother with PWS will be subject to the judgments of others; how the judgments of others are perceived will contribute to the concept of self. Some siblings may be vulnerable to the development of negative self images and/or carry a sense of guilt, but others will be affirmed in a positive way for qualities such as compassion, service, and leadership.

Responsibility to help

Having a sister or brother with PWS usually places responsibilities on the other sibling(s), particularly in the areas of supervision, socialization, and food access controls. While still at home, older siblings often share the role of caring with the parent, and in some cases inherit it or assume it when parents are no longer able. One mother commented that her daughter had three brothers "who adored her," and as a consequence she was "very well protected."

Older siblings may also take on a teaching or mentoring role, helping to guide a younger child's development. Tammy wrote:

> As the oldest of three children in my family, I have naturally always felt a sense of responsibility for my younger brother and sister as most first-born children do. I have strived like many older siblings, to be a role model and teach my younger siblings what I have learned in the process of growing up.

As with any relationship, there were reciprocal benefits. As a young adult she goes on to say:

> Now that I have matured, I have realized the impact that my brother has had on my life. Stephen has taught me lessons about having patience, being sensitive to others and their needs, and taking the time to enjoy life for all that it brings. He has shown me the importance of having a positive attitude, a sense of humour and the value of being myself. I will always be grateful to my brother, Stephen, for the lessons he has taught me. (James, 2006).

Future care

As parents advance in years, they often look to siblings to continue to provide care for the child with PWS. There are examples of siblings taking a brother or sister with PWS into their home to provide care, or functioning as guardian or trustee. Brenda stepped in to care for her brother, Bill, after their mother was seriously injured in an automobile accident and their father was no longer able to provide the level of supervision needed. Peter and Mary assumed guardianship of their sister after the death of their father and they had concerns about their mother's advancing years. Of course not all siblings may be able, or have the interest, to assume such responsibility. Distance, family relationships, and personal circumstances sometimes prevent involvement.

Despite preoccupation with the future care for their child with PWS, some parents are adamant about protecting siblings from inheriting what they perceive as the burden of care for the brother or sister. Thankfully, there are more options today than in the past for future care.

Grandparents

Like parents, grandparents agonize over the birth of a grandchild with special needs. While they don't share the concerns which come from the immediacy and constancy of daily parenting, they do experience their own feelings unique to the grandparenting role.

Accepting the disability

It is not unusual for grandparents to initially reject the prospect of their grandchild having special needs. Depending on the geographical or emotional distance between the parents and grandparents, communication may contribute to the issues.

Grandparents may have difficulty bridging the generational gap. Remember, when they were young, children with special needs were placed in institutions. There was little community understanding of special needs. The announcement of the arrival of a child with special needs may conjure up images of institutions and archaic treatments. Grandparents may deny the existence of a problem, or insist that it will be outgrown. They may be adamant about treating all grandchildren equally, delight in providing special treats and refuse to deny the child's appetite. At best their denial and lack of cooperation may leave a tenuous status quo, but it delays the inevitable reality. Usually it creates strained, or in some cases, broken relationships.

Family pride can also interfere with initial acceptance of a diagnosis. It may take time to adjust, particularly if the parents' announced intentions are to have no more children or if the child is the only male heir and therefore unable to carry on the family name. Family pride may deny the disability; fear of the unknown may create avoidance. Some will expect a cure and hang all hope of normalcy on an impending medical breakthrough.

Grandparents need to understand. They benefit from inclusion in meetings with medical doctors so that they can get the information first-hand, where they can have "their" questions answered. Some attend other meetings to support their children, including conferences. Not surprisingly, they engage in their own dialogue and ask their own questions. For example, they are concerned about whether they passed on defective genes. They want to understand the latest medical news.

They are interested in the prospects of growth hormone treatment. They want to know the hope for the future. They need reassurance, information, and more reassurance.

Grandparents, too, will experience an emotional response to the news of possible special needs or the diagnosis. Emotions may range from anger, grief, and self-pity to love and concern. There is often a period of grieving and then acceptance. If geographically and emotionally close they will want to be there to support their own children in their new role as parents of a child with special needs.

Bavis (2003), a grandmother asks "Do I feel sorry that [my granddaughter's] parents have a child with special needs?" She then answers, "Yes, but more than that I am proud of the way they are meeting the challenge and rejoice in the strength of their family."

Protecting and supporting children

As Heinemann (2000) reminds, "the natural instinct of most grandparents is to protect our children from pain..." (p. 4). Pain, once inflicted, however, needs to be treated with comfort and support. The immediate fears for the future need to be assuaged with love and reassurance for the parents. Grandparents can be helpful in facing the uncertainties by being proactive, researching, and learning about PWS,

Table 2 lists some of the ways in which parents have been supported by grandparents. By far, the most appreciated help from grandparents is support for the dietary requirements and food access controls. Knowing that the grandchild can visit and be subject to the same standards and supervision is a comfort to parents. Grandparents have attended doctors' meetings, workshops, camps, and association meetings. They have provided reliable respite. One grandfather took his PWS

Table 2
Grandparents have been praised for

- accepting the disability
- researching PWS
- enforcing diet
- preparing non-food treats
- maintaining behavioural consistency
- encouraging the grandchild
- providing respite
- offering emotional support
- accompanying to doctors' visits
- attending family camps
- participating in vacations
- joining a PWS association
- going to conferences and workshops
- providing transportation when needed
- enjoying 1:1 time with the grandchild
- teaching vocational skills
- sharing recreation activities

grandson regularly on Saturday mornings to his job site, giving him simple responsibilities, and teaching him basic work skills. Certainly support is easier to provide when living in the same community. Even from a distance, however, visits and family holidays, can be supportive, meaningful experiences.

One mother, having single-parented two children with special dietary needs for 13 years, applauded her parents for the support they provided. Weekly for almost 20 years, they had the grandchildren over for a meal on Thursdays. They were there to pick up the children from school and support special events at the school or in the community. Grandpa established special routines, annually taking his granddaughter to the Remembrance Day ceremony and participating with her in planting the community mile of flowers. Grandma took her to TOPS, a meaningful social activity that continued for more than ten years, as a teen and young adult.

Grandparents not only provide support, they also provide memories. This same mother told how grandpa provided daily transportation during his granddaughter's time at the child development centre and kindergarten. She laughed about the time her daughter jumped out of the car before grandpa got around the car to open the door for her. In doing so she also pressed the lock button, locking him out of the car with the engine running. And then there was the time in kindergarten when she wanted to get out the car early and walk down the hill to the school. He insisted on driving her all the way to the parking lot. Having a strong will, she got out of the car and headed back up the street so that she could walk down the hill. Grandpa then drove back up the road and tried to pick her up again. A watchful neighbour, not knowing the sequence of events, reported him to the police for trying to pick up a little girl on her way to school. These events were humourous, happy memories of better times - grandpa now has Alzheimer's disease.

Spoiling the grandchild

Grandparents sometimes assume that they have a right to "spoil" a grandchild. This refers to special indulgences that children receive from grandparents, often with a wink and a smile. Spoiling the child is a tangible way of showing love for many grandparents. Most often these indulgences are in the form of treats, which parents would not provide or allow (e.g., an extra cookie between meals, or an ice cream on an outing), or they may take the form of special outings, going places that the parents perhaps would not take them (e.g., fast food outlet, the zoo or a hockey game). Unfortunately, many treats do involve food. This is perhaps strongest in some ethnic groups where grandmothers seem to have a mission to satiate the child.

Grandmother's kitchen is often a place of bonding with a grandchild - food is the glue which keeps the bond strong. In fact, the grandmother who delights in preparing special treats for her grandchildren, simultaneously enhances her own quality of life. Many grandmothers feel valued and special when they cook and bake treats for grandchildren. They have been culturally prepared for this stage of life. "She just doesn't get it!" is a criticism often directed at indulgent grandmothers who don't recognize the need for food access controls.

Grandparents, however, must adjust their approach to spoiling the child. Indeed, if spoiling is to occur it must manifest as love in other forms, for example as gifts which encourage academic learning (books, videos), problem solving (board games, cards), physical activity (exercise equipment, activity outings), and cultural learning (special performances, trips to cultural or historical centres).

In some cases grandparents only get to see their grandchildren on special occasions, and often these events are centred on sharing a meal together (e.g., Christmas, Thanksgiving, birthdays, anniversaries). Unless there is awareness and cooperation, attending functions in grandparents' homes can be awkward and embarrassing. Some parents have admitted that they simply don't visit the grandparents as much anymore because of food-centred activities and resultant behaviour issues. When grandparents desire to see their grandchild, and are prevented from doing so, their quality of life is diminished.

On the other hand, there are grandparents who embrace the situation, providing welcomed supports. Parents have acknowledged grandparents baby-sitting, visiting regularly, sharing vacations, attending conferences, and spending quality one-on-one time with grandchildren. In each instance the grandparents have accepted the need for food access controls and have worked with the parents to maintain standards, regardless of the environment. Their quality of life is enhanced through learning, providing support, and maintaining relationships.

Bavis (2003), writing about her three year old granddaughter with PWS asked rhetorically, "Is she manipulative?" and then went on to answer:

> Yes, she bats her big blue eyes at Grandma, smiles her imp-
> ish smile, says please and gets almost anything she wants.
> Surprisingly, this rarely is food. Usually, it is the Grinch

video or another squirt of the sweet smelling liquid soap in grandma's guest bathroom.

Spending time with Grandma does not need to focus on food; there can be many other types of treats at Grandma's house. It is essential for grandparents to learn that:

- to spoil the child with food can affect the long-term health of the child
- to spoil the child by overlooking behavioural issues will undermine parental ability to manage the behaviour of the child.

Parents have lamented the fact the grandparents will not respect these two essentials. In some cases, parents have limited or prevented visits in order to avoid the consequences of grandparent misbehaviour!

Cultural issues

Grandparents often provide the context for passing on cultural values and traditions. Most often, however, family gatherings centre around food. Parents of Ukrainian, Yugoslavian, Chinese and other ethnic backgrounds have expressed frustration about taking a child with PWS to a traditional family function. They complain that foods, usually high in calories, are attractively presented; the buffet presentations imply an "all-you-can-eat" smorgasbord; and the gracious hostess wants everyone to feel satiated.

The first parent strategy is one of education, trying to teach grandparents about the requirements for food access controls and restricted caloric intake. While some learn quickly, others are slow, reluctant or completely unwilling to change. In these situation the parent strategy becomes one of avoidance, for example feigning illness, citing conflicting dates, rejecting the invitation, or simply not showing up to family gatherings.

Language is an important part of culture. Canada is a bilingual nation and supports minority language rights. Some children with PWS acquire two languages from birth as two languages are spoken in the home. Others are exposed to a second language at an early age through day care, nursery school or public school. Some, because of speech and language difficulties, struggle with only one language.

Bilingualism is a family issue for Francophone families living outside of Quebec and Anglophone families within Quebec. Given the difficulties with communication experienced by some children with PWS (93% have speech and articulation defects according to Gunay-Aygun et al., 2001), parents have questioned the importance of bilingualism for their child. Cheryl and Marc Andre, living in B.C., made a very difficult decision:

> Prior to the arrival of Isabelle, our first language was French...though we live in a predominantly English speaking area. We only spoke French at home and both of us also happened to work in French... me exclusively and my husband about 60% of the time. Our son, Maxim, at the time of Isabelle's birth was almost 2 1/2 and we spoke French at home and he had English, as well, from his daycare. My whole life revolved around languages...at the time I was working on my Masters in...the French language. I teach French and about French speaking areas... in French. One side of our family does not speak any English.
>
> Then Isabelle was born. I researched a lot about PWS and a lot more about languages. I am very pro-bilingualism... not just from a linguistic point of view, but for all around brain development, problem solving skills, ultimate mastery of a first language...this is what I study and what I teach. I believe it is the best choice and I still don't sway from that opinion...for most children and even for some with learning disabilities. Yet, once Isabelle was born...after looking into PWS and the typical challenges with language...we opted to switch our entire household to English. Drastic, yes... and we have been judged (by family, friends, colleagues...). We have been made to question our decision, in the beginning...but now, as Isabelle is three and a half years of age... we know in our hearts we made the right decision....
>
> We knew we were taking away an excellent opportunity from one child (our son), from a very young age, to become completely bilingual. We knew, too, that to give one language, to give a chance for Isabelle to understand and communicate well, in an area where we were planning on living, we had to switch. Though she will never be able to communicate with part of her family (unless they choose to learn English)...we are hopeful she will one day be able to communicate with the people who live around her and with whom she is in contact daily.

The bilingualism question does not only involve English and French. Any ethnic minority families wishing to retain their languages face the same dilemma.

Can children with PWS become bilingual? From the author's experience, there are examples of children with PWS who have acquired minimal second language skills and some who parents consider to be functionally bilingual. As in the case described above, however, decisions about bilingualism must be made based on the unique characteristics of the child and the family circumstances.

Grandparents have an important role to play in the life of their grandchildren. The adjustment to the presence of PWS, however, may not be easy for them. The PWSA-USA provides an eSupport Group where grandparents provide support to each other, discussing issues, sharing information and grandparenting strategies.

Diagnosis of PWS

In 1987 Greenswag reported that only 2% of cases were identified soon after birth and that 36% were not diagnosed until after age 16. In a Canadian study in 1992, James and Brown devoted several pages to the topic of diagnosis, reporting the average age of diagnosis for males as 3 years 10 months, and for females as 10 years. The discrepancy in age between the sexes was consistent with the literature of the day. Improvements in diagnostic techniques, however, have dramatically changed in the intervening years. Most children are now diagnosed as infants, within weeks or months of birth. Receiving a diagnosis of PWS immediately affects the quality of life of family members.

What's wrong?

The PWS birthing experience varies. Some mothers give birth prematurely, others go full-term. Some births are breech, others aren't. Some require a Caesarean, others don't. Regardless of how the birth occurs there is often an immediate sense that something is wrong. Susan recalls:

> After a 4 hour long breech delivery, he came into the world with just a soft whimper, not the lustful wail you expect from a newborn. Stephen was as floppy as a wet noodle and he did not have a sucking reflex. My husband and I knew something was terribly wrong.

Having a floppy infant who is unable to suck does not necessarily mean a diagnosis of PWS. These symptoms will, however, cause doctors to initiate further testing. In Stephen's case:

he was immediately transported to the NICU [Neonatal Intensive Care Unit] at McMaster Children's Hospital in Hamilton. There they did numerous tests but could not give us a diagnosis. After 14 days at McMaster, we had learned to naso-gastric (NG) tube feed him, and we took him home.

It was not until three years of age that Stephen was finally diagnosed. This was in 1987. Many mothers have told similar stories about sensing that something was not right. In some cases the premonitions began during pregnancy with little fetal movement, with others it was at birth with the lack of cry or ability to nurse.

Early identification

While there was only a single case diagnosed at birth in the original study by James (1987), most are now diagnosed, with genetic confirmation, in infancy. Thirty years ago, the average older ages at diagnosis were also skewed by the backlog effect, that is to say the identification of older individuals within the community and institutions who were finally being diagnosed.

Today there are still some older individuals receiving a diagnosis. In recent months an 18-year-old was diagnosed in B.C. But this is the exception rather than the rule. A mother reported how some years ago, in 1998, a friend referred her to the PWSA-USA website where she was able to download the diagnostic criteria, which she then presented to her general practitioner. This action led to a genetically confirmed diagnosis by the 17th doctor! Hopefully such an odyssey would not occur today.

More recently, Berall, Allanson, and Desantadina (2004), in a two-year Canadian surveillance study found 69% of new cases were genetically confirmed before two years of age. With exclusion of patients over nine years of age, the mean age was 1.1 years. It should be noted that there is no national registry for PWS in Canada. The provincial health surveillance registries are only as good as the information that is provided to them and likely reflect under-reporting. Horvath (2006), in a survey study in the Central West Region of Ontario found disparities in the pattern of identification. It may be that regional disparities in patterns of identification still exist in other jurisdictions as well.

Figure 1, using data from the author's files, illustrates a trend to earlier diagnoses. Since the mid 1990s there have been an increasing number of infant diagnoses within the first few months and a decline

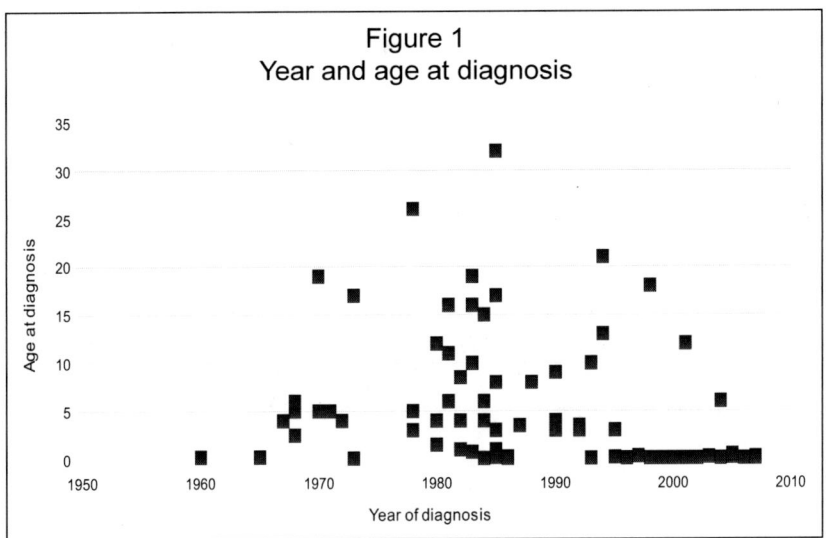

Figure 1
Year and age at diagnosis

in diagnoses at older ages. This coincides with improvements in, and availability of, genetic testing. One B.C. parent recounted receiving a tentative diagnosis of PWS within 24 hours of birth, and genetic confirmation within three weeks, back in 2004. Some older parents question whether early identification is really a blessing or not. Early identification should lead to early intervention. It won't stop the child's food cravings but it should lead to availability of professional supports, better management practices, and more normalized growth and development. Some older parents feel that they really got to know their child without having all of the negatives associated with an understanding of PWS, which they received at a much older age. Today, however, early identification is linked to early intervention with multi-disciplinary resources. There is an optimistic sense that early intervention will lead to a better quality of life for everyone.

Manner of diagnosis

With earlier diagnoses by specialists there are now fewer complaints about the manner of diagnosis. Younger parents are generally receiving the diagnosis more appropriately delivered by medical specialists. They are less likely to learn about the diagnosis over the phone in a rather clinical way from the doctor or accidentally from the dietitian (James & Brown, 1992). This does not mean to suggest that all doctors have mastered the art of diagnosis delivery. Even in 2007 one mother described receiving the diagnosis in a traumatic way, incidental to a well-baby check-up and without her spouse present.

Today there is no need for parents to be given poorly understood articles from medical journals, with naked pictures of grossly obese subjects with PWS. Rather, parents are likely to receive attractive brochures from local PWS associations, with pictures chosen by parents for their normalcy. The diagnosis is accompanied by offers of multidisciplinary professional supports, such as infant stimulation, community nursing, physiotherapy, and occupational therapy. Parents are provided with support group literature and encouraged to network with the local PWS association. The initial telephone contact with the association usually leads to a visit, beginning friendships, and group support. Parents soon realize that they can access regional, national, and international information and support with the click of a mouse or a telephone call.

Parental feelings

Generally, receiving a diagnosis is appreciated by parents. In the past, while the nature of the diagnosis may have led many to questions and uncertainties about the future, the receipt of the diagnosis at least acknowledged the problem and provided some relief and vindication for parents who had been struggling with the management of their child, often over a period of years. Pat describes her sense of release from years of emotional strain when a doctor finally suspected PWS when Sara was 4 years and 4 months old:

> He seems to feel she is suffering...from something called Prader-Willi Syndrome.....Just what all this means, I am not sure...Perverse as it seems, I feel only relief - not that there's something wrong, heaven knows I don't feel that, or want that, but just that I really haven't been wrong all this time. All the years (yes, years) of depression and guilt and anxiety and fighting with Rick, and making excuses for her slowness - they've all been vindicated. I was right. She has had a problem all this time and, at last, we can learn about it and deal with it. (Johnson, 2004, p 42).

The sense of exoneration, or freedom from blame, implied here has been described by many mothers, particularly those who endured years of difficulties. For pioneer families often it was not until others, usually educators, made observations and expressed concerns, that a medical diagnosis was pursued. For the pioneer parents a diagnosis most often brought a sense of relief ("I was right" - "I'm not just an over-concerned parent" – "No, I'm not going crazy") and a sense of hope ("We can learn and deal with it"– "We can normalize the rest of our life").

Vindication has been particularly sweet for some mothers who have had to cope with the daily management of their child while father worked away from home, or for some who experienced a marriage separation or divorce. Having to deal with the management of a child with PWS is one thing, but having to deal with an absent, doubting, or unsupportive husband as well just compounds the stress.

Donna's story echoes a similar theme of relief and hope. Her son received his diagnosis in a unique manner, from Dr. Cassidy at the 1989 PWSA-USA conference in Calgary:

> For the first nine years, we had alternately fought with doctors about the possibility that there was something very wrong or that I was just an unfit mother. What a release to finally realize at the conference that we had not lost our entire set of marbles, or that we were not alone!....although this is definitely not what we had hoped for, the label opened up a world of hope and help.

As she points out, the diagnosis not only provided hope, it also paved the way for help. Having a low incidence label brought eligibility for multidisciplinary resources that would not otherwise have been available.

In contrast, today's parents are receiving the diagnosis in infancy, in some cases before the child leaves the hospital. They hardly have time to enjoy the birth of their child when they are given the diagnostic news. Whereas most pioneer parents came to a gradual realization that they had a child with some special needs, today's parents may receive this realization in a more traumatic way:

> We were fortunate that the pediatrician at his birth recognized the symptoms and suspected Prader-Willi syndrome almost immediately.... initial chromosome tests came back as normal and although we were all very hopeful, it was very obvious that there was something seriously wrong with our son. DNA studies were done...that diagnosed PWS. I was devastated by the final diagnosis although my husband and other family members had already accepted the situation and felt relieved that we could put a name to the problem.

The sense of devastation described here has been echoed by many others. Mothers have described being "numbed" and "left in shock." Their expectations suddenly dashed, they have had to adjust to the uncertainties of hypotonia and feeding difficulties. Despite the passage of many months, one mother admitted that she still had not completed grieving her loss of a normal child.

PWS subtypes

While the pioneer parents simply received the PWS diagnosis based on physical and behavioural characteristics, today's parents receive a diagnosis based on differentiated genetic subtypes. There is increasing prognostic information becoming available based on subtypes.

As many parents and professionals have observed, all people with PWS do not look or act in the same way. In 1981 a deletion associated with chromosome 15 was first identified as a causative factor in PWS (Ledbetter et al.). In 1989 maternal uniparental disomy (UPD) was identified as an alternative causative factor (Nichols et al.). Research into causation has identified three major subtypes:

- paternal deletion of the proximal long arm of chromosome 15 (15q11-13) (approximately 70%)
- maternal uniparental disomy (approximately 25%)
- genetic imprinting errors affecting paternal gene expression (5%) (Butler & Thompson, 2000).

The subtypes do not show the same maladaptive behaviours. Those with the paternal deletion, for example, have been shown to have greater rates of skin-picking, nail-biting, hoarding, over-eating, sulking, and withdrawal (Dykens et al., 1999).

More recently, Butler et al. (2004) reported a finer discrimination of chromosome 15 deletions as:

- Type I (larger deletion), and
- Type II (smaller deletion).

Those with Type I deletion "generally have more behavioural and psychological problems" when compared to those with Type II or UPD. The research into subtypes will help to better understand behaviours associated with PWS. It underscores the variability within the syndrome and should be a caution against generalizations about PWS.

PWS-like

What happens when there is not a genetic confirmation of PWS? Initially, a child presents with clinical characteristics which lead to the exploration of a possible PWS diagnosis. Thirty years ago, clinical presentation would have been sufficient for a PWS diagnosis. Today, however, the diagnosis is confirmed on the basis of genetic testing. So when the tests do not confirm a diagnosis, the child may be described as "PWS-like." This recognizes that the child displays many of the symptoms of PWS without the genetic confirmation. It is possible for an individual to have PWS even though the genetic tests have come back negative in the past. The sophistication of testing techniques has increased the accuracy rate for diagnoses in recent years.

The descriptor "PWS-like" usually creates anxiety for parents. The hope for a firm diagnosis has been at least temporarily dashed. Will there be a need for more tests? More doctors? Meanwhile, will eligibility be denied or services cut? And what are the implications for the future? Will the child develop more PWS symptoms? Or will the situation be compounded with symptoms from another syndrome as well?

It is possible to have PWS-like symptoms that have been acquired. For example, a head trauma affecting the hypothalamus can result in hypothalamic obesity. Likewise, radiation or surgical removal of brain tumours can result in severe obesity (Christensen & Hainline, 2001). Regardless of whether a child has been PWS-like since birth or has acquired PWS-like characteristics, the individual shares some behavioural characteristics with others with PWS. It may be helpful for parents to identify with a PWS organization for support.

The case of Bob. An adult male displaying food foraging behaviours (raiding the fridge, taking food from the garbage containers, taking food from others), obesity (BMI >35), and excessive daytime somnolence (sleeping after eating, sleeping when riding in a car) was treated by the house parents as having PWS. For 12 years, from ages 30 to 42, interventions included restricted access to food, daily exercise, diet control and supervision. His weight reduced from 260 to 210 pounds over this time. However, there was never a medical diagnosis of PWS. He was in good health and seldom needed medical attention.

Today, at age 66, Bob no longer resides in a group home. His caregivers do not think that he has PWS. He has a placid personality, not displaying what they understand as common PWS behaviours. He no longer requires oxygen for his sleep apnea. He has a healthy appetite, does not obsess over food, and weighs 220 pounds. He is described as having a healthy constitution and takes medications only for high cholesterol and his thyroid.

His younger years were spent in Woodlands and Tranquille, B.C. institutions for the "mentally retarded" of the day. There is insufficient file information to retrospectively apply the diagnostic criteria and no urgency to do genetics testing at his current age.

Does this individual have PWS or is he just PWS-like? Because he is six feet tall some have discounted the possibility of PWS - but is he just an atypical case? Because his behaviour is less problematic now some think he does not have PWS. But could it be that his behaviour has just mellowed with age?

Tall stature

While short stature appeared as one of the prominent features of PWS in the original work by Prader, Labhart, and Willi (1956), it is only a minor criterion in the consensus diagnostic criteria for PWS published in 1993 (Holm et al.).   Although relatively rare, tall stature can be an atypical characteristic in children with PWS (Harty, Hollowell, & Sieg, 1993).   Greenswag (1987) noted that 27 taller-than-average children with PWS had taller parents.

Tall stature should not rule out the possibility of PWS if other clinical characteristics are present.   Hall and Smith (1972) reported the case of a young man of 22 years who was 71.5 inches in height.   One young man from Alberta in the current study, with UPD confirmation, was short when compared to sibling height, but measured just over six feet tall.

Twins

The occurrence of twins is rare.   A 2005 update survey of the PWSA-USA database found only 3 sets of identical twins and 19 fraternal twins in the data on 1141 respondents (Heinemann & McManus, 2005). There are no figures available for Canada.

The parents of fraternal twins experience all that any new parents experience... and more.   Coincident with one baby failing to thrive there is another baby who thrives well; while one infant crawls the other 'bumscoots,' as one child progresses normally at school the other requires special education services, while one wants attention the other demands a disproportionate share of the parents' time.

Joanne and Gordon have fraternal twins, a girl and a boy.   The challenges began at birth.   The daughter with PWS wouldn't nurse and had to be gavage fed.   She had to stay in hospital while her brother was home in nine days.   Joanne was expressing her milk and visiting the hospital daily.   With no extra help at home, older siblings had to take on extra responsibilities.   After two months an extended trip to Vancouver's Children's Hospital was required.   An older sibling looked after her younger brother while the sister went for further testing.   Her diagnosis of PWS was received at four months.

From a developmental perspective, it is thought that the presence of a twin achieving normal milestones can be an incentive for the child with PWS.   On the other hand, the presence of a twin with special needs might be detrimental to the other.   While both need attention, one demands more.   The challenge is to be fair without necessarily being equal.

Elementary school presented some challenges for the family. Their son felt pressures at school to be a problem-solver for his sister. Her behaviours caused him embarrassment. With the support of a behaviour consultant he learned how to ignore things. The parents noted that he was absent from school for 30 days in his grade 2 year. The following year the twins were separated. Their son was placed in a different school and didn't have a single absence that year. The change allowed him to be his own person for at least five hours each day.

At home there is always a sense of competition as their daughter constantly makes comparisons, especially for food portions and privileges. Diet is strictly controlled and their son only gets to eat junk food at friends' houses. Family activities are often dictated by their daughter's behaviour and tolerances.

The family is fortunate to have a behaviour consultant provided by the Association for Community Living who is available to come into the school and home to assist with training and case management.

Prognosis with PWS

The early PWS literature was not very optimistic. At the time little was known about lifespan development. Today there is emerging information that paints a more positive outlook. Unless there are complications, the prognosis is much more encouraging. Those with PWS will remain with their family, attend neighbourhood schools, reside in the same community as their family and friends, and enjoy greater longevity.

Life expectancy

The early PWS literature suggested a reduced life expectancy due to complications from gross obesity (Hoefnagel et al., 1967; Zellweger & Schneider, 1968). While longevity has increased in the last 40 years, survival past the 5th or 6th decade has been described as unusual (Eiholzer & Lee, 2006). Today a near-normal lifespan is a possibility. However, this statement should be qualified – providing there is early identification and appropriate interventions. The oldest PWS subjects in the literature are 65 (Alexander & Greenswag, 1988), 68 (Butler, 2000), 69 (Goldman, 1988) and 71 (Carpenter, 1994) years of age. The upper ages in survey studies are beginning to reach into the fifties and sixties.

A review of the Canadian sample studied by James (1987) identi-fied several young people who died in their teens or early 20s, but this is certainly not the rule. At least 18 per cent of the original subjects are now over age 40, the oldest being 57 at the time of writing. Given that the health adjusted life expectancy for Canadian males is 68.3 and for females is 70.8 (Statistics Canada, 2007), some individuals with PWS may, with appropriate lifetime interventions, have a near normal life expectancy.

Support

Today, a diagnosis of PWS will kickstart support services that weren't around for the pioneer parents.   Early diagnosis is accompanied by better services and a more optimistic outlook. Susan reports that

> Evan was diagnosed at birth [three weeks] so we were lucky
> to have supports put in place for him right away, including
> O.T., Physio and Speech Therapy (initially for help with
> feeding).

Additional early supports identified by others included infant develop-ment consultants and home care nurses.

Support also comes from family and friends. While professionals provide expertise related to the condition of PWS, it is those close to parents who can best provide the emotional support. The devastation, depression, guilt, and anxiety mentioned earlier, may only be part of the picture. Initial denial may turn into anger focused at the doctor, spouse, self, or even friends with normal babies. Such negative feel-ings can interfere with bonding with the new baby, or even dealing with the other children. Recognizing the negative impact on quality of life, some will try to repress or deny these feelings. It is important, however, that feelings be confronted in a constructive way. Confession to a trusted friend or family member, someone who is a good listener and non-judgemental can be helpful. In some marriages the spouse is also the best friend. Where this is so there seems to be a strength for coping. For those with faith, a minister, priest, rabbi, or imam may receive the confession and provide assurance of normalcy, as well as resources to help. For those with computers, complete strangers, parents who have gone through similar feelings, can be found through PWS websites.

3

Self-concept

The experiences of early childhood, particularly while in school or other group contexts, are important in helping to formulate an individual's view of self. Unfortunately, in childhood there is often a pecking order established, and some get picked on more than others. While some children can be very accepting of peers, others tend to bully and over-assert themselves. As a consequence, many children with special needs experience aggression, bullying, and humiliation from peers. Parents and teachers are not always aware of the isolating and abusive actions. Some of this goes unreported, as the child doesn't want to get the "friends" in trouble. Parents anguish over incidents of taunting, ridicule, and name-calling; they know there is more that goes undetected. Using descriptors such as "immature", "naive," and "childlike" they explain the need to protect their child. They ask "What do such incidents do to a child's self-concept?"

For adults with PWS there is more protection. Supervised residential and day programs insulate against inappropriate actions of others. The majority of adults with PWS are very accepting of their daily routines and express satisfaction with their quality of life. They have accepted the conditions imposed by PWS. However, as Christa emphasized, "look at me as Christa, not as Prader-Willi." In other words, PWS is something that they have, not who they are.

Thoughts about self

Self-concept is how one views oneself. It is determined by personal characteristics and the feedback from others. Being able to fit in, to have things that others have, or do the things that others do, gives people a feeling of acceptance and helps them to feel good about themselves. In children, providing opportunities for success is essential for the development of a healthy self-esteem (Chedd et al., 2006).

Eternal child

Individuals with dependent level handicaps are often viewed as "eternal children." Because of the level of cognitive development and support needed there is a tendency to treat them as children, despite their adult age. Some parents of adults with PWS similarly have this tendency. Despite cognitive levels which can be in the normal range, they are kept in a state of perpetual childhood because of the supervision and support requirements. As one 34-year-old woman with PWS stated, "I will always be my mother's little girl."

The challenge for parents is to see their child as an adult with all of the inherent rights and privileges guaranteed in Canadian society. The preservation of the eternal child status often has more to do with parent needs than those of the adult with PWS. Some parents have a need to retain control, deriving their self-worth from a feeling of importance or commitment to their child. There is a concern, however, that promotion of eternal childhood might become a self-fulfilling prophecy, stifling opportunities for growth and development, and denying human potential.

Need to belong

If belonging is an essential need of humans, then it follows that it would be a measure of quality of life. To the degree that individuals experience rejection, separation, or isolation they will have some unhappiness about their life.

The sense of belonging begins in the family, with the mother –infant bonding, but expands quickly to include the other family members. For those infants with prolonged stays in neonatal intensive care units the need for belonging, or bonding, is now recognized with the involvement of the parents in daily feeding and care routines, and in a special way with "cuddle" time.

Children, teens, and adults with PWS have the same need to belong as anyone else. To the degree that they are limited in joining group activities they may have restrictions on their quality of life. Sometimes they are limited by their own interests, which parents must expand. At other times they may be limited by parents and caregivers who are unwilling to risk the consequences of the social environment. All too frequently, the parents' and caregivers' need to protect trumps the individuals right to risk. As a consequence, teens may live without friendships and adults may live without intimacy.

The need to belong is not something that will be well articulated by the individual with PWS. Parents need to be looking for the symptoms of lack of belonging as they are more likely to surface as issues. For example, rejection by peers may lead to acting out or withdrawal. Whether an individual is quietly shunned, or otherwise socially isolated, or unmercifully targeted for ridicule, it is undeniably rejection.

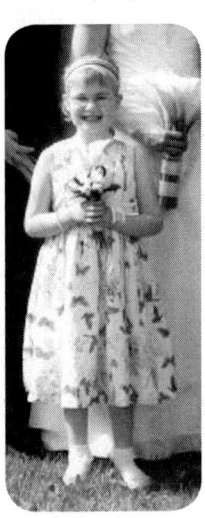

The lack of peer acceptance imparts a deeper message about worthiness to belong. If a child is experiencing such alienation from peers at school then intervention is needed. No child should have to endure this type of torment. In the event that it does occur, the support from other circles of belonging, for example the nuclear and extended family, the church or other special activity group, is important to counteract the rejection.

Janine as a
flower girl

The need to belong is satisfied by the inclusiveness demonstrated by others. Welcomed participation in regular activities and invitations to participate in special events make an individual feel included. This has been demonstrated powerfully when siblings or relatives have honoured the person in a special way, such as inclusion in a wedding party. Janine was a flower girl. Others have been a maid of honour or an usher.

Personal power

Personal power comes from having control over one's life. To have no control means that others make all the decisions. Without choices, the concept of self will suffer. How can anyone feel valued and of worth if they are not permitted to make personal decisions?

Adults with PWS who speak positively about their quality of life value their ability to make decisions over their life – for example, decisions about where to live, workers to hire, social activities to participate in, vacation trips to take, and relationships to pursue. The improvement in relationship with parents, as noted in the residential chapter, which occurs once the young adult with PWS moves out of the family home is at least in part a function of personal power. Under social services guidelines, which support personal empowerment, individuals with special needs are encouraged and supported to make decisions for themselves.

But what happens if an individual with PWS has no personal power, that is to say that he or she cannot exercise choices in their personal life? If those in control remove all choice-making there will be behavioural confrontation.

Independence

For most young people, the teen years represent a growth toward independence. Like their siblings and peers, most teens with PWS want to move toward a greater independence from their parents, to be able to exercise more personal control over their lives. When asked about their hopes for the future, PWS teens often describe a more independent lifestyle, free from the close personal supervision that they have always known. They often talk, like their siblings and peers, about leaving home, getting married, having children, and getting a job. The exercise for parents and caregivers is to empower choice making while at the same time providing an orientation to reality and the protections deemed necessary. There are many instances of personal empowerment in the context of semi-independent living, discussed elsewhere in this book.

Realistically, the emphasis of the family and the school system should be on "inter-dependence" and not "independence." Preparing the individual with PWS for the realities of supported independent living, group living, sheltered employment or day program is a focus often missed. Inter-dependence emphasizes the importance of such things as: support networks, service levels, social relationships, community involvement, and family dynamics.

Physical appearance

The short stature and "pear-shaped" body traditionally associated with PWS make those with the disorder stand out amongst their peers. Many parents have reported that physical appearance is a factor leading to teasing. At age 40, John wrote about his school experiences:

> The kids at school were cruel and mean....I did not have any friends and at recess I was teased and kicked. I had no one invite me over to their house or to play with during or after school....In High School the students did not understand me either. I continued to be without friends, although I tried hard to be accepted. The students did not understand that my glands were different, I did not get hair on my face or body as they did, I was short and fat. I still have hard times dealing with the memories that haunt me today (James, 2010, p. 91).

Clearly, John saw his physical appearance as a contributing factor to the rejection that he was experiencing by his peers.

According to Dykens, Hodapp, Walsh, and Nash (1992), being overweight may have a psychological impact, contributing to difficulties in peer relations. Preoccupation with body image is common for teens. Why should it be any different for those with PWS? While wanting to belong, acceptance by peers can be prejudiced by body characteristics. All with PWS, however, do not look the same. Appearance may be affected by the genetic subtype. Those with PWS due to maternal disomy are less likely to have the typical facial characteristics (Cassidy et al., 1997).

For children, the alteration of body height and shape is one of the possible benefits from growth hormone treatment. There are many on growth hormones now who have increased height and more lean body mass, making their body proportions more similar to their peers.

Weight loss

Most of the older individuals whose names appear in this book have experienced dramatic weight reduction at some point. They have survived gross obesity and with the help of caregivers have been able to maintain more appropriate weights. In the following examples each has dropped more than 150 pounds:

- At 26, a young man weighed 368 pounds and was near death; at 47, he leads a very active lifestyle and maintains his weight at 140 pounds. He walks six kilometres each day and curls with Special Olympics.
- A woman, age 45, weighed over 300 pounds in her early thirties. Now in a very structured semi-independent living situation her weight is 123 pounds.

- At 24, a young woman weighed 280 pounds when she left an institution. At age 55, she lives in her own apartment in an agency-operated building and maintains her weight at 140.

These examples are testimony to the fact that adults with PWS can survive obesity, are capable of significant weight loss, and can live a higher quality of life as a result. It is noteworthy that in each case a change of residential environment and commitment of new caregivers were precursors to weight loss. This should not be viewed as a criticism of parents or previous caregivers. Excessive weight is a cumulative problem that takes place over time. There are many individual circumstances which contribute to weight gain. Sometimes a fresh start is necessary in order to break old habits, change routines, establish new goals and foster increased cooperation.

Clothing

Being in style, helps a child to fit in. As early as preschool children want to be like their peers; they want to look like them and have the same things as they do. Some parents have described the difficulty of finding stylish clothing which fits their child if they have put on too much weight. For others it is simply finding clothes which fit, regardless of style. This is a dilemma which can remain across the years if weight is excessive.

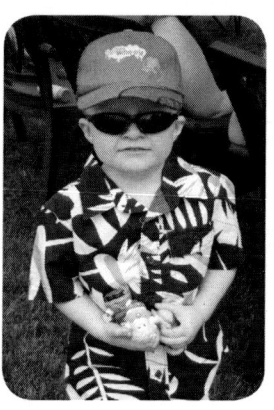

Cool Cody

Awkward sizes. For those who are overweight, standard clothes sizes seldom fit. Combine short stature with excessive body fat in the midsection and thighs and clothes will surely need adjustments. One mother described resorting to denim maternity pants at one point for her son when everyone else was wearing jeans, but acknowledged the inappropriateness of the choice. She quickly found sweat pants to be more acceptable. To have pants made was too expensive.

The options for clothing are better in larger centres and better for girls than boys. In some communities there are seamstresses who specialize in making clothes for people with disabilities; some also advertise their "adaptive clothing" over the internet.

Rack shopping. Most of the woman who had experienced significant weight losses identified clothes shopping as one of the benefits of weight loss. At 34, and after losing 169 pounds, Carrie proudly talked about enjoying shopping because she could now find more and cheaper clothes. Similarly, at 45, Margaret said that she enjoys buying off the racks now, after dropping about 170 pounds. Previously her clothes came from The Salvation Army or were home-made. After losing about 100 pounds Lindsay, too, enjoys shopping for clothes. She enjoys finding a stylish bargain.

Self and work

Self-image is how we view ourselves. Self-worth is related to how we value ourselves and whether we feel valued by others. Having a job and disposable income contribute to one's self-identity.

Most adults with PWS receive some form of income assistance for people with disabilities, a guaranteed income which is really "minimal" income. They generally participate in individualized or group day programs. Some may get a supplement, or an incentive allowance under a work training program. Others have taken an entrepreneurial approach, earning supplemental income from the sale of crafts or personal services. A small number earn minimum wage or a competitive salary. How adults with PWS spend their days contributes to their sense of self-worth.

Value of work

Most teens and young adults with PWS express a desire to work. They grow up believing that they will be able to work. School reinforces the expectation to work and the value of good worker characteristics. Having a job is a parental hope and a cultural expectation. Parents feel justifiably proud when their child gets a job.

The adult with PWS has a different feeling of self-worth when working. After Sara got a job in the hotel laundry, her quality of life improved. According to her mother,

> since she got into the working world, she has been WAY happier with her life. Her coworkers treated her with a respect she had never known before, and her self-confidence and self-esteem just blossomed when she was appreciated for her contribution to the workplace every day.

The vast majority of adults with PWS do not work in competitive employment. Most are in supported employment programs, sheltered workshop situations, or individualized day programs. These options, too, can contribute positively to the view of self. Regardless of remuneration, work provides meaningful activity, a chance to learn new skills, and the opportunity for social contacts, friendships, and status.

In Calgary, Madeline sets her own volunteer work schedule each week. She has a number of non-profit agencies (e.g., Red Cross, Alzheimer's Society, Kidney Foundation) where she does volunteer work. She works with donor lists on the computer, prepares mail-outs and assists with other clerical tasks. At age 47, she feels good about her contribution, enjoys the variety of places and tasks, and is disappointed if no help is needed.

Erin works in a pet store in the West Edmonton Mall. She receives token pay for caring for puppies and birds, a job that she really likes. Her new job skills have transferred to her living situation. She shares an apartment with another young woman, in a supported living model, and enjoys the responsibility of looking after two cats of her own.

In Kelowna, Ben works full-time in a school library where he repairs books, handles check-out procedures and assists students. Work has also allowed him to move into more independent living, sharing a condo with his sister, without any agency

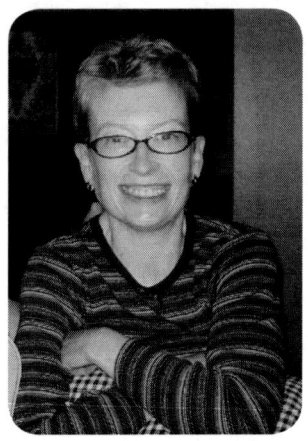

Erin enjoys her work
and independence

support. Ben contributes his full share for all of the expenses. He is pleased with his lifestyle and proud of his independence. (Employment options and successes are considered in detail in Chapter 10.)

Control of personal finances

There are relatively few ways to obtain food – buy, barter, beg, or steal. Someone without money might try any or all of the last three. With access to money, however it is logical to buy food. From a parent's perspective, having access to personal finances creates risk of excessive spending on food, or other items, and needs to be prevented. Here, again, there is a dilemma. Is it better to support autonomy and run the risk of obesity, or take away the right to manage personal finances in order to prevent weight gain?

The government system supports personal autonomy. In B.C. a high functioning young woman with PWS was considered unemployable and was receiving a monthly support cheque from the Ministry of

Human Resources. She lived in an apartment on her own. Her mother assisted her with cleaning and laundry and lamented the amount of food that her daughter was able to have with independent control of her finances. There was nothing that she could do to change the situation without her daughter's consent. Unfortunately, the young lady died from a heart attack at age 24, weighing 289 pounds.

In Victoria, on the other hand, a man has accepted that he cannot handle his own finances. In the past he would spend any money he had on food or other items he wanted. He had learned how to order things through the catalogue and not pay. Whenever there was a shortage in cash at his work site he was suspected of taking it. Now his caregiver handles his finances and he only handles the money that he needs for a specific occasion or purchase. He must produce receipts for all transactions. He likes the system. He proudly produces his receipts and helps his housemates to do the same. He acknowledges his difficulty with money and expresses appreciation for the present arrangement.

In most cases the independent control of finances is problematic. Generally, some controls are necessary, for example: producing receipts, joint accounts, co-signing cheques, no credit cards, minimal allowance, and no pocket money. The exercise is to allow access to money for legitimate expenditures but to minimize the risk of food purchases.

Self-expression

A quality of life approach necessarily requires listening to those with PWS. On an individual basis this may be hard to do, as the busyness of the day or the emotion of the moment takes priority. As a group, those with PWS seldom have a collective voice of their own.

Voice of young people with PWS

At the 1989 PWS-USA national conference held in Calgary, Marlett shocked some parents and professionals as she worked with a group of 10 teens and adults, facilitating the expression of their personal success stories to the parent audience. During the preparation she reported that:

> these young people supported, censored, and encouraged
> each other; they laughed together and became convinced that
> they had something worthwhile that they could tell people.
> They determined that they could contribute, not only to their

> parents, but particularly to the parents of younger children
> that were at the conference (Marlett, 1991).

They spoke about their successes with independent living, friendships, employment, weight control, depression, relationships, service to others, and entrepreneurship. Interestingly, the official transcript of this conference session included an editorial comment from the Executive Director of the PWS-USA who was critical of the session. She acknowledged that "as the parents left the session, many were beaming and stating, 'Yes, our young people can live independently, and yes, they can work out in the community.'" She then went on to express her personal opinion:

> We want the most and the very best for our children, but
> is that independent living and working in the community?
> Right now, it is my opinion and the answer is no. Until we
> can develop supported independent living that is truly that,
> and until we can "train" the community to accept our young
> people as they truly are, what their capabilities truly are, I
> do not feel working in the community can be successful.
> (Wett, 1989)

The session had been titled "Voices of young adults who live with Prader-Willi syndrome: A beginning." In retrospect, it may truly have been the beginning. The criticism Marlett received failed to acknowledge her years of experience in facilitating dialogue with people with disabilities. It also failed to hear and accept the voice of those with PWS who were speaking. At the time, the predominant U.S. model included large PWS-specific group homes and attendance at vocational training centres. The PWS-specific residential model was not a viable option in Canada. With a sparser population there had never been a sufficient concentration of individuals with PWS wanting this type of accommodation. Also, with a social services system attuned to the philosophy of normalization, adults with PWS were already living and working in the community in Canada.

More recently, Kinash (2007c), a professor at the University of Calgary, has produced a book that is quite unique amongst PWS publications, which focuses on the voices of those with PWS. It profiles the story of Angela, a woman with PWS, and includes illustrative material from interviews with 24 families from Alberta. Kinash asserts that self-advocate voices

> are seldom heard in the research literature and in the public
> sphere. Research is about, rather than by and for, those
> experiencing disabling conditions. People with disabling

conditions are usually cast as the patients or subjects, and re-search is done to them and on them, rather than asking them what they would like to know and how they can inform the responses. Even though the phenomenological experience of disability is deeply personal, and the diagnosed person and his or her parents live the day-to-day reality, their voices are discounted (p. 8).

However, a quality of life mind-set requires listening to those with PWS. While there is no body in Canada which represents the collective voice of individuals with PWS, parents and professionals must not assume to speak for them. It is encouraging to see that the PWSA (USA) now has an Adults With PWS Advisory Board, although its role and accomplishments are not clear.

Self-advocacy

Self-advocacy has to do with people speaking up for themselves or the group to which they belong. Advocacy is necessary when a voice cannot be heard. There are a few people with PWS who have taken on the role of PWS self-advocates. In Alberta, Angela values the opportunity to speak to human service worker students at Red Deer College, and speaks proudly of advocating for the release of a man with PWS from a provincial institution. In Ontario, John received a standing ovation for his speech in front of 400 people at the 1997 People First Conference. He was posthumously recognized by the Association for Community Living as a "self-advocate who has demonstrated a commitment to the goals of people identified as having an intellectual disability."

One parent attributed her son's new-found success at advocacy to a move from home to a residence run by an Association for Community Living. "We saw a profound change in him," she said. "The support workers actually taught him how to speak in public, and now he is an advocate for people with Prader-Willi syndrome" (Hornsey, 1997).

Self-advocacy requires self-knowledge and self-confidence. While few may have the skills to engage in self-advocacy, even fewer have the opportunity. Yet who can better speak on issues related to PWS than those with the syndrome? Self-advocates do not like to be silenced; they desire opportunities to be heard.

Voice of PWS parents

Not all PWS parents are keen to affiliate with PWS organizations. Some parents, wearied by daily management struggles, say that they do not want to go and listen to others express their problems. For others, it is precisely the support and encouragement that they get when they share their problems that makes the group attractive.

Sometimes organizations seem fractured by age group interests. For example, more senior parents are concerned with residential and vocational matters and younger parents are interested in behaviour and school issues. One parent saw a further split, between those who accept the label of PWS and those who aspire to overcome the PWS label:

> I suspect that all PWS associations have two types of parents; those that use the PWS Badge to excuse behaviours with statements like 'Oh, they're so sweet,' or 'They just can't help it – they have Prader-Willi,' and those parents who struggle not to use this 'badge.' Our 'anti-badge' group want to, and do, stay away from meetings because they get frustrated listening to the 'badge' group, who dominate and stereotype.
>
> I've been encouraging and supporting the 'anti-badge' group to get more vocal and direct about their needs, but they feel very uncomfortable disagreeing with the 'know-it-all' older person. Unfortunately, they (like myself) were thought/conditioned not to question – suggest change – fight the elder wisdom! It is very challenging trying to get recognition and respect for the anti-badge group! I know that that is where hope for their children is and so I continue to challenge!

Many parents, unable to easily attend local or regional PWS parent meetings, do become affiliates of larger groups, particularly the PWSA-USA or IPWSO organizations (see Appendix A). These larger organizations offer websites, eGroups, newsletters, and conferences.

Parents not wanting to attend meetings can vent and listen to others in the comfort of familiar surroundings at home. The PWSA-USA offers eGroups for ages 0-5, 6-12, teens and siblings (www.pwsausa.org). A Canadian eGroup is available for parents, caregivers, service providers and professionals (PWS Canada@yahoogroups.com). Some parents are now using Facebook as a way to connect with other PWS families on a more personal basis.

PWS conferences

The largest annual conference in North America is the one hosted by the PWSA-USA. Their Eleventh Annual PWSA Conference was held in Calgary, Alberta, in 1989. This was the first and only time that this conference has been held outside of the USA. Many Canadian PWS families have attended one or more of these annual American three day conferences which feature specific sessions for scientists, parents, group home staff, and PWS children and young adults. Some make this conference an annual trek.

The largest annual conference in Canada is hosted by the Ontario PWSA. While there may be other regional conferences from year to year they do not offer the scope of sessions or number of attendees.

For parents of infants with PWS attendance at a conference can be "a two-edged sword," as one father of an infant described it. On the one hand, there is the opportunity to learn and meet other parents; on the other hand, there is exposure to problematic characteristics which are inconsistent with their own early parenting experience. Such parents have described PWS post-conference sadness and depression as they wrestle with what they saw and learned. At the same time they describe a special bond which they immediately established with parents of other young children. This response is in contrast to parents of older children attending a conference for the first time who often describe a reassurance from knowing that there are other families experiencing the same difficulties. Either way, parents learn about self and family.

Few Canadians have experienced the International Prader-Willi Syndrome Organization (IPWSO) world congresses. The last triennial PWS International workshop and conference was held in Cluj Napoca, Romania, in June of 2007, and registered 348 participants from 38 countries. In reflection, Dianne Rogers, Past President of The Canadian Prader-Willi Syndrome Organization (CPWSO) wrote:

> My husband and I attended the international conference held in Cluj, Romania, in June 2007. What struck me most about this conference was the effort people of different languages made to speak with one another. There were many small groups of people speaking amongst themselves with all of them knowing only a few words in common. I met a lady from Spain. She couldn't speak English and I couldn't speak Spanish , so we talked in the broken French we knew. You would hear people greeting one another in their own language. It made for a very cohesive group, even if we didn't always understand one another. For me, international conferences now feel like a huge, happy, yet informative, family reunion.....The people at international

conferences come from diverse cultures and backgrounds. There is always something new to learn from someone in the group.

Conferences can have a big impact on families with a PWS member. While some parents have expressed disappointment, the majority of participants say that they would return. And some do, year after year, looking forward to the workshop sessions, networking, and the opportunity to feel encouraged in their parenting role.

Relationships

It is natural for young people with PWS to desire friendships and for some to eventually seek more intimate relationships. There are both subtle and overt pressures to engage in relationships. At school, they see peers flirting with the opposite sex. Television and DVDs bring the teaching about relationships into the comfort of one's home. Most powerfully, older siblings may model interest in the opposite sex.

Hopes and aspirations

Teens with PWS often express age appropriate hopes and aspirations about relationships. Like their peers, most say they want a girlfriend or boyfriend, and get excited about a date and anxious about how to act. They may express a desire to marry and have a family. Influenced by siblings, peers, and media, they may also consider cohabiting or living common-law. Relationships are part of the social norm, just like moving out of the family home and having a job. People feel good about themselves when they are in a relationship.

Marriage and common-law relationships

Should children with PWS be allowed to marry or have a common-law relationship? In the past, the thoughts of marriage or cohabitation and independence from family protection conjured up fears in the minds of parents. Much, however, has changed in the last quarter century. There is now legislation protecting the rights and freedoms

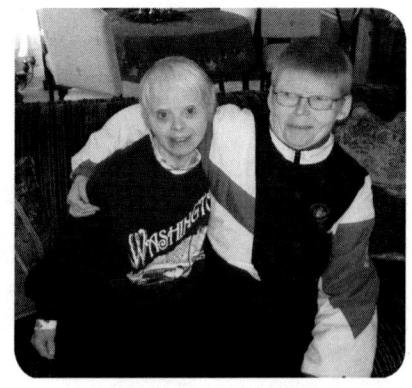

Bill and Maggie - happily engaged

of individuals, including those with disabilities. Social services systems are required to have policies which support client rights and personal empowerment. While the family is a partner in providing supports, it no longer makes decisions for the individual receiving services (unless the individual is proven "incompetent" as defined by law). Hence, parents should be aware that despite family values an adult with PWS could find social services support for an expressed desire to marry or or live in a common-law relationship.

Relationships provide the chance for self-growth. While parents may have reservations about supporting the possibility of a relationship, they need to consider the opportunity for growth, meaning and self-confidence. (Relationships are considered further in Chapter 5.)

PWS conference relationships

Amongst families who have attended major PWS conferences, where there have been programs for youth and adults, there have been stories of relationships that have developed. The memories of new boyfriends or girlfriends have lasted for years in some cases. The knowledge that someone gave them attention or expressed an interest in them contributed to feeling good about self.

For others, conferences provide the opportunity to make new friendships or renew old acquaintances. According to Harriet, her son Trevor "was only able to attend two conferences, but those were highlights in his life." In Trevor's words, "It is always neat going to conference, because I know that I am not alone." Having peers who share common experiences helps to validate feelings and contributes to self-worth.

Rites of passage

Rites of passage are those milestone events that mark the transition between important stages in the lives of people. In indigenous cultures around the world rites of passage involve the passing on of cultural knowledge, the cultivation of self-knowledge, and personal development. In contemporary North American culture these are often religious events (e.g., baptism, confirmation, bar mitzvah); relationship events (e.g., first date, engagement, marriage); life stage events (e.g., menses, retirement, death); or achievement events (e.g., obtaining a driver's license, graduation). Some rites of passage reinforce religious views, others cultural or family values. Usually they involve some ceremony or celebration which is shared with relatives and friends. These events affirm one's place in a social context and mark the passage of important milestones. However, children with special needs may lack a progression through certain rites of passage and consequently they may experience an incompleteness which may diminish their self-worth and quality of life. To this end it is important to affirm their social role through the celebration of rites of passage.

Birthday celebrations

It is important for children's self-esteem for them to have the opportunity to be honoured at a time of celebration, and to honour others by attending their festivities. Birthday parties are the most common type of childhood celebration.

Mothers, more than fathers, have shared fears and frustrations related to birthday events. Birthday party invitations commonly begin at the preschool level and may continue throughout the school years. Some PWS mothers have reported stories of bad experiences, for example embarrassing food over-consumption and tantrums. Others have described keeping their fingers crossed and praying, with acceptable results. The two biggest concerns seem to be:

- inability to control food (type and quantity)
- lack of understanding by other parents.

At younger ages parents usually chaperone their child and supervise what they eat. They cannot, however, control the presentation or type of food, or the actions of others. Birthday foods are often of a high caloric type, for example: cake, ice cream, cookies, candies, pizza. Often a smorgasbord type presentation allows children to eat at will with little regard for volume consumed or wasted. Some parents, lacking an understanding of PWS, indulge the PWS child's immediate wants with no regard for the dietary or behavioural consequences.

Mothers have reported declining future birthday invitations after negative experiences. Unpleasant episodes also reduce the likelihood of future invitations. Some mothers have lamented the lack of invitations as a reflection on friendships, while admitting that the lack of invitations makes life easier for them in some ways. This is an example of where the quality of life for the child and quality of life for the parent may be in conflict.

As children grow older, it is common for parties to be hosted at favourite food venues such as McDonald's or Pizza Hut. Here the temptations are many and the controls few. There is no substitute for supervision. Loot bags are problematic at all ages, as they usually contain unhealthy treats.

Certainly, when hosting a celebration a parent has more control over the situation. A primary concern is who to invite. Some children with PWS cannot name their school friends. Others will name popular students who they would like to have as their friends, but with whom they really have few interactions. Parents may need the perspective of the teacher or educational assistant to verify the names of appropriate invitees.

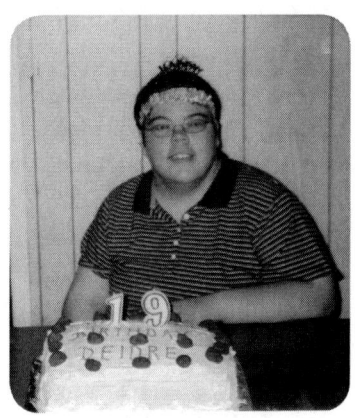

Deidre's 19th birthday

What to eat is the second major concern. The consensus is to keep a low caloric focus with controlled portions. By serving individual portions rather than allowing children to help themselves some of the regular strategies related to plate presentation and quantity control can be employed. For example, serving individual cupcakes instead of a slice or a slab of cake allows more control of the quantity and reduces the visual comparison of whose piece is larger.

What to do at the celebration is the third consideration. Increasingly, parents are opting for special group experiences such as bowling, swimming, or movies. Such commercial options help provide time parameters and allow for activity without food present.

Personal birthdays are a special time of celebration in adulthood as well. The birthday cake is the most recognized symbol of the celebration. Some families have encouraged low-cal alternatives, others allow the person with the birthday some choice and extra latitude for the special occasion.

Brenda threw a surprise party for her brother Bill to celebrate his 50th birthday. He came home from work to a house that was decorated on a Pirates of the Caribbean theme. His housemates and guests were all in pirate attire. As for food:

> the cake was a fruit torte layer with low sugar and pure chocolate curls and so absolutely delicious and amazingly decorated. It wasn't totally low cal but it was a 50th after all and we had a ton of veggies/dips/fruit bowl (watermelon scooped out and various fruit "cannonballs" inside it) and legal "befores," i.e., fruit punch and then with dinner -

"Bones" for the Pirates - baked chicken legs, and veg chili
with mugs of "Grog" (diet Root beer).

Brenda suggests substituting "things" for food. in order to redirect the
anxiety that could be increased with a party such as this:

the Karaoke was a fantastic diversion and kept everyone
busy for hours so I could keep an eye on portions and
amounts that could have proved to be just too hard for them
to handle without assistance.

She concluded by saying, I guess it was as much my celebration as
Bill's...remembering the days of yore!

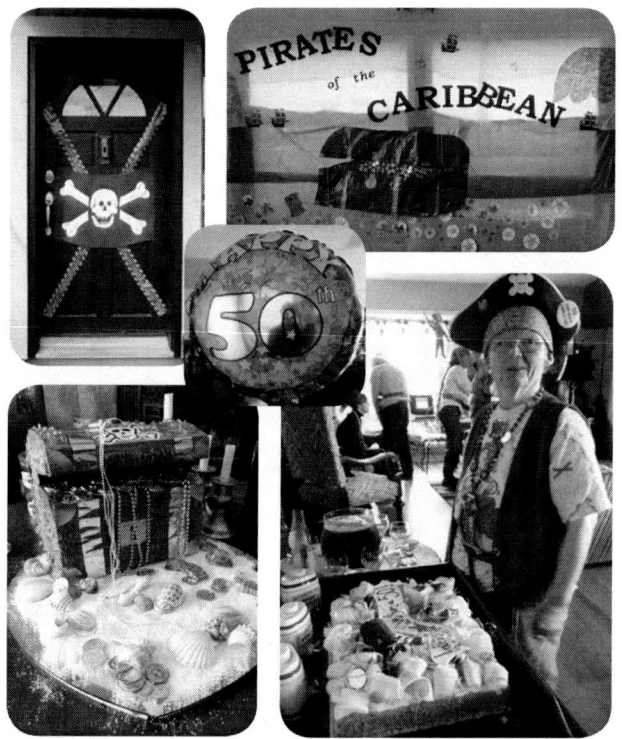

Summer camp

Summer camping experiences are part of Canadian culture. Attending a summer camp is often the first step of independence from the
family. For young people with PWS this is particularly true. Where
else can they have the sense of freedom from the family while parents
can feel confident about the level of supervision provided? In fact,
participation in a summer camp experience may be the greatest degree

of independence from the regular levels of supervision that a child or adult with PWS may ever get. This is not to suggest that there is a lesser level of supervision, but rather that it is a change from the daily supervision routines. There are many integrated and disability-specific camps across the country. (Camping experiences are discussed in more detail in Chapter 8.)

While some with PWS attend camps for children with special needs, such as Easter Seal Camps, children in Ontario may have the privilege of a holiday at a PWS-specific camp. An article on the PWS camp week at Shadow Lake describes the "home away from home" for a veteran camper, and the opportunity for the first time camper "to be with friends and enjoy his independence." The activities are described as "awesome," with a schedule that leaves "no time or even inclination to nap." The campers "cry when they go home" because they "miss the camaraderie, the high fives and the group hugs." Parents are assured of an active program with a strict 1200 calorie a day Red Yellow Green diet (Ferenc, 2007).

Driver's license

The acquisition of a driver's license gives any teen a sense of accomplishment and self-worth. It is a recognition of adult responsibility and a symbol of independence and freedom. Not surprisingly, few individuals with PWS obtain a driver's license. Most parents are fearful of the potential freedom factor, and the ability to make driving judgments.

Two women with PWS in British Columbia have obtained motor vehicle licenses. In both cases they reside in smaller, somewhat geographically isolated communities. Both obtained their license at age 17. One has been driving for 8 years, the other for 26 years. The first lives at home and uses her mother's car upon request for going to college classes and appointments. Her mother feels that she has not abused the privilege of using the car, and there have been no incidents of poor driving behaviours. The second similarly borrows her parents' car to go to special activities. Her parents are pleased with their daughter's driving record. She has only had one ticket in this time, for exceeding the speed limit in a school zone.

Certainly others with PWS do drive. Kevin lives in a coastal logging community and has been driving a pick-up truck since he was 14. He drives at his grandfather's logging company yard, where he collects and hauls rubbish on Saturday mornings. At about the same age, he was given his own quad (all terrain vehicle). He is permitted to drive alone and with friends on the forest trails adjacent to his home. He also enjoys operating his father's crew boat on the lake and can operate some of the logging machinery. However, while he has demonstrated his physical ability to operate vehicles his parents have not given consent for him to obtain a learner's license. Being able to drive and operate equipment is important to Kevin's self-esteem and quality of life. Another young man has had his own quad for eight years. He was given this as an alternative to a driver's license.

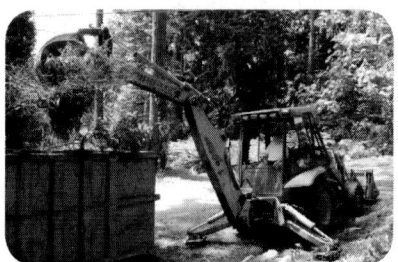

Kevin operating a backhoe

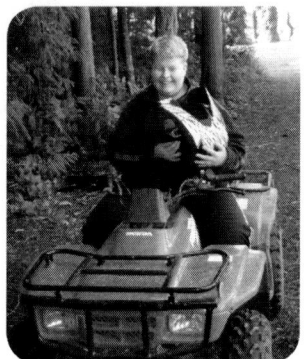

Kevin on his quad

High school graduation

Graduation from high school or secondary school is an accomplishment to be celebrated. Schools sponsor the graduation ceremony and "dry grad" activities, but there are always other events as well leading up to the graduation day. Today students with special needs are allowed to walk across the stage and receive a diploma along with their peers. This was not the case for some of the older generation with PWS who never had the opportunity for 12 years of schooling, or who completed their special education program but weren't eligible to graduate.

Graduation is a milestone which touches the hearts of parents. It is often the culmination of years of frustrations and heartaches. Seeing a son or daughter walk across a stage and receive their acknowledgement brings tears to parent eyes. Graduation is a formal affair with most boys wearing suits or tuxedos and girls wearing the latest in dress fashion. Formal "cap and gown" photos taken in

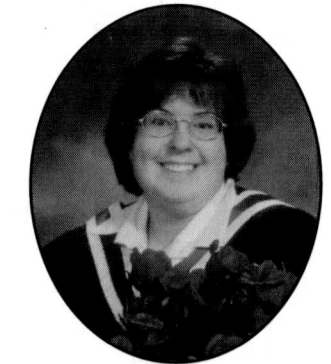

Lindsay

the grade 12 year are cherished memories of this important rite of passage.

Some families have planned alternative activities or augmented graduation with special family events. David's family threw a block party and extended the invitation to friends and neighbours. Trevor's family planned a weekend of activities which included a party, to which two teachers came. They then made an out-of-town trip which included a night, and a midnight swim, at a hot springs resort. When they came home he enjoyed an out-of-town visit from his grandparents. Special gifts and photographs always help to make grad a memorable occasion.

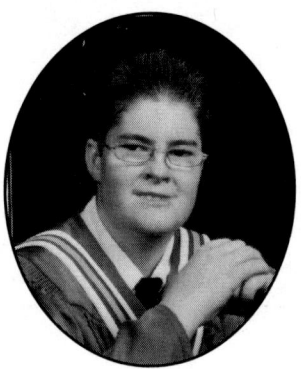

David

Moving out of the family home

As mentioned earlier, young people with PWS usually express the same desire for independent living as their siblings and peers. Parents often have difficulty even imagining the conditions under which a move out of the family home would be acceptable to them. Some parents feel indispensable. Perhaps they have not done enough homework, that is to say that they haven't visited other settings, talked to other parents or had serious discussions with agencies and social workers. Unfortunately, the pain of separation is often stronger for these parents than it is for the PWS adult when the move finally happens. There is considerable anecdotal evidence to suggest that a timely, proactive approach to moving out of the family home can be a positive experience for everyone. Just as families might celebrate a child going off to college or university, or out of town to take a job, or to leave home to travel or get married, so too can a family celebrate the move of a PWS child or adult into an alternate living situation.

Of course, the move from the family home isn't always done under ideal circumstances. As Johnson (2004) asked: "How do you tell a 14-year-old, going on 10, that she is tearing up the family and has to move out?" He goes on to describe the anguish leading up to the decision: "We put our first-born out of our home and into the care of strangers, though it broke our hearts to do so."

In contrast, consider the move from the family residence under more ideal circumstances. Lindsay initiated the discussion with her parents, asking when she was going to get foster parents, like some of her peers. When the opportunity came to move into supported independent living she was ready to move from home, at age 22. And Vodia relates how David, at age 30, came home and announced "you can start packing my bags, mother. They have a place for me at Headon House on Friday."

Being ready to meet the challenges of a residential move requires a high degree of self-confidence. The readiness for such a move will depend on individual preparation and family circumstances.

Rights

Since *The Charter of Rights and Freedoms* was introduced in 1984, provincial legislation has mirrored federal initiatives protecting individual rights. The legislated protections are now reflected in policies and practice in all areas of services to people with special needs. When individuals understand their rights and are empowered to make personal decisions they are more likely to feel good about themselves.

Why talk about rights?

Section 15 of *The* Canadian *Charter of Rights and Freedoms* prohibits discrimination on the basis of race, national or ethnic origin, colour, religion, sex, age, or mental or physical disability. Every Canadian is "equal before and under the law," having the right to "equal protection" and "equal benefits" of the law (Government of Canada, 1984).

Families must understand the importance placed on the protection of rights for people with mental and/or physical disabilities. While some parents naively assume that they have the right to control aspects of their child's life, even in their adult years, this assumption will likely bring them into conflict with social services and agency policies. Simply put, adults with disabilities have the right to make decisions about their own lives, and will be supported by government and agency personnel to do so.

To have one's rights violated suggests that quality of life would be diminished. When an adult with PWS lives in the family home, for example, there are often issues of control which impact everyone's quality of life. To deny an expressed choice might be viewed as a violation of rights resulting in less than optimal quality of life.

Parent responsibilities and rights

Parents have both rights and responsibilities with respect to the care and upbringing of their children. For example, they have a responsibility to register their child for schooling and a right to educational reports; they have a responsibility to participate in individual educational planning and a right to appeal educational decisions of staff. Parents have the right to determine the approach to care and management of their child and a corresponding responsibility to provide an adequate level of care for a dependent child.

To not provide adequate care could be negligence; it could also be abuse. The widely publicized story of Christina Corrigan, a 13-year-old American girl who died of congestive heart failure at 680 pounds, underscores the parent responsibility to care. The mother was found guilty of misdemeanour child abuse and received a 100 dollar fine, three years probation and 240 hours of community service. Her's was a crime of inaction, of not obtaining the necessary medical help for her daughter. Prosecutors said that the mother should have seen her daughter's bed sores and other obvious signs that her daughter was suffering. The mother said that she didn't see the bed sores and evidence of uncleanliness because her daughter was increasingly shy and ashamed and never showed her body (BBC News, 1998).

Any parent of a young teen can identify with the parental dilemma - the child's right to privacy versus the parent's need to know. In the Corrigan case, the Judge clearly expected more parental responsibility. While this is an American example, the underlying principle to care would likely play out the same way in Canada.

Child's right to know

Parents generally acknowledge that their child has a right to know about PWS, however they wrestle with when, how, and how much to say. There is no script or time line for this matter; each family circumstance is unique. In the present study some children understood that they had PWS and could talk openly about their issues; in a few instances the interviewer was asked not to mention the name of the disorder.

By the teen years, most have come to understand and accept PWS; as adults, they cope with varying degrees of success. One man, who was managing his weight and coping very well, seemed to be representing the sentiments of many when he said: "PWS is a pain in the butt!" A few, however, have more difficulty. One woman in her thirties was described by her mother as being "in denial about PWS." She refused to accept any limitations that would come with this diagnosis.

Choices

Being able to make choices is important for self-worth and an important aspect of quality of life. Adults and teens with PWS have emphasized the importance of being able to make their own decisions. Wise caregivers understand how to give choices rather than ultimatums.

Offering choices

The manner of presentation of choices is important. The basics are simple. It is better to offer a dichotomous choice (e.g., Would you like to do A or B?), rather than ask an open-ended question (e.g., What would you like to do?). It is better to offer two, or more, acceptable alternatives rather than leave the door open for an unacceptable answer to an open-ended question. Do not give a choice which cannot be lived with.

Choices empower self-control. Along with the power to make choices, however, is the responsibility to live with the consequence of the choices. Children and adults should be taught principles such as cause and effect, and logical and natural consequences. Accepting responsibility also includes making restitution and apologizing, if necessary.

On the negative side, someone skilled at choice making may want to engage in bartering or negotiating. One young woman engages in an easy banter with her worker, bartering for preferred foods. According to the worker, they have a strong trust relationship and the bartering works in their case. Other parents, however, have reported being fatigued by the incessant nature of negotiating. Parents and caregivers should be clear that some things (most things) are not negotiable.

When the individual has no choices

If all choices are removed, that is to say that an individual's life is so structured that he or she is not permitted to make any decisions, there will be problems. There will be issues of control. By the teen years, there will likely be rebellion against authority. If opportunities to make meaningful choices are consistently denied, teens and adults may revert to very base behaviours. The one area over which parents cannot exert control in their child's life is in the area of bodily functions. In worst case scenarios, individuals may resort to fecal or menstrual smearing. Such behaviour is offensive and immediately draws the ire of those in control. However, once the behaviour is understood as a protest against a lack of personal decision making there is a path for intervention. Allowing more personal control through the provision of choices is important.

Choice to drink alcohol or smoke

The right to drink alcohol is a simple rite of passage conferred at the legal age of majority by each province. With it comes the right to enter pubs and bars, and to order alcoholic drinks in licensed premises or at licensed events. For some, the first legal consumption of alcohol is scarcely noticed at a family meal, for others it has been a new experience at a pub or a bar. For many, alcohol is simply avoided in a precautionary way or because of family values.

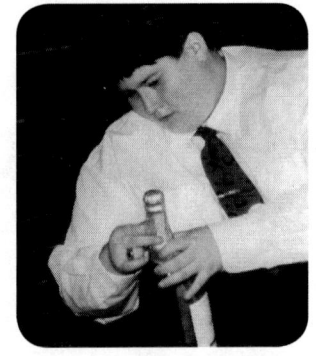

Trevor celebrated at grad

Some families permit an alcoholic drink on a special occasion. Trevor wanted to celebrate his grad with a bottle of champagne at a family party, which he did with the permission of his parents. Others enhance a celebration with non-alcoholic sparkling beverages, "soft" ciders or mixed fruit drinks. The specialness of the occasion is remembered with a new drink experience or a fancy bottle.

Angela, a woman of 40 years, described how she did not like to be told that she could not have a glass of wine with a nice meal. She maintained that as a mature adult that she had a right to make the decision whether or not to have a drink. Others, like Angela, feel that they can make the choice to drink or not. Several adults from small communities liked to go to the Legion, a social event in such communities. Men with PWS reported having a beer with a worker on occasion.

There was only one negative report of alcohol consumption amongst adults with PWS in the current study. That involved a young woman who became belligerent and non-compliant while visiting the family home for a seasonal celebration. The already strained relationships may have been a precipitating factor. There were no other reports of excessive drinking or other inappropriate alcohol related behaviours.

A small number of adults with PWS have chosen to smoke. Shelagh began smoking at age 20 and consumed a half pack daily until age 45, when she decided to quit. It was "my decision" she says. "I wanted to be healthier." Now she chews sugarless gum and eats sugarless candy. She also gets strong encouragement from her new living environment to be a non-smoker.

A fundamental message

Adults with PWS simply want to be treated as adults. This is one of their primary messages. Like other adults, they feel good about themselves when others treat them with respect and allow them to have some choices in their life.

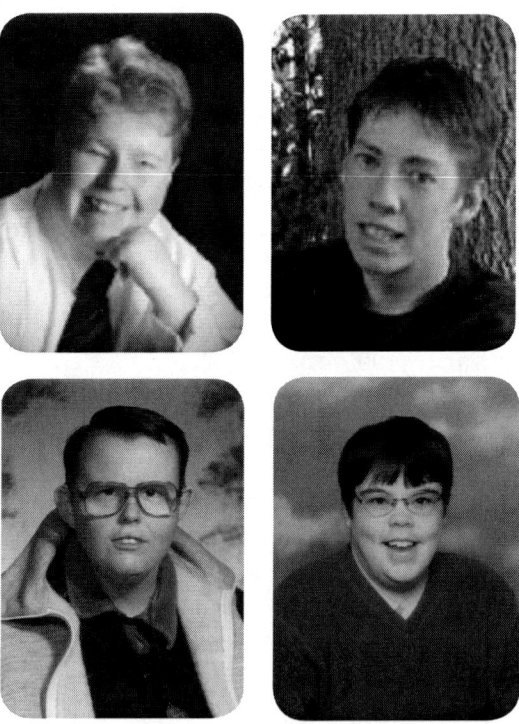

Teens

4

Behaviour

The quality of life of parents is affected by the behaviour of their
child. Many parents find themselves just coping, living a lifestyle
that is less than optimal. Drained by the constant demands of behaviour management, they experience stress in marital and other family
relationships, and have less interest and energy for social activities.

The management of behaviour begins in infancy. When the first
stage concerns for thriving abate parents are initially relieved that their
child has an appetite. Establishing routines and limits at this stage is
important for future management of behaviours. To try to impose
stricter sanctions at a later point, after a child has been given more
latitude, is a difficult task that will most often meet with opposition.

Food is the primary trigger for behavioural issues. For example,
denial of food, removal of food, change of meal times, reneging on
food commitments, or forced sharing of food can result in oppositional
behaviours. Responses can include: immediate gorging, hiding of food,
physical resistance to food removal, escalation of verbal response,
verbally abusive comments, aggressiveness, or a full-blown tantrum.
Some of these behavioural responses may occur many times in a day.
However, such behaviours, while often portrayed as characteristic, are
not universal.

Food is not the only trigger for behaviour difficulties. Sibling
rivalry, issues of fairness and equality, expectations of compliance,
forced participation, lack of personal autonomy, paternalistic attitudes,
influence of peers, transgressions in the community, amongst others,
do occur. There is often confusion between behaviours which are a

normal part of child and adolescent development and those which are specific to the syndrome. Most families seek, or are offered, the assistance of professionals with behavioural training in order to better manage their child.

The home receives the brunt of behavioural issues which arise in the school or community. As other family members might do, the child with PWS lets down in the security of the home. Sometimes it is difficult to be consistent with behavioural expectations across environments when the parent is dealing with emotionally charged situations without the benefit of the full knowledge of what has triggered the behavioural response.

Behaviour management

The management of behaviour is likely the most stressful part of raising a child with PWS. Individuals and families vary considerably in their abilities to manage the often difficult and irritating behaviours. Parent personality, previous parenting experience, personal childhood experiences, state of emotional well-being, and tolerance to stress are some parental variables which influence the quality of parenting. Beyond these, all parents can acquire a knowledge of PWS and learn behaviour management skills that can enhance their parenting role.

Parent anguish

It is normal for parents to experience anguish over the behaviours of their child. These are perhaps greatest when parents must make tough decisions about the care and treatment of their child. One mother, in describing the stresses on her son during the Christmas season (Beddoe, 2000), revealed her own anguish as she made a number of "I" statements in the article:

- I ask myself hourly, if we made a wise decision.
- I often blame myself and feel that my management style leaves much to be desired.
- I get caught every time and I feel I should know better by now.
- I wish I could help him find some peace in his heart.
- I feel for him terribly.

These statements reflect the type of self doubt, blame, and frustrations that many PWS parents feel. Parents typically worry about the potential consequences of behaviours, and feel distress with the outcomes of behaviours.

Sibling issues

Parents often have to deal with sibling issues amongst their children. Having a sister or brother with PWS complicates lives for siblings. As parents wrestle with equity in time and treatment, siblings may compete for love and attention. Some, close in age, have described rivalries at their worst during the teen years when parents have created behavioural expectations that limit freedoms. While sibling rivalries are normal, they can be intensified by the emotional instability of the child with PWS, the increased expectations for behavioural support and compliance by the parents, and the degree of sibling social embarrassment and alienation from peers. Parents may find themselves dealing with sibling rivalries that manifest in negative engagement, such as competition, disagreements, and hostilities. Other siblings may choose to avoid, disassociate or even reject their sister or brother. Parents must take time to understand the sibling issues and not simply blame the syndrome.

While there are encouraging testimonies of siblings changing their attitudes as adults, there are also some adults with PWS who must endure long-term estrangement from their brothers or sisters. They don't know where their siblings are or what they do, This leaves a void in their life. In contrast, siblings and their families are very important to others. Several women with PWS delight in their nieces and nephews and show their love by knitting, crocheting and sewing gift items for them.

Family resilience

Resilience has to do with the ability to bounce back to normalcy after a negative event. It is a characteristic of individuals and of families. Some families are more resilient than others. Some have to cope with many other stressful life events in addition to raising a child with special needs. For example, families in this study experienced stressors such as: diagnosis of a terminal illness, untimely death of a family member, auto accident, permanent disability, broken marriage, mental health issues, conflict with the law, residential moves, or changing provinces. In some cases families stumble under the weight of concern, in other cases they seem to come through relatively unscathed. What makes the difference? There are many individual and family factors which contribute to resiliency. Important amongst them are a knowledge of PWS and behaviour management skills.

Understanding behaviour

Some parents are more intuitive at understanding behaviours, others are more analytical. Some anticipate behaviours, others react to them. Regardless, all parents can "try" to understand their child's behaviours by:

- careful observation
- asking the right questions
- listening to the answers
- reversing roles to see the PWS perspective
- soliciting or accepting the input of others.

Not all scientists agree on the origin of behaviours commonly associated with PWS. While behaviourists argue that all behaviours are learned, and can therefore be changed or modified, others believe that there is a behavioural phenotype for PWS, that is to say a set of common behaviours associated with PWS by genetic predisposition. Still others believe that there are elements of truth in both positions.

Behavioural phenotype

A question often asked by those first working with someone with PWS is "How much of the behaviour is due to the syndrome, and how much is learned behaviour?" Some researchers have tried to define the PWS behavioural phenotype, that is to say the set of characteristic behaviours for the syndrome. Consistent with earlier studies, Holland et al. (2001), found an almost universal eating disorder along with an increased propensity for temper tantrums, skin picking, mood fluctuations, repetitive questioning, and obsessional traits. They suggest that PWS involves multiple genes and a complex behavioural phenotype "with at least some characteristics that are not universal" (p. 152). For example, possessiveness, lying, and argumentativeness were not found to be significantly more prevalent in PWS.

Some parents explain all aberrant behaviours as being part of the syndrome. They reason that if the behaviour is genetic in origin, then there is nothing that can be done about it. PWS then becomes an excuse for all unacceptable behaviours. Of course another fear is that knowledge of PWS can become a self-fulfilling prophecy. Poor behaviour becomes expected. By taking such a stance, parents may lose focus on behaviours that can be changed or modified.

Learned behaviours

Some behaviours exhibited by children with PWS are learned. Like other children, they will learn from their environment and those in it. Learned behaviours are amenable to behavioural interventions. Desired behaviours can be encouraged with praise and other reinforcers; undesired behaviours can be reduced by the use of strategies such as the reinforcing of alternative behaviours, introducing a response cost, or a time-out procedure. These are techniques of behaviour modification or applied behavioural analysis.

By attributing "all" behaviour to the syndrome parents may absolve themselves of responsibility for behavioural training. Visits to the homes of PWS children confirm that there is a considerable range in parent behaviour management skills and the observed behaviours of children with PWS. This is not meant to be a criticism of PWS parents. Some have more experience, support or training than others. It is important, however, to focus on possibilities. By attributing all behaviour to the syndrome there is an implicit denial of the possibility of behavioural training techniques to assist the situation.

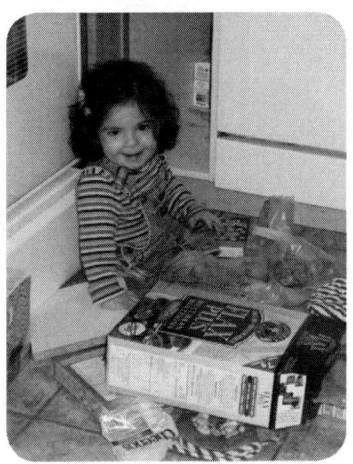

Normal or PWS behaviour?

Observing and documenting behaviours

From the point of view of a behavioural consultant, one of the first tasks is to try to define the behaviour of concern, its frequency, intensity, and duration of occurrence. The following two approaches are useful to help parents in dialogue with consultants.

ABC analysis. ABC refers to "antecedent," "behaviour" and "consequence." It is a simple form of recording in order to analyse behaviours (Figure 2). The first column notes what happened immediately before the behavioural incident. The second column describes the problematic behaviour. The third column specifies what occurred as a direct result of the behaviour. The ABC process assists parents in describing behaviours objectively and provides background for behaviour specialists to look for patterns of behaviour and flaws in management procedures.

Baseline measures.
Noting the frequency, duration, severity and timing of
a particular behaviour is
important if seeking professional assistance. Recording this data for a period
of a few days or a week
establishes a baseline for

Figure 2

ABC Analysis		
Antecedent	Behaviour	Consequence

future comparison. Behaviour specialists can then assist with the
design of interventions that can be measured against the baseline.
Without a baseline there will be no objective way of knowing if an
intervention is successful. An advantage of collecting such data is
that they can be graphed so that there can be a visual representation
of progress of the intervention. Figure 3 illustrates the frequency of
occurrence of a behaviour during baseline and with intervention.

Figure 3

EDS of a grade 7 student

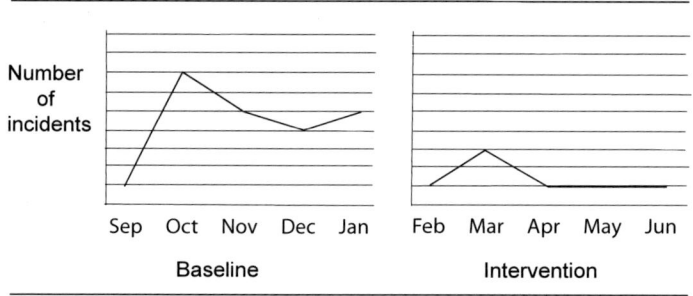

The baseline indicates the frequency of excessive daytime sleepiness (EDS) incidents of a grade seven student during the fall of the
school year before intervention. EDS was defined as "falling asleep."
This behaviour was neither consistent with the events of the previous
school year nor at-home behaviour. During the fall months the focus
of the school program was on full inclusion. At the end of January the
program was adjusted to include some out-of-class activities: public library, community mall, weight room, recreation centre, and therapeutic
riding. The incidents of school EDS dropped off dramatically.

Graphic representation can be an encouragement to a child or
adult with PWS. It can be a visual reminder of targets and progress.
It can work for behaviours, weight, calories, test scores, or anything

else that is easily measured. With younger children the use of stars and stickers can enhance the visual presentation.

Maintenance and generalization

Individuals with PWS are capable of some behavioural self-control. Most often this is demonstrated while under supervision. The measure of real success, however, is whether or not the self-control can be generalized across environments when not under supervision. Behaviour training must seek to maintain positive behaviours and their generalization. Maintenance refers to continued demonstration of a positive behaviour over time (e.g., does the child always remember to say please and thank you?); while generalization refers to demonstration of the desired behaviour across environments (e.g., does the child remember to say please and thank you at home, in school, and elsewhere in the community?).

Authoritarianism

Experience with crisis management and anecdotal comments by parents and teachers suggest that an authoritarian approach does not work very well with most teens and adults with PWS. One father said that telling his teen-aged daughter to go to bed would only result in her getting her back up and staying up all night. A teen ignored a grounding edict and left his house; another young man became angry, berating and pushing his widowed mother when she told him what he was to do. And several parents described their child "trashing" their room after being ordered there for time-out.

Recognizing that all aspects of their lives are either supervised or regulated, it is understandable that individuals with PWS might resist being "told" what to do and how to do it. Parents, teachers, group home staff, and employers, amongst others, are all recognized as authority figures. All expect compliance to schedules, routines, or standards of performance. Unless there is freedom to make personal choices, to have a sense of control over some aspects of life, there will be resentment and eventual rebellion towards the demands of authority.

Demanding an apology or admission of guilt requires a submission to authority. As one parent explained, it is better to assume guilt on the basis of the evidence and then move on, simply expecting restitution for something taken or damaged, or an adjustment to calories if food has been consumed. Children are often embarrassed or ashamed of their transgression and will be remorseful. Insisting on an apology, however, should not occur during the height of emotion.

A parent of an older woman in her fifties said that she has learned that all things should be negotiable - she has learned not to say "this is not negotiable!" Negotiation *may* work for some, but not for all teens and adults. Parents of younger children, however, report that negotiation does not work well with children. Once a child learns that negotiation is possible, the scene is set for a continued pattern of negotiation. Even with only occasional successes this will be difficult to change.

Parent behaviour management principles

Professionals working with clients exhibiting severe behaviours have usually been trained in behavioural psychology. They have a theoretical understanding of behaviourism, applied behavioural analysis, intervention design, and behavioural measurement. They can be a great resource for school or home, often mentoring parents in the process. Joanne has high regard for the behaviour consultant provided by the local Association for Community Living. He has been available to assist the family in the home and the staff at school. She even recruited him as a workshop presenter for her PWSA group. However, not all families have access to, or need, a behaviour consultant.

The following principles have been utilized by PWS families. While they may not address all issues, they do provide a solid platform from which to work on behaviour management:

- *empower with choices:* The presentation of structured choices (i.e. alternative acceptable choices) empowers the individual to have some control over life. When all choices are removed, behaviour will become confrontational or will regress. For example, when the group home prescribed a bath on Friday night there was opposition; when the mother stepped in and gave the choice of a bath on Friday or Saturday night there was no conflict. When able to make choices individuals are much more likely to be happy. Without choices it might be said that there is no quality to life.

- *provide structure (schedules/routines):* Most children and adults with PWS do not do well in chaos and disorganization. While they might like their hunger to be resolved on demand, the reality is that food must be apportioned according to a schedule of meal times. As children they soon learn the importance of the food schedule. When they get to school they take classes according to a daily or weekly schedule. When they relax at home they watch television according to a schedule. Schedules are predictable and reliable. They provide order to life and in so doing avoid at least some stress.

- *minimize change/ease transitions:* Transitions occur across most environments. The most consistent transitional issues, however, probably come from the educational environment. Here children experience change between levels within the system. At each level there is change involving location, administration, staffing, classmates, bussing. Transitions bridge the changes. They can be structured in order to introduce the change slowly and ensure a level of comfort.
- *insist on consequences:* Consequences can be natural (e,g,, touch a fire and you get burned) or logical (if you take something you must replace it). Laws demonstrate that society is based on principles of consequence. Without the consequences of law in society there would be anarchy. Without consequences for behaviours in home, school, and community there will be a self-centredness that will be out of control at times.
- *provide time-out:* Provision of a space for time-out is a respectful way to allow a child or adult with PWS to cool down, regain composure, and then re-enter the activities of the family or group. It is important that the right to return be open-ended. Time-out should not equate to "jail." The rules of time-out should be pre-explained without the heat of emotion.
- *be fair and consistent:* There is a strong sense of fairness and justice which is shared by many with PWS. It is often heard with respect to food, but it also applies to fairness in other situations as well. Fairness and consistency are cornerstones to effective management and are most effective when applied consistently across environments. This requires good communication amongst team members.
- *choose your battles:* Many battles are simply not worth fighting. Being able to remain objective, dealing with issues without emotion is helpful. Chronic supervision necessarily creates opportunity for friction or confrontation. Knowing how best to de-escalate a situation is important. There is wisdom in counting to ten, saying a prayer, or walking away from the situation for a few minutes of composure.

- *use graphic reminders:* The use of visual reminders utilizes a PWS strength that has been recognized in both research and anecdotal reports. Parents, like teachers and job bosses, tend to rely heavily on verbal communication. The auditory modality is over-worked. The chances of retention are greater if more than one sense is involved.
- *provide praise:* James (1987) identified praise as the most powerful motivator for children with PWS. Praise reinforces the likelihood of a preferred behaviour being repeated. It can be delivered easily by any one across any environment. It is a respectful way to encourage desired behaviours. Conversely, scolding, criticizing, arguing, threatening, and other coersive behaviours seldom work.
- *maintain communication amongst team members:* Maintaining communication is particularly important across home, school, and community environments and essential in order to maintain consistency. Communication amongst the team members is a group responsibility which should not be left to the leader to initiate.

Parents need to be affirmed in applying a common sense approach to managing behaviours. Many families have weathered a multitude of storms without professional guidance - and done well in the process.

Maladaptive behaviours

"Mal" implies poor or bad behaviours; "adaptive" relates behaviour to the social norm. Maladaptive behaviours are those which prevent an individual from meeting the standard of personal performance expected by the community. Characteristic behaviour problems listed as minor diagnostic criteria include: temper tantrums, violent outbursts, and obsessive/compulsive behaviour; tendency to be argumentative, oppositional, rigid, manipulative, possessive, and stubborn; perseverating, stealing, and lying (Holm et al., 1993).

Maladaptive behaviour studies

Over 180 families and group home providers responded to a questionnaire from Dykens and Hodapp (1995) which helped to clarify the high prevalence of behaviour problems often encountered in PWS. Problems that occurred in 50% or more of persons with the syndrome included: temper tantrums, impatience, impulsivity, problems relating to others, sadness, and highly repetitive thoughts and behaviours. Their work also correlated these common problems with IQ and weight. Three findings are particularly noteworthy:

- behaviour problems were not generally related to IQ scores. People with relatively high IQs showed just as many (and as intense) behaviour problems as persons with relatively low IQs....
- behaviour problems were related to obesity, but not as .... expected. Individuals who were less obese (who had lower weight to height ratios) showed more problems than those who were more obese. Thinner people generally showed more problems in thinking and in sadness, fearfulness, and anxiety....
- very high rates of non-food related obsessive thoughts and compulsive behaviours [were found]. These included hoarding and collecting, the need to tell or ask, checking, concerns with cleanliness, and repeated rituals....(p. 4).

In the United Kingdom, Holland et al. (2003), in a population-based study of children and adults, reported "further evidence for a distinctive behavioural phenotype in PWS" (p. 149). Compared to a learning disabled group (of various causes), those with PWS had significantly higher rates of: skin picking, temper tantrums, compulsive behaviours, mood fluctuations, and were weaker on socialization. Studies have continued to examine behaviours by developmental stages, and in comparison to other disability groups.

Children.   Parents begin to notice more maladaptive behaviours once a child enters the pre-school or school setting where they must socialize with other children and are required to conform to conduct codes and adhere to time schedules.

A number of behaviours have been noted to increase with age in childhood: skin-picking, compulsions (such as hoarding and ordering), food theft, lying (predominantly about food), anxiety, sadness (Dykens, 2004). There is also insistence on sameness and "just right" behaviours (Greaves et al., 2006), and rituals (Wigren & Hansen, 2003) which appear in childhood. Maladaptive behaviours generally increase from childhood to adolescence (Dykens, 2004).

The present study suggests that childhood generates the greatest number of outside referrals for behavioural assistance, often at the initiation or encouragement of the school system, for example, referrals to counsellors, psychologists, and behaviour consultants.

Adolescents.   In a study of adolescents and adults with PWS,

Dykens, Hodapp, Walsh, and Nash (1992) found strengths in daily living skills and weakness in socialization, particularly in coping skills. Externalizing behaviours, particularly associated with adolescence, also persisted into adulthood (e.g., temper tantrums, arguing, irritability, stubbornness, lying, skin-picking, obsessions, and defiance). Levine, Wharton, and Fragala (1993) described adolescence as a challenging time which may present dramatic difficulties at school due to "increased demonstrations of anger, resistive behaviours and out of control appetitive behaviours" (p. 8).

The intensity levels of behaviours, as described by parents and service providers, appear greatest during adolescence. Teens with PWS can become very assertive or resistive. Verbal anger may include yelling and the use of vulgarities; physical actions may include throwing and hitting, or passive resistance. This does not mean to suggest that all behaviours during this stage of development are intense.

Young adults. Young adults have been shown to be at high risk for maladaptive behaviours. Dykens (2004) suggests that young adulthood may be a period of new psychosocial adjustments which create new stressors. For example, the transition to adulthood means leaving the comfort of the school system; beginning new work, training, or day program; exploring new social/recreational activities; and perhaps moving into a different residential setting. They know that they can't be like their siblings or non-handicapped peers who are driving, getting married, having children, and living independently.

The testimonies of older Canadian adults with PWS supports the idea of increased stressors and psychosocial adjustments during young adulthood. Most individuals over the age of 40 (James, 2010) had been morbidly obese, had health issues, and had left home during their twenties. As will be seen in the next chapter, conflicts in the community increase in young adulthood.

Adults. In the United Kingdom, Clarke, Boer, Chung, Sturmey and Webb (1996) compared 30 adults with PWS to 30 adults with non-specific learning disability and suggested that temper tantrums, self-injury, impulsiveness, lability of mood, inactivity, and repetitive speech are characteristic behaviours in PWS in adult life. Holland et al. (2003) noted that aberrant behaviour increased with age for PWS adults, but decreased with increased IQ.

Interview data from parents and caregivers of adults in the present study suggest that maladaptive behaviours vary considerably with individuals with PWS. While a few become more aggressive with age, a greater number seem to mellow with age (i.e., attitudes and behaviours become milder and easier to tolerate). Those living at home are more likely to exhibit anger and tantrums; those living in alternate residential situations are generally described as being more stable.

Older adults.   Maladaptive and compulsive behaviours diminish "to an astonishing degree" in older adults with PWS according to Dykens (2004). She noted "less skin-picking as well as significantly fewer externalizing symptoms, social problems, total maladaptive behaviours, and number of compulsive symptoms" (p. 149). Older adults also showed less ordering and arranging. James (2010) similarly found those over 40 to be "generally more mellow" than in earlier years.

Maladaptive behaviour and genetic subtypes

Advances in genetic testing have lead to more refined differentiation of the PWS behaviour phenotype. Dykens, Cassidy, and King (1999) compared the maladaptive behaviours of individuals with PWS due to paternal deletion to age and gender-matched subjects with maternal UPD. They found "a milder behavioural expression among Prader-Willi individuals associated with maternal uniparental disomy relative to paternal deletion" (p. 73). The deletion group were more likely to skin-pick, nail-bite, hoard, overeat, sulk, and withdraw.

Butler, Bittel, Kibiryeva, Talebizadeh, and Thompson (2004) presented a paper on the assessment of clinical differences in individuals with a Type I (longer) or Type II (shorter) deletion of chromosome 15. Those with a Type I deletion scored significantly worse than those with Type II or UPD on psychological, behaviour, and academic achievement measures. "Maladaptive difficulties were coupled with a reduction in independent behaviors, suggesting a requirement for closer supervision" (p. 567) for those with Type I deletion. The average age of subjects in this study fell within the young adult range, so the observations may not apply to children.

Behavioural impact of growth hormone (GH) treatment

How does growth hormone therapy affect behaviour in children with PWS? Whitman, Myers, Carrel, and Allen (2002) conducted a two-year study involving 54 children, aged 4 to 16 years, with genetically confirmed PWS. Data was gathered from parents and teachers at 6-month intervals. The authors reported a significant positive effect, the reduction of depressive symptoms for those over 11 years of age, and "no apparent behavioural deterioration associated with GH administration." Interestingly, parents reported a number of areas of improvement in daily life activities which had not been covered by the structured questionnaire, including: "more willingness to participate" and "more normal participation in sports and physical education" (p. 7). Eiholzer, Gisin, Weinmann et al. (1998) earlier described similar benefits when they noted that PWS children on GH had increased physical activity and performance. They were described as "more attentive and lively, which made them more independent, more self-assured, and less anxious" (p. 374).

The study by Whitman et al. (2002) also reported that the improvement in physical appearance of the sibling with PWS reduced the embarrassment to the other siblings. Parents benefitted too, reporting fewer "snide remarks" from the public. The authors suggest that these improvements may be important from the perspective of "family pain." They also point out that the two-year time span of the study was insufficient to unequivocally attribute the improvements directly to GH treatment.

It is difficult to assess the effects of GH on behaviour as it is a relatively new treatment received by only a small number of children, and even fewer teens and adults. One mother of a three-year-old, whose daughter had been receiving GH for over two years, pointed out that GH didn't stop the hunger or the "interesting" behaviours that her child exhibited. The mother of a teen reported that her daughter had been on GH since age nine and that her behaviour had "improved dramatically" as a teen. But can improved behaviour be directly attributable to GH? Behaviour can be affected by a host of personal and environmental circumstances. More research is needed in this area.

Obsessive-compulsiveness disorder (OCD)

OCD involves recurrent obsessions or compulsions that are time consuming, excessive, or unreasonable. Dykens, Leckman, and Cassidy (1996) examined non-food obsessions and compulsions in 91 people with PWS (5 - 47 years) and found prominent symptoms in 58% of the sample, including: hoarding; ordering and arranging; concerns with symmetry and exactness; rewriting; and needs to tell, know, or ask. They found moderate to severe symptom severity ratings in a high proportion of the participants and similar levels of symptom severity and number of compulsions when the PWS group was compared with age and sex-matched "non-retarded" adults with OCD. They concluded that there are increased risks of OCD in individuals with PWS. Dykens and Shah (2003) later asserted that "compulsivity appears intrinsic to the Prader-Willi genotype" (p. 170).   Compulsivity begins to appear during the pre-school years according to Dimitropoulos et al. (2000).

OCD has been observed in home interviews.   One young teen had an invariable three day rotation for crackers (stone wheat, graham and soda).   He also ate the same breakfast daily - oatmeal and toast with jam and peanut butter.   When his mother cleared his dinner dishes from the table he insisted that she bring them back as it was his routine to do it.   According to his mother, the OCD is more difficult to contend with than the food issues:

> Our biggest challenge is his obsessive behaviour - we call him our freighter as it takes a long, long time to get him moved in any direction.   He has a very difficult time with change in routine.

One positive is that he is equally compulsive about an active daily exercise program and at age 14 weighs 93 pounds.

Autistic tendencies

Some parents have queried the link between autism and PWS. They observe behaviours such as hand-flapping, hand clapping, and body rocking which they associate with autism.   One mother noticed that her son spontaneously does these activities at home but is able to control himself in public as she has explained that the behaviours would make people think that he is odd.   She permits the behaviours at home as he seems more relaxed when permitted the freedom to act as he would prefer.

Children with autism spectrum disorders (ASD) have deficits in social interaction, verbal and non-verbal communication, and demonstrate repetitive behaviours or interests.   Often, they will also exhibit unusual responses to sensory experiences.   These symptoms can range from mild to severe.   They can also range from what is referred to as classic autism to a milder form known as Asperger syndrome.   In some cases a child might have some symptoms of one or the other of these disorders, or be on the continuum in between, but does not meet the specific criteria for diagnosis.   In these cases a diagnosis of pervasive developmental disorder (PDD) is likely.   Certainly there can be overlap between PWS and autism.   In a British study, Greaves et al. (2006) asserted that the range of repetitive behaviours in PWS, including insistence on sameness and 'just right' behaviours, showed a surprising overlap with those of children with autism.

It is possible to have a dual diagnosis of PWS and autism.   Boyle (2007), a parent of a 20-year-old son with PWS (UPD), sees two groups, those with PWS and autistic-like behaviours who do not look classically autistic, and those "who would be recognized as autistic by any community" (p. 10). The PWSA(USA) sponsors an on-line support group for families with this dual diagnosis (http://health.groups.yahoo.com/groups/pws-autism/).

Self-injurious behaviours

A survey of 62 families from 20 states and one Canadian province revealed self-injury for 81% of the PWS subjects, aged 3 to 44 years (Symons, Butler, Sanders, Feurer, & Thompson, 1999). Skin-picking (82%) was the most common form of self-injury. Other forms included nose-picking (28%), hand-biting (17%), head-banging (14%), hair-pulling (9%) and rectal-picking (6%). Self-injury sites were disproportionately located on the legs, head, and arms. Males and females had similar rates of self-injury. Those with paternal deletion were more likely to self-injure than individuals with maternal UPD. The authors noted that their method of reporting may have been more sensitive to readily visible body areas and suggested that future studies should consider that some individuals may pick areas of the body that are not easily or clearly visible. Dykens (2004) found skin-picking to be more frequent amongst girls than boys, with the severity of symptoms predicted by gender and living status. Males had higher significant severity scores than females and individuals living "in programs" had significantly higher severity scores than those still residing at home.

In a Swedish survey of parents of 37 individuals (12 to 30 years of age), Wigren and Heimann (2001) found that two-thirds displayed skin-picking, ranging from chronic to transient episodes. Of the skin pickers, 73% had started to show the symptom before 7 years of age, all but one had displayed the behaviour before age 11, and that once having started, no one gave up the behaviour. The majority of skin pickers (70%) displayed the behaviour in private contexts (e.g., during bedtime or bathroom routines). Skin-picking seemed to be independent of gender and level of intellectual disability. A study of Dutch children (Didden, Korzilius & Curfs, 2007) found skin-picking present in 86 percent of the sample. Severity was reported as mild (37%), moderate (36%) and severe (25%). The mean age at which skin-picking was observed to begin was 6 years. Most common picking areas included arms, legs, and feet.

There was only one report of serious self-injurious behaviour in the present study. One woman previously had to visit a wound clinic on a regular basis to treat the open sores on her body. This behaviour was now controlled with the use of gloves which were held in place with tape. Other reports of "skin-picking" included such descriptors as "rubbing sensitive skin," "creating sores," and "picking at scabs." In some cases they were described as intermittent, others were lifelong. Some were move evident under times of stress. Preventive measures such as long-sleeve shirts and activities to occupy the hands were commonly employed.

Psychotic behaviours

In a U.K. report, Clarke et al. (1998) described six adults with PWS (ages 20 to 46) who had developed psychoses. They suggested that PWS is associated with a vulnerability to psychotic symptoms in adult life. In a study of people with PWS over age 16, Clarke (1998) gave a "crude estimate" of 6.3% for possible psychotic disorders amongst adults with PWS. A Japanese study found that "adolescents and young adults with PWS showed symptoms of psychiatric illness and that the prevalence rate increased with age" (Hiraiwa, Maegaki, Oka, & Ohno, 2007, p. 539). They suggested a rate of 27.6% for psychotic symptoms amongst young adults with PWS.

Of particular interest, is a British study (Boer et al., 2002a), which explored the prevalence of physical and psychiatric disease, comparing the characteristics of those with different genetic make-up. The rate of serious psychiatric illness in this study was 28%. However, they found that only 8% of adults with deletions had psychotic illness compared to 62% for those with disomy.

It was difficult to determine the number of people with PWS in the present study who had ever been under the care of a psychiatrist. In some cases caregiver knowledge was incomplete, in other cases the topic of mental health was difficult to discuss. While there were reports of psychiatrist visits, psychiatric ward admissions, and the use of psychotropic medications, the numbers were low.

Running away

Several parents reported issues related to running away. Not knowing where a child is or when he or she will return is a great worry to any parent.

In a letter in *The Gathered View,* a mother from Alberta described how her 9-year-old son had taken off from home, school, neighbours, and day camp, in excess of 25 times in the previous two-year period (Nicholas, 1999). His favourite get-away method was to hop on the public transit. With insights gained by attending a PWSA national conference she began to help both members of the transit system and police department to better understand PWS, resulting in fewer suspicious looks and unkind comments and a more supportive response. The pattern of taking off has continued through his teen years.

The mother of a 19-year-old in the Okanagan area updated her son's escapades, saying:

> after three months he was off and running again. Unfortunately this time his destination was Vancouver Island. We had him brought back twice but after his taking off three times in one week I stopped putting out Police calls on him and decided I'd wait till he got it out of his system.

Eighteen years later, the mother reported that his "running away stopped when he grew up."

These examples suggest that running away can be a pattern of behaviour and not a one-time event. While running away is not a characteristic which is reported in the literature, it is included here because it may be problematic in a small percentage of the PWS population. Other examples are cited in the next chapter under the topic of "missing persons."

Food and behaviour

Food is the trigger for many behaviour issues. It is not just the sight of food. It can be the smell, the sound, pictures, or other reminders as well. Those unaware of the food craving in PWS may feel that it is simply a matter of self-control. John, a man with PWS, described his hunger thusly:

> I sometimes become rather terrified. The hunger is so overwhelming type of feeling, it sometimes takes you unconsciously. The hunger grows and grows and grows and becomes so big that it starts to rush you in your thoughts and you have to rush to the fridge so as not to lose consciousness. The only thing that you are able to concentrate on is the taste (PWSA-BC, p. 4).

Understanding food-related behaviours is central to the management of PWS, whether in the home or community.

Problematic food-related behaviours

There are a two food-related behaviours which are frequently reported as annoying, usually by mothers. They are:

- *preoccupation*: where everything revolves around food. Before the completion of one meal there are questions about the next. The daily schedule revolves around food times.
- *perseveration:* where there is a persisting preoccupation with thoughts related to food. Often it is the incessant repetition of questions related to when the next meal will occur, or what will be prepared. Parents have described it like a short-circuiting in the brain.

Then there are behaviours related to obtaining food. These are the behaviours which dictate the need for supervision, and include:

- *food-seeking:* the searching for food, usually within the context of familiar, controlled environments. Many are food-seekers but do not go to the next level of foraging.
- *foraging:* the searching for food, usually within the community. In the worst case scenario, foraging can lead to the eating of food remains from garbage cans or items otherwise considered inedible.
- *stealing*: most frequently it is food that is taken illicitly, how ever the stealing of money for the purpose of procuring food is also a concern. Cafeterias, corner grocery stores, coat rooms, and teachers' desks are examples of where stealing often occurs.

And then there are those behaviours having to do with what happens when the individual has obtained the food. Often these result in confrontation:

- *hiding/concealing:* food gained illicitly may be concealed in clothing until able to be devoured in private. Food may also be cached or hidden in bedrooms for later consumption.
- *clandestine consumption:* the consumption of food in a way that is not allowed, that is to say the clandestine eating of stolen food or simply the eating of food beyond the diet restrictions. When illicit it is often gorged.
- *gorging:* gorging refers to eating gluttonously, or greedily eating too much. This usually occurs when there is fear of being caught in the act of eating.
- *regurgitation:* this is not a frequent complaint, but it is a most annoying one. It is the return of partly digested food to the mouth to be enjoyed again. One father explained this as a bad habit that could be avoided by providing coffee or gum.

Again, it must be emphasized that not all individuals with PWS will exhibit all of these food behaviours. Most children, teens and adults have learned appropriate table manners and can behave in a socially acceptable way when supervised in the presence of food.

Food and self-control

Are individuals with PWS capable of exercising self-regulating behaviours in the presence of food? Many parents will say an emphatic "No!" Yet others believe that it is possible under certain circumstances.

Parents and caregivers have provided examples of self-control for children, teens and adults. Most of these occur in the presence of witnesses, for example, while partaking of a smorgasbord or buffet. In such circumstances, however, someone is usually providing supervision. Some homes do not have locked refrigerators or food cupboards, and some even have food visibly available. For example, in one home there was always a bowl of fruit available on the counter for all family members to enjoy whenever they wished. Parents say that self-control is evident when food is not taken or consumed without permission. And there are examples of adults being left at home for a few days, responsible for all food preparation. In order for food to last, some self-control must be exercised.

Parents usually suspect the worse when they know that food has gone missing. The following humorous anecdote definitely illustrates self-control:

> Vera had baked cookies and, forgetting that she had left them on the counter to cool, left her teenaged daughter alone in the house while she went out. When she returned the cookies were gone from the counter and there was evidence of crumbs around her daughter's mouth. When questioned, she explained that she had put all of the cookies into the cookie tin to help her mother, and that there was one left over. To solve the problem of the extra cookie she ate it.

Vera reported that the cookie tin was full as described. Her daughter had found a solution to the dilemma of an extra cookie.

Should teens with PWS be enrolled in foods classes at school? Again, there are parents who would say an emphatic "NO!" Jill, however, grew up without food locks at home, took foods courses, and worked in the school store selling snack foods. When questioned about the temptation she emphasized that "the food was for someone else." She went on to explain that the food had to be bought and that she didn't have any money. Her parents maintain that she will not take others' food and will only eat what is designated for her. She has a strong sense of right and wrong and gives evidence of self-control.

Food seeking. Individuals with PWS, regardless of age, are commonly described as engaging in "food seeking." This aspect of the syndrome is often sensationalized in the media, with reference to the eating of garbage or other inedibles. An American study, however, concluded that "individuals with PWS are able to discriminate the appropriateness of eating items in more or less contaminated areas" (Young et al., 2006) They found that the amount of time spent seeking food and the amount of food covertly consumed depended more directly on younger age and lower BMI. In other words, younger children on very restricted diets were more likely to engage in food seeking. This was a small study conducted in an artificial situation, however, and warrants further investigation. Testimony of some parents would challenge this finding.

Kitchen privileges. Should individuals with PWS be permitted kitchen privileges? There are examples of teens being responsible for making their own school lunch, preparing tea and snacks for guests, and cooking a full meal for a guest. Adults living in semi-independent living usually have some kitchen privileges and responsibilities. In some cases they are totally involved in meal planning, shopping, and food preparation; in others they may have their meals prepared for them and they may only have drinks and snacks available to them in a small fridge. For some parents it is simply easier to keep the child out of the kitchen than have to cope with monitoring behaviours in the kitchen.

Eating out. Some parents have described eating out as highly problematic. To avoid waitresses who offer too many choices or try to push desserts one father would choose a small restaurant and pre-visit to educate the waitress. Several parents described patronizing a favourite restaurant and pre-determining the meal choice before leaving home. Others described limiting the choices, or getting prior agreement to share a "large" order. Rose, a caregiver, described herself as a "companion eater," only eating what Lindsay eats when they go out together.

Eating out requires more than menu strategies. Parents have described choosing or reserving a table away from the line of traffic to the kitchen and not within view of the smorgasbord or buffet tables. Positioning to take advantage of a window view can be helpful to provide a distraction. Being closer to the washroom can be helpful too. However, one woman with PWS was still observed taking sugar packets from empty tables as she made the short trip to the washroom.

Food preferences

An American study examined food type preference in 12 PWS subjects in comparison to obese and normal control groups. Those with PWS preferred high carbohydrate foods over high protein foods, and high protein foods over high fat foods. This was a different food preference profile from either of the control groups (Fieldstone, Zipf, Schwartz, & Berntson, 1997). In the U.K., Hinton et al. (2006) reported that "individuals with PWS expressed relative liking of different foods and showed preferences that were consistent over time, particularly for sweet foods" (p. 633). There was a "lack of a strong preference for a particular macronutrient (protein, carbohydrate or fat)." There was, however, "a significantly greater preference for sweet-tasting foods over salty, bland and sour foods in the PWS group" (p. 639).

In another American study of visual processing of food images in adults with PWS the authors reported differences between the deletion and UPD groups. "The deletion group appeared to group the stimuli based on the quantity of food, while those with UPD focussed more on the quality of food" (p. 543). This food stimulus analysis happens in an immediate and automatic fashion with "little or no direct cognitive involvement" (Key & Dykens, 2008).

There is testimonial evidence that children and adults do have food preferences. One three-year-old, on a strict 800 calorie diet, demonstrates definite food preferences according to her grandmother. "When there is broccoli on her plate, she will push it away and say 'Yuck!' Like any other young child, she has her definite likes and dislikes when it comes to eating" (Bavis, 2003). A senior with PWS thoughtfully identified his favourite foods, which were corroborated by staff: steak, hamburger, kipper snacks, sardines, hot sauces, and mustard. When permitted, individuals with PWS can make choices based on food preferences.

Hunger or food salience?

In a Canadian study from Alberta, involving 24 families with a PWS member, Kinash (2007c) points out that the distinction between the "physiological state of hunger" (i.e., the hunger drive) and the "psychological trigger of food salience" (i.e., the presence of food) is an important consideration. She cites the testimony of adults with PWS and their parents which indicate that there are times when individuals with PWS can be occupied for hours without the preoccupation of hunger. Rather, they are only drawn to eat if food is present. She asserts that the distinction between hunger and food salience matters because understanding the difference will help to determine the best way to support persons with PWS. She goes on to explain:

If persons with PWS are constantly hungry, then intervention must include frequent low-calorie high nutrient foods, distraction from the unpleasant sensation interceding these meals and snacks, and training in coping strategies such as progressive relaxation and visualization, as is facilitated with those persons who have chronic pain.

If food salience is the primary triggering factor, then the most effective intervention is to construct and stay within environments where there are minimal food sights, smells and sounds (p. 37).

Given the uncertainty as to whether one or both factors determine the food behaviours she concludes that perhaps the best approach is "to rigorously apply both types of intervention."

Food "brilliance"

Some stories of food acquisition behaviour demonstrate what some parents describe as "brilliance" and what psychologists refer to as "executive planning" abilities, that is to say the ability to make longer-term plans to obtain food. This is in contrast to the need for immediate gratification so often associated with PWS. Some individuals can plan multi-step sequences with delayed gratification. For example, one article described how a young man

would go through the garbage outside a local confectionery and bring rotten eggs to the IGA, saying he was returning them for his parents. With the money the supermarket gave him he would go back to the first store and buy two cartons of chocolate milk. [He] would drink half the milk and complain that the cartons were half-empty when he bought them. The storekeeper would give him another two cartons.

In another incident, the same young man

went into his mother's purse, stole the keys to the basement where the food is locked up and took two bottles of ginger ale, four tins of beans, cans of grape juice and four bottles of Italian sauce.

He then "locked the cellar, hid the food under his bed, and returned the keys" (Dickson, 1987).

Sometimes the brilliance is not only associated with planning but also with the execution of the plan. One couple related how their overweight teenaged son adroitly tiptoed down creaky wooden stairs from his second floor bedroom and then took the key for the refrigerator padlock from their headboard while they slept. He then unlocked the padlock, removed the bicycle chain, got the food he wanted, replaced the lock and the key and returned to his room. Food brilliance was implied when parents and workers described such uncanny ability to procure food.

Hunger and satiety

In the U.K., Hinton, Holland, Gellatly et al. (2006) used brain imagining to investigate the neural basis of the abnormal eating behaviour associated with PWS. Thirteen adults were measured with positron emission tomography in three sessions, following an overnight fast and after energy controlled meals of 400 and 1200 kcal of similar volume and appearance. They concluded that

> there is a dysfunction in the satiety system in those with
> PWS. These findings suggest that brain regions associated
> with satiety are insensitive even to high-energy food intake
> in those with the syndrome. This may be the neural basis
> of the hyperphagia seen in PWS (p. 313).

Comparison of neural activity after the different energy-value meals suggested that some with PWS are able to detect an increasing fullness, yet others do not experience fullness in the same way as individuals without the syndrome.

Food and safety

For a small percentage of individuals with PWS the consumption of "inedibles" is a concern. This is particularly so for those who forage in the community. There is the fear that they might ingest tainted products or liquids containing poisonous ingredients. Vigilant parents have warned neighbours as a preventive measure. There were no stories of illness resulting from foraging, although there was obvious parent discomfort and fear associated with this behaviour.

Vigilance is also essential in the home. Parents have expressed concern about the eating of decaying meat products and kitchen scraps, and the drinking of alcohol and household cleaning fluids. Even edible products can pose a safety concern. In a sad case, a three-year-old boy with PWS died after choking on marshmallows. Left alone in the kitchen for only a few minutes, he opened a barred kitchen cupboard to find the marshmallows, something he had never eaten before (Halifax Daily News, 2001).

Crisis intervention

Parents should anticipate that there will be times of crises in the management of a child or adult with PWS. With this recognition, the best approach to crisis intervention is a preventive one. Key to this approach is the identification of:

- professional resource people with a knowledge of PWS who can become familiar with the individual and family
- personal friends who will listen with a non-judgmental ear
- the closest local PWS association
- Internet resources (websites, chat rooms, Facebook) where help can be found.

Where should parents get their help in times of crisis? There is often the parent quandry: is it better to utilize a qualified professional with no experience with PWS or rely on non-professionals who are at least knowledgeable about PWS? Unlike Americans, who have the PWSA-USA organization with a crisis counsellor available for families, Canadians rely on health and social services professionals or peer help through their local association in times of crisis. Because of the low incidence nature of the syndrome, in many communities there may not be a professional with experience with PWS.

Word-of-mouth is one of the best ways to find help. It can come directly from other parents of PWS children or through a PWS parent organization. Recommendations might also be sought from social services agencies, other care providers, or professional associations. There are a small number of behaviour specialists who are now beginning to emerge with experience with PWS.

Elements of crisis management

During crisis parents are desperate for help. In most cases, they have not anticipated the problem and are suddenly searching for assistance. What can be expected in the way of professional assistance?

- *Reassurance to parents:* During times of crisis parents need to be reassured that they are doing the best that they can under the circumstances. It usually helps when they hear that others have gone through similar situations. They need to have their concerns validated and be reassured that things will get better.
- *Reassurance to person with PWS:* When in crisis people with PWS need calm reassurance that they are not "bad." They need to recognize that "we" have a problem that needs

to be addressed. An objective third party can be helpful, particularly if the person is not a stranger inserted at the height of crisis.

- *Professional intervention:* Professional intervention can be many things: assistance with designing a behaviour plan, provision of resources, writing letters of support, providing networking contacts, advocating for new or increased service levels, conducting staff in-service or community workshops, counselling family members, and providing research updates. Usually it will be a combination of approaches.

- *Follow-up:* As parents are usually at wit's end and desperate for help it is important that they not be left unsupported after the initial intervention. Unfortunately, government and agency service workers tend to focus on immediate intervention and have little time for follow-up. In some cases, the crisis dissipates quite naturally or the intervention doesn't work. In such cases there needs to be feedback to the professional. Minimally, a consultant should remain available via telephone.

Some families have evolved their own strategies for crisis management which do not include professional assistance. Time-out, whether a period of time alone in the bedroom, or a weekend away in respite, can be helpful to break the immediacy of the issue. The use of trusted third parties such as siblings, grandparents, or friends to provide required supervision ensures consistency of approach and safety of the individual. Personal support to the parent, from a spouse, relative, or friend is helpful for reassurance and to reduce stress.

PWS Associations

Members of the local, regional, or national PWS associations are as close as the telephone. They may simply provide an understanding ear, or they might assist with information, resources, or referral. The parent of a toddler praised her provincial association, saying that she valued "the parent-to-parent help." She was also thankful for access to "lots of information that hasn't been published."

The PWS Canada e-group is also a source of support to parents. A review of posts to this group indicated some which are behavioural and might be considered urgent or of a crisis nature. This is a supportive network which can be quickly accessed and helpful to both avoid and address crises.

Respite

Respite is a period of temporary relief. It can be either informal (i.e., provided by family or friends) or formal (i.e., agency or government funded).

While the pioneer PWS parents seldom had the benefits of formal respite programs, they did utilize friends and family. Even today, not everyone who is eligible takes advantage of respite services. Some parents are strongly independent and don't want to initiate a relationship with the government or an agency. Or they may not have a need when their child is young as they utilize relatives or share babysitting with friends in order to create breaks for themselves.

Value of respite

Parent testimony suggests that respite assists in three important ways, providing:

- temporary parent relief from PWS concerns
- parent time for other family members, and
- socialization of the PWS child.

In reflection, one mother wrote: "one of the biggest mistakes I made when I look back on our 13 years of living with PWS is not accepting and pushing for more respite care." She went on to say:

> I would really recommend to young families to push hard for it - even when you don't think you need it....I had good family support (and thought I was Wonder Woman) so I turned down respite several times....Now he is attached to me like glue and I really think it would have been much smarter for us to have had him in respite at a young age.

In many jurisdictions, however, today's young parents begin to get respite while their child is still an infant. Cheryl, mother of two year-old Isabelle, said that respite:

> likely saved our sanity, marriage, family life. We take scheduled time as a couple to talk things through and goal plan without having to do this with kids around or house chores calling us. We also use the respite to give us quality time with our son ... time where we can do things he wants to do without his sister around, time to give him 100% attention without having to worry about her getting into something. The time has helped create the balance in our lives.

Respite not only benefits the parents and siblings, it is usually a positive experience for the child as well. Several children delighted in going to spend time at their grandparents' home or the home of their cousins. Spending time with extended family usually resulted in special attention (and sometimes treats and permissions that parents would not give!).

Contracted workers have been used to provide after school, weekend, and summer relief for children, teens, and adults. Often they provide enriching social and integrated experiences. They facilitate participation in community recreational activities, cultural events, or other day activities.

Long term respite workers become valued members of the team. One worker, providing respite in her own home, included the teen with PWS into her own circle of friends. Another, similarly provided respite in her own home, where the young adult with PWS developed a close friendship with her daughter. The young woman always looked forward to respite time with anticipation because of this special friendship.

Lack of awareness

Not all parents are aware of the availability of respite. If the family takes pride in its independence and is not involved with social service agencies, then they may not be aware of the services available, including respite. Sometimes it is not until there is a crisis that services suddenly become available.

In one unusual case, a charge of child abuse became the catalyst to get respite services. With the mother in the hospital and the father charged with child abuse, the child was provided temporary care by social services. The judge recognized the child's injury as the result of an accident and dismissed the charge against the father. In the parent's words:

> Oddly, there was a very positive outcome to us as our son went in to a respite situation, which continued (was offered twice a month and we accepted). If this had not happened, we would not have known about respite, which was a godsend.

Changing policies and fiscal management may increase or decrease the budget available for respite to families. A recent province-wide reorganization of services to children and adults with developmental disabilities in B.C., along with requirements to trim expenses, has left some families without services, including respite. Whenever there are system-wide changes there is the possibility that some families will be left uninformed. Families have complained that social workers do not tell them what is available. Parents need to regularly ask what resources and services they are eligible to receive, and push for respite.

Response to need

The availability of respite varies across provinces and regions within provinces. Parents are reminded that the level of respite available will depend on the assessment of the child. The more severe the need, the more time will be available. A single parent of a pre-teen described her personal crisis which resulted in an increase in respite. In addition to dealing with her daughter's puberty, she was coping with menopause, job loss, loss of social supports, rheumatoid arthritis, her own new disabled status, and the murder of a relative. Recognizing her need for help, the respite was increased from four hours per week and four weekends per year to six hours per week and two weekends per month. As mentioned earlier, in some jurisdictions parents have been offered the service, in others there has been a need to seek out the service.

Respite may take the form of after-school care, relief for a day or weekend, or for a longer period if required. In some regions parents are provided a certain number of hours or days per month, or year. This allows for planning to meet family circumstances. In some locales, however, it seems to be a service given only in response to a crisis.

It appears that services are easier to establish when children are infants. That is to say, if a family is able to survive without services when the child is younger it will be more difficult to establish the need for the service later. Formal respite is generally more available for children and adolescents than adults. Parents caring for an adult with PWS have lamented the lack of respite services available to them.

Most respite is self-administered. that is to say that parents must identify and hire their own respite caregiver. The problem, according to one mother, is that "I can't find anyone to hire." She described a need for trust and not being able to give her daughter to a stranger. With individualized funding, it is now easier to hire a trusted relative or a friend. Contact with local Community Living Associations, special needs support groups, or other PWS parents has been success-ful in locating respite workers in some cases. Parents have also hired teaching assistants from their child's school to provide respite. These people are trained to work with children with special needs and usually have proven behaviour management skills. Because they are hourly paid employees and only work school hours they are often open to supplement their income with part-time contract work.

A lack of respite is one of the factors that most affects parents' quality of life. As a mother of a 22-year-old expressed, "I have become envious of my friends going off and doing their own things, whatever and whenever they want to." Without respite the long-term drain on physical and emotional stamina can ultimately affect the health and well-being of a parent or family.

It may not be easy

Utilizing respite may not be easy. Children may not be accepting of the idea, particularly when they think that they will be missing out on something. Pat wrote:

> Even our respite time isn't working anymore because she is always terrified the rest of us will do something without her, and she is right. But, to take her along with us every time almost guarantees a major tantrum over something, then the point of the excursion is, more often than not, totally lost.

And then there is the reality of time and energy. Sometimes it is easier to avoid something than face the inevitable. She continued:

> Getting her to agree to go with the respite worker has become a huge ordeal. It's usually simpler to just stay home.
> A half day battle to get her out the door so we can enjoy a couple of hours with our other two kids just isn't worth it any more (Johnson, p. 142).

It seems important to establish the routine of respite in early childhood and to structure and monitor it to ensure that it is an enjoyable experience for the child. To try to utilize respite at a later stage, as just described, may not be easy.

Even for experienced caregivers, respite may not be easy. One educational assistant accustomed to providing weekend respite for teens, described her sleepless weekend providing care for a teen with PWS. In addition to the daily food vigilance, night time supervision was draining. She resorted to pushing a double bed against a wall and sleeping on the outside edge of the bed in order to thwart the young lady's nocturnal wanderings.

Some respite caregivers have found the challenges too demanding; in other cases parents have not been satisfied with the level of supervision provided. Finding suitable respite workers has been cited as a problem by many families.

The Children's Institute of Pittsburgh

The PWS program at The Children's Institute of Pittsburgh is the only hospital program of its kind in North America. Since its inception in 1981, the Institute has treated more than 1000 children and adults with PWS. Since 1999, a dozen Canadians with PWS have been admitted. Eleven of these referrals have been from the province of Ontario. Eight individuals were between the ages of 19 and 25, three were under age 19, and one was over age 25 (K. Smith, personal communication, March 27, 2008).

Prader-Willi Syndrome Program

The Children's Institute employs a medically supervised multi-disciplinary approach to individualized treatment programs to address weight control, motor development, nutrition awareness, social skills, and self-motivation. The team includes: pediatricians, physiatrists, dietitians, psychologists, teachers, and occupational, physical, and speech and language therapists. While patients learn behavioural self-control, families and caregivers receive training to maintain the program after discharge (For further information visit www.amazingkids.org).

One family's story

At age 30, and after exhausting all of the resources available within her province, Sara became the first individual from western Canada to go to the Institute. The following notes from her mother's updates provide a glimpse of what Sara and the family went through:

> *June 28:* ...a year's worth of planning and begging from us, her social worker, 3 doctors, psychologist, psychiatrist, endo, dietician, various agency people, and some politicians has resulted just this week in the... government finally deciding to fund Sara to go to Pittsburgh. . . .
>
> *July 8:* The head of her agency will be one of the people going down for training before Sara comes back. There will be him, plus the case manager, the house manager, her social worker, dietician, behaviour specialist, and us, all going as part of her team. Every one of us knows this is Sara's last chance, so we have to get it right.
>
> *July 21:* Sara is on 600 calories a day, and they set her goal weight at 129 lbs. ...She is 242 now. Sara has to save milk from her glass if she wanted to have some in her coffee....

They're testing her for type 2 diabetes.... They work on a point system and everything is based on earning points and privileges with behaviour modification.... There is a psychologist and a psychiatrist on the floor at all times.

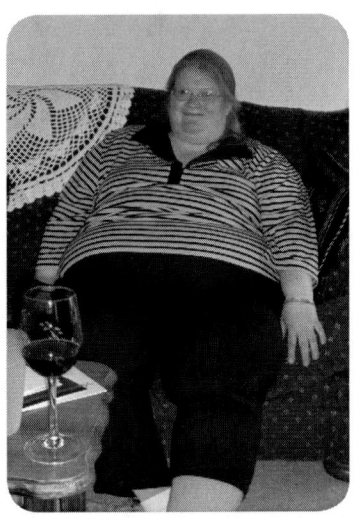
Sara before going to Pittsburgh

Sept 30: She's doing just awesome. She has lost 35 lbs and is off oxygen for 2 hours each time, twice a day. She's doing stairs, walking her laps in the gym, playing running games, all activities we once thought she would never be able to do again. For this family who once believed we were going to have to plan a funeral, there are no words to describe how this feels.... The staff 'get it.' They're all on the same page, they're calm, professional, and inspiring. They've helped her to blossom....

They gave us their assessment of the plans we have set up for her return home, and living situation, and they made suggestions as to what will work and what might need to be tweaked. And we got a written report of all of her health issues and the progress she's made. Best of all is that Pittsburgh promises to be available to any of us, any time in the future, if we have concerns and need some advice....

Sara's quality of life improved as a result of her stay in Pittsburgh. She was restored to better health and given a fresh start when she returned to Canada. Her parents similarly found hope and encouragement with the Pittsburgh resource. At the beginning of January, 2008, Pat wrote:

Our Sara, age 31, who went to Pittsburgh this past summer for 3 months in the Prader-Willi clinic, has lost... drum roll...103 lbs in the past 18 months!!! She started at 299, and now she's 196. Isn't that just fabulous? Pittsburgh set 130 as her goal weight and even Sara herself can actually see it as a real possibility in the next year or so.

She has improved her health so much she no longer has to wear her oxygen all the time, just when she is exerting herself. She still needs her Bipap for overnights. But she has way more energy and her thinking is so much clearer. She's not falling asleep at all like she used to, not even in the car. We can go for walks and she keeps right up. She even runs from time to time!! She was home over Christmas for 3 days and not one meltdown! She could whup us all in Scrabble before, but we haven't a hope of winning now. And she's funny when she sees past photos of herself, and says things like "Whoa ...I HAVE lost weight!!" Or "Boy am I ever skinny!" It's hard for us to believe this is the same Sara, who we feared would not even be here this Christmas.

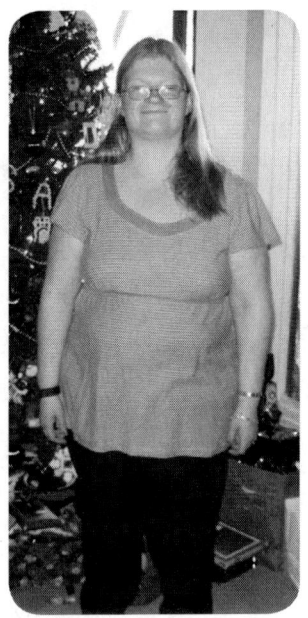

Sara six months later.

∽

The range and variability within PWS is most evident in the area of behaviour. Parents are cautioned not to attribute all maladaptive behaviours to the syndrome, nor to buy into the "self-fulfilling prophecy" with the expectation of maladaptive behaviours. While a behavioural phenotype may statistically exist, it does not mean to say that all individuals will exhibit all of the behaviours, and most certainly not all of the time. Observations of children and adults with PWS in home, school, and community settings affirm the normalcy of behaviours for most of the individuals, most of the time.

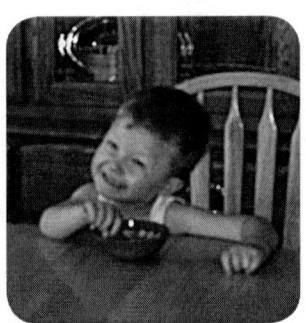

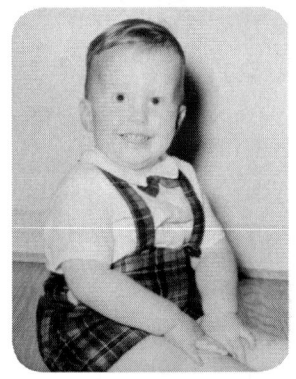

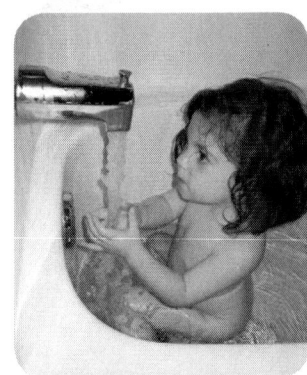

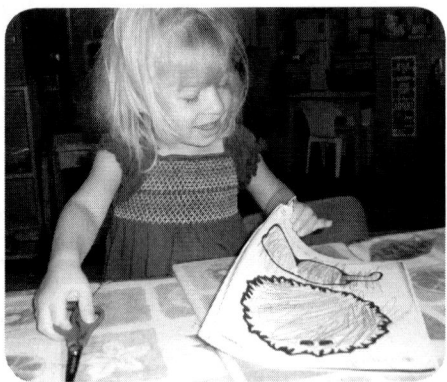

Toddlers

5

Socialization

Friendships and social activities are important aspects of quality of life. Unfortunately, having disabilities may limit social opportunities for children and adults with PWS; at the same time, having a child with disabilities may restrict the social life of parents.

Social skills

Social skills are specific behaviours that are deemed important for social competence; they are important across all environments and throughout life. As Hughes (1990) points out, there is confusion between the use of the terms "social skills" (specific behaviours leading to judgments of competence) and "social competence" (evaluative term referring to overall effectiveness of social behaviours).

Educators often talk about "social skills training," recognizing the need for teaching how to operate successfully in a social context. Chedd, Levine, and Wharton (2006) maintain that "a social skills/ pragmatics program should be a priority in any IEP" [individual education plan] (p. 317). Most importantly, parents should assist the team to identify and prioritize the social skills which need to be part of the individualized program.

But social skills training is not just the mandate of the school system. Parents begin the process with their infants in the home, and hopefully, with the assistance of family and friends, the training is reinforced in other settings. Once a teen leaves the education system social skills goals usually form part of the individual program plan in adulthood. Improving social skills reduces interpersonal problems such as peer conflict, ostracism, loneliness, and bullying.

Poor social judgment

A 2004 American study (Koenig, Klin, & Schultz, 2004), measuring the ability to make appropriate social judgments from an ambiguous visual display, compared a PWS group to a group with pervasive developmental disorder (PDD) and an IQ matched group with no known syndrome. Those with PWS performed significantly more poorly than those with comparable intellectual ability and similar to the PDD group, suggesting that those with PWS have an "underlying difficulty interpreting social information that is presented visually" (p. 573). If there is a basic problem with understanding social situations, it follows that there will be difficulties with appropriate social responses.

Regression in social skills

From their work with various disability groups, Brown and Hughson (1993) pointed out that regression in behaviour can be expected when an individual experiences new tasks or situations. Young people with PWS, for example, have demonstrated changes in behaviour in response to having to learn new tasks at school or on the job, or when having to cope with a family separation or rejection by peers. Parents describe regressive behaviour such as: "tuning out," avoidance, a lack of cooperation, irritability, and moodiness. Such descriptors may also be viewed as a decline in social skills. Under the circumstances described, however, regression in behaviour is to be expected and should not necessarily be attributed to the syndrome. When social skills seem to regress it is important to look at the stressors in the life of the individual. In some cases social skills deficits may be situation-specific and time limited.

Transferable skills

Recognizing the tendency to poorer performance in new situations, it is important to teach for transfer of learning. While social skills may be learned and demonstrated in a classroom setting, it is important to give the opportunity to transfer the learning to new or less structured situations. Structuring for success is essential. This is one reason why it is important for the home and the school to communicate about social skills goals.

Social skills curriculum

There is a wide range of social skills which are considered desirable for adequate social functioning. Table 3 illustrates some of the deficit areas that parents have cited as concerns. There are common themes of politeness, respect, and safety in this table. Some of the skills relate to peers, and others to inter-generational relationships. The list is not exhaustive. There may be social skills which are unique to ethnic groups, for example, how to behave in certain religious and cultural celebrations. Still others may relate to expectations in residential, work or day programs. Social skills are required in all settings; some will be generic in nature and others may be specific to the environment. While some schools and agencies develop their own generic skills lists, there are also established curricula which can be used.

Table 3
Some social skills deficit areas identified by parents

Child	Teen	Adult
taking turns	arranging a date	public display of affection
acknowledging guests	responding to a social invitation	understanding consent
remembering manners	using the telephone appropriately	invasion of personal space
answering questions	respecting time limits	computer safety awareness
interrupting others	listening to answers	dominating conversations
playing nicely with peers	respecting quiet times	appropriate questions
ignoring strangers	table manners	
	acknowledging friends	
	respecting authority	

Social competence

There is not a universal definition of social competence, nor even a common set of behavioural standards by which to judge competence. What is expected within families, ethnic groups, or local communities may vary.

Competence requires a subjective judgment of the sufficiency or adequacy of social behaviours. It is more than just a knowledge of appropriate skills; it considers the application of the skills. To be considered as socially competent implies that one has acquired the skills necessary to cope successfully with daily social demands. It suggests that the individual will be able to demonstrate socially appropriate behaviours across settings. It is important that children and adults have an adequate level of social skills to function without embarrassing themselves and their families, or coming into conflict with authorities.

The characteristic problems identified as minor diagnostic criteria for PWS predictably will affect social competence and social acceptance. Social competence is further restricted by social isolation and the limiting of social experiences. It is, however, increased with the reinforcement of social skills training from the school, and taking advantage of "teachable moments" in the home. Parents do not require a social skills curriculum; they simply need to remember the positives of what they were taught as kids, and what they expect of the other siblings. Addressing good manners such as politeness, turn taking and respect for elders will help to address social skills and hence the judgment of social competence.

Why talk about social competence?

Have you ever felt embarrassed by the actions of your child? Have you ever chosen not to participate in a particular social event because of the possible misbehaviour of your child? Or have you ever simply wished that your child could behave more appropriately? If so, then you have had a concern for social competence. Likewise, if you have agonized about the social rejection of your child, tried to mediate a peer conflict, or even warned others about your child's gullibility, then you have tried to address issues of social competence. If you have ever rehearsed appropriate behaviours with your child before attending a function, prompted the appropriate use of "please" and "thank you," or cautioned which behaviours to avoid, then you have tried to engage in social skills training to increase competence.

There is considerable evidence which suggests that problems with peer relationships in childhood are predictive of a variety of negative outcomes in adolescence and adulthood, most notably peer conflicts and lack of friends. It is easy to rationalize poor social behaviours such as stubbornness, selfishness, and bossiness as personality variables. But are these irreversible characteristics or learned behaviours? Each of these can contribute to a judgment about social competence. Without specific interventions, an individual may be left quite incompetent in social settings.

Competence is not a term that parents like to hear or use. After all, parents are advocates for their child, and do not want to hear the negative judgments of others about their child's performance. On the other hand, it is a term which is commonly understood. It is important to talk about social competence because we are all social beings and we place value on competent functioning.

Social inappropriateness

Incidents of inappropriate social behaviours were cited by many parents. Some children and adults were described as "having personal space issues" and being "in the face" of others. A boy who was befriended by girls in the primary grades was abandoned by the same girls in the intermediate grades, in part because of his persistent and annoying behaviours. They had outgrown their interest in nurturing and set their limits, but he didn't understand the boundaries. His behaviours were not socially appropriate for the school yard.

The mother of a young woman who was no longer living at home, described how she dropped in to visit her daughter and learned that she was about to be dropped off by her worker at a boy's home in order to deliver a Valentine card and a rose. The mother felt it necessary to intervene, to save her daughter from embarrassment. The young man was a friend of the brother and he had no relationship with her daughter. According to the mother, the card was more appropriate to give to a spouse. While giving a card might be appropriate on February 14th, the choice of card, the rose, and the recipient were not appropriate in this case.

Other examples of social inappropriateness cited in interpersonal relations included: domineering, commanding, controlling, badgering, interrupting, ignoring, and swearing, Issues of judgment involved: harmful relationships, running away, and contravention of laws.

Dimensions of competence

Competence has several dimensions, For example, there are intellectual, behavioural, physical, and social aspects to competence. There may be others as well. All are inter-related. A limitation in one area may interfere with competence in another. A limitation in intellectual ability, for example, might interfere with social awareness and ability to communicate. A physical disability might be a handicap to social opportunity. Of course, behavioural competence is important to PWS parents. Behavioural extremes push the limits of social acceptability.

The frequency and severity of more aberrant behaviours unfortunately help to define the degree of social competence. Rosner et al., (2004), in examining social competence across three disability groups, found that "the Prader-Willi group fared worst in behaviour with others and was the least active in social organization" (p. 214). Also, compared to the Down syndrome and Williams syndrome groups, the PWS group did not increase in social competence as they got older.

Community tolerance

Community tolerance refers to the degree to which a community will allow the existence of differences without interference. Communities are not always tolerant of behaviours associated with PWS. Without an understanding of the syndrome the public may be critical of gross obesity or behavioural inappropriateness. Tolerance is stretched as behaviours move from being socially bearable to socially offensive. Ultimately, formal societal intervention may be required when behaviour exceeds the limits of social acceptability.

Levels of community intervention

James (1995) followed 34 children and adults with PWS from western Canada over an eight-year period to determine the type and level of community interventions required. Three levels of community tolerance were conceptualized: socially bearable, socially offensive, and criminal. The incidence of the latter two increased during the late teens and twenties. Examples of maladaptive behaviours can be seen in Table 4.

Most of the characteristic behaviour problems associated with PWS are socially bearable. It was speculated that the tolerance of childhood deviance may be related to greater supervision levels, family advocacy, and social leniency during the school years. Community tolerance was a greater issue for teens and adults. Socially offensive behaviours such as foraging, skin-picking, and aggression were cited as problematic during the teen years and requiring specialist intervention. It was suggested that without appropriate interventions aggression might lead ultimately to charges of assault.

Trouble with the law

People with PWS do run afoul of, and suffer the consequences of, the law. This reality underscores the importance of educating professionals

Table 4
Summary of maladaptive behaviours

Socially bearable	Socially offensive	Criminal
attention seeking	aggression	arson
arguing	eating hair	assault
deviousness	fecal smearing	panhandling
disobedience	foraging	property damage
distractibility	masturbation	shoplifting
dominance	running away	theft
irritability	self-abuse	
lying	skin-picking	
manipulation	urinating in public	
moodiness	violence	
obsessive-compulsiveness		
perseveration		
stubbornness		
swearing		
tantrums		
wandering		

Adapted from James (1995)

and the public about PWS. Without professional awareness of PWS those with the disorder will be treated like anyone else when they transgress - as lawbreakers. Unfortunately, the justice system is a very black-and-white system. One is either guilty or not guilty. If guilty, the consequences of crime are prescribed. The judicial system is not very well equipped to operate in shades of grey.

Difficulty with the law creates undue stress on all those involved. Unfortunately, stress is often increased by the time factor, the interval required to get resolution. Anxiety is also heightened by the uncertainty of the process and consideration of special needs. Quality of life is certainly diminished when having to contend with the judicial system.

Shoplifting. There have been many reports of young people with PWS shoplifting. Usually the temptation is related to food items. Some parents and caregivers find it important to advise the corner grocery or convenience store about their child and provide some education about PWS. They have introduced the child or taken in a picture. This proactive approach has likely averted shoplifting charges in some instances as parents have been called when the child has taken off without paying.

Shoplifting can begin at an early age. One elementary-aged student took cookies from a corner store. The proprietor forced him into a back room to contain him until the police arrived. The lad lashed out and bit the store owner and then did damage to the back seat of the police cruiser. A west coast parent wrote that there were "shoplifting charges periodically" between the ages of 12 and 17. At least twice her son was "banned from going into specific stores for a period of time." At one point charges were laid for shoplifting some donuts, which resulted in probation.

One young teen and two friends went into a music store to check out the CDs and tapes. One friend wanted to steal a music tape and proceeded to remove the cardboard wrapping so that it would not alert the scanner as she left the store with the tape in her pocket. The teen with PWS didn't want to leave the cardboard garbage on the shelf so she put it in her own pocket. As they tried to leave the store her action activated the alarm and both girls were arrested for shoplifting when mall security and police were called. Her father went down to talk with the mall security officer. The daughter was very remorseful and embarrassed and offered to pay for the tape. Thankfully, the security officer did not press charges and she learned a great lesson about the consequences of stealing.

The consequence for adult shoplifting is usually more harsh. In Victoria, a man "who has stolen food all of his life" was caught taking food and tapes from a nation-wide drugstore chain. The police were called and with the guardian's permission, took him to the police station and took finger prints, in order to scare him. He was not required to go to court, but he was banned from the drugstore. This seemed like a reasonable response when compared to a similar shoplifting incident some years earlier in Alberta. In an incident with lesser dollar value, a 31-year-old mildly mentally handicapped woman with PWS was taken to court for taking cookies, chocolates, and spaghetti, worth $4.50, from a drugstore in a mall in Calgary. Her lawyer argued for a discharge considering the unusual circumstances associated with PWS and the fact it was a first offense. The judge, however, told the woman to "follow the law instead of her stomach" and fined her one hundred dollars for shoplifting (Lunman, 1990).

In another case, 20 years ago, the Alberta PWS Association was called to assist with an untenable situation when shoplifting resulted in probation and community service hours, which were to be served at the Food Bank. It is unlikely that this type of sentence would be given today.

The matter of shoplifting is particularly troublesome in situations where stores have a zero tolerance policy, that is to say that "all" shoplifters will be prosecuted without exception. It is not unreasonable to assume that for every case of shoplifting that is brought to the attention of authorities there are numerous other cases that go unreported.

Theft. Shoplifting is theft from a store. Theft, however can occur in many other settings as well. While inappropriately taking the possessions of others will not likely bring a child into conflict with the law, the same action as a teen or adult may bring charges. Table 5 illustrates the types of theft that have occurred across developmental stages.

Table 5
Some examples of theft

Child	Teen	Adult
car keys	ice cream treats	till cash
teacher's lunch	diamond ring	neighbour's car
pens/pencils	student lunches	parents' money
fast food	restaurant food	kids collectibles
jewelry	freezer food	grocery store food

In an effort to teach the serious consequences of stealing, some parents have appealed for police assistance. One mother reported her daughter to the police and insisted that they confront her after she learned that her daughter had stolen money from a gymnasium locker in a recreation facility.

With increasing urbanization and the proliferation of fast food restaurants there are now reports of incidents of "dine and dash," that is to say eating and not paying. Actually, there is very little dashing as the individuals are usually easily apprehended. Parents are then called and left to pick up the tab.

Assault. When physically confronted or challenged, some teens and adults with PWS have pushed back, resulting in charges of assault. Usually the assault occurs in reaction to physical contact or restraint and during a time of emotional agitation, often involving food. According to the Criminal code of Canada (1985), assault occurs when "without the consent of another person" someone "applies force intentionally to that other person, directly or indirectly."

In Calgary, two young women with PWS, living in shared accommodation, were both charged with assault, in different incidents, on the same staff person. The staff person was new to the job, and only lasted three weeks. In the words of one of the parents, "I believe the staff person was totally unsuitable, but it doesn't make facing a court case any pleasanter." The girls pleaded "not guilty." The preliminary hearing was in March and they had to wait until July and August for their respective cases to come up. The young women each received one year of probation.

One of the women, aged 33, was subsequently charged with another assault on a new social worker as the worker tried to stop her from taking her word search books in her bag when she was going bowling. She swung the bag, hitting the worker, resulting in a charge of assault and another court appearance. This time she received two years probation. A male with PWS in another province similarly received two years of probation after he had hurt a female staff person.

While the above cases fit the letter of the law, one is left to wonder if the assault charges would have materialized in the same way with better trained staff.

Mischief. A charge of mischief can mean many things. It is a charge that allows for more discretion, as illustrated in the following case of an 18-year-old, a case which gained more national media coverage in Canada than anyone else has ever had for PWS.

The young man was sent to jail after his food-seeking behaviours had led to eight arrests in eight weeks for theft and assault. While he had been well-managed as an adolescent, after he turned 18 he was too old to stay in the group home. The Association for Community Living helped him to rent one-half of a duplex and he received one-on-one support from 8 a.m. to 8 p.m. He stayed with his parents during the evening. However, the duplex arrangement did not stop him from begging and stealing food, which ultimately lead to his arrest.

After 26 days in confinement, and a guilty plea to a charge of mischief, he was released into the care of a Windsor hospital psychiatric ward. In the words of the judge, "this young man should never have set foot in jail. We don't deal with disabled people by putting them behind bars" (Mandel, 2003a). The judge urged that he be sent to the Children's Institute in Pittsburgh, the top American facility for treatment of PWS. The Ontario government subsequently approved care up to $80,555 US for a 90-day program (Mandel, 2003b). Charges were subsequently withdrawn upon satisfactory completion of the program (Van Wageningen, 2004).

Panhandling. Panhandling is a nuisance behaviour, referring to the practice of begging from the public. The parent of a high school student described an incident of panhandling while her son was under the supervision of the school:

> He was on 'work experience' through the school. The program required a student to travel to and from the workplace on his own. Although it was not considered wise by those involved, there was no alternative – if he was to participate he must go and return by himself. On the way, he was knocking on doors 'panhandling' and the police were called and picked him up.

In this case no charges were laid. Other parents have described how teens with PWS have an "uncanny ability" to get money while on the streets.

Arson. Arson may not have any particular connection to PWS, but it is included here to illustrate that individuals with PWS may commit other misdemeanours which result in trouble with the law. One young man at age 18 began to set dumpsters on fire and admitted to setting a car on fire. He was charged with arson, but the charge was later reduced to mischief resulting in damage exceeding one thousand dollars. There was an out of court settlement and payment for the car. The sentence required 75 hours of community service, probation, and counselling. At age 19 he set fire to a wastepaper basket in a bank's automatic teller enclosure. Again the original arson charge was reduced to public mischief and the young man voluntarily agreed to a forensic assessment before sentencing. He and his parents understood that this would occur in a hospital-like facility and were shocked when he was incarcerated with criminals.

In another situation, a young woman with PWS set fire to the family home. This resulted in a period of hospitalization in the psychiatric unit.

Fires aren't only set by teens. One mother reported that when her son was 9 or 10 he went into a neighbour's house, through an unlocked basement door, found matches and started a fire. "There was a fair amount of damage caused to the house." The Fire Department sent firemen out to talk to the boy about the seriousness of the offense. The real consequence was the neighbours saying that he could no longer go to play with their children.

Missing person. Running away sometimes poses a problem for PWS families. With a concern for child safety, police are usually involved. Families in Alberta and Ontario related how they had to inform the neighbourhood and the police about their child's tendency to leave the yard to explore the community. In one case, a pre-teen in good physical shape would run away and go for several kilometres. In another case the parents of a 14-year-old shared that they had called the RCMP 46 times to report him running away. They considered his running to be purposeful food-seeking. He had been away up to eight hours, but never overnight.

One young woman from Vancouver ran from her group home and went to Victoria. She was gone one week the first time. She ran a second time and the police advised the parents that she had been picked up living on the streets. When her mother retrieved her the daughter's leg was so badly infected that she had to be taken to the hospital. A young man from the Okanagan was reported as missing several times by his parents. He repeatedly ran to Vancouver Island, and was ultimately placed in a group home.

In another case, an 18-year-old woman with PWS ran away from her mother's home to move in with her boyfriend. The mother called the police for help, although the daughter was not technically missing. The police said that they could do nothing as she was an adult and could make her own decisions.

The story of a young man from B.C. illustrates the creative capacities utilized in running. At age 28, and weighing 200 pounds, he left his well-supervised home in the Fraser Valley, walked for an hour to the freeway and then hitchhiked. He had run away several times before but had always been easily found. This time was different. The police were called immediately. Leaving without money or identification the young man made his way to a neighbouring community where he stayed with a friend for three nights, then he rode the SkyTrain to downtown Vancouver and walked to an east-side church that feeds the homeless. With a high-pitched voice and dark, almond-shaped eyes he found it easy to pose as a battered woman. A charity found him a bed in a women's shelter and gave him a dress. He lived there for 11 days before heading to Seattle. There, wearing a long black dress and a thick sweater, he panhandled for food and cigarette money. He always said that he was trying to get out of an abusive situation. For three weeks he lived in a Seattle shelter. When his caregiver finally caught up to him he had been gone six weeks and had gained 18 pounds. (McLellan, 1998).

Facing charges. Parent testimony suggests that conflicts with the law increase individual and family stress and negatively impact quality of life for all concerned. Several issues continue to be generic stressors:

- lack of knowledge about PWS by those in authority making decisions
- confusion between judicial and social services mandates and responsibilities
- lack of system resources to meet PWS needs
- policies which place supreme value on the individual right of choice.

Unfortunately, parents and advocates often seem destined to fight each offense anew. Support and intercession from parent organizations can be very helpful in times of such conflict.

Social acceptance

Social competence, that is to say, the ability to perform adequately in a social situation, is not the only measure of social acceptance. How others respond to the appearance and personality characteristics of the individual are at the heart of acceptance.

Appearance

How a child appears to others is important. There is no doubt that North American culture is too focused on Hollywood stars and runway models. The short stature, obesity and behavioural issues often associated with PWS make those with the disorder stand out amongst their peers. As a result, parents have reported children being teased, bullied, and physically abused. Earlier in Chapter 3, John described how he had been "teased and kicked" because of his physical appearance. Not surprisingly, acceptance is easier at the elementary level. By pre-adolescence the differences in physical characteristics become more apparent. The teen years are the most difficult.

Growth hormone treatment is helping to eliminate the physical differences, and will result in more social acceptance by peers. When a child is similar to peers in physical appearance parents may also be more likely to seek integrated programs rather than those for children with special needs.

Bullying

All schools are concerned about bullying. Unfortunately, there is often a pecking order that places children with special needs at a disadvantage and at risk to be bullied. While children can be "rough" and "mean" they aren't necessarily bullying. And much of what adults might find of concern between children would not necessarily be described as bullying by a child. There are aspects of child play, however, which make some children a victim.

There has been increased awareness in recent years of the tragic consequences of bullying, such as teen revenge or suicide. While this may not be high profile in the PWS community, one has to wonder about the long-term affects of bullying on the self-concept of the victim. Bullying can be viewed on a continuum, beginning with teasing and progressing through social isolation and eventual targeting for abuse. An Ontario mother wrote:

> I know from firsthand experience the damage that short stature and obesity from PWS can do to a child. [My son] was the target of bullying too many times, and it has definitely psychologically damaged him. It would be great if all our PWS kids could be treated for hormone deficiencies, so they could grow up as normal as possible and avoid the teasing that goes on in schools today. Maybe if GH [growth hormone] had been around earlier, [my son] could have avoided a lot of bullying and physical abuse he received from the other kids because he stood out as being different physically.

After the death of her son, another mother wrote: "My first words after hearing that he was gone, were 'he'll never be teased again!'" Her son had been plagued by teasing throughout his young life.

Parents and teachers are not always aware of the abusive actions toward a child with PWS. Signs of bruising (from pokes), reluctance to go to school, and behaviour outbursts at home after school may be clues to victimization taking place. "Bully-proofing" is a term describing a process of giving children skills to guard against their victimization. While there are school-wide initiatives to address the problem of bullying, parents must have awareness and help their child to be able to express what they are experiencing.

Fitting in

Most children, teens, and adults want to be able to fit in with their peers. Parents recognize the powerful influence of peers when they try to encourage or discourage certain relationships. Fitting in may be difficult, however, if one lacks social perception and judgment.

Educators have observed students with PWS playing with children from younger grades, suggesting that they often fit in better with playmates of a similar cognitive level rather than age level. In some cases this has been viewed as a strength and individualized education plans have encouraged them as tutors, to assist with younger students.

Fitting in with same grade peers means sharing common experiences. This is often a challenge to children with PWS who have more limited opportunities. One mother related how her daughter, wanting to fit in with middle school classmates, talked about going to a boy's house. The teacher, overhearing the sharing, believed the girl was fabricating the story and subsequently discussed it with the mother. The story, in fact, was true. In the pre-teen's desire to be socially accepted, however, she had related an incident which had actually occurred six years earlier when she was in grade one!

Fitting in is difficult for teens at the best of times. Parents need to understand the importance of, and changing trends in: clothing styles, accessories, electronic gadgetry, musical experiences, movies, video games, popular hang-outs, and use of slang. This may be difficult where the child with PWS is an only child or the oldest child in the family. Fitting in requires a knowledge of what is current. Some teens with PWS are keen to be like their peers; others, perhaps because of past rejection or lack of social awareness, don't seem to care. Parents, if aware themselves, can play a facilitative role. Some parents related how they purchased fashionable clothing, tickets for popular concerts, and the latest in CDs and DVDs to help their child. There were also examples of other families who seemed to over-protect, thereby limiting the opportunities for their child to fit in.

Social support

Social integration is part of normalization. It begins with an integrated placement at the pre-school level and follows through elementary and secondary education, where there is a philosophy of inclusion. Even when a student is placed in specialized classes, individualized education plans should contain social goals. At the adult level individual program plans similarly include social aspects. Integration does not occur, however, without social supports.

Peer supports

The involvement of friends in providing support to those with special needs is not really a new concept. Living in community, it is natural to care for each other. In recent years, schools have encouraged the formation of networks of support from non-handicapped peers.

However, while teen friendship circles may work for awhile, they seldom translate into on-going support in the adult years. Of course, there are exceptions.

Alexa and Meghan met Robbie when he was in fourth grade. He was just standing beside the office door "hoping for a new friend to come and say hello ... before we could stop to think, we were standing in front of Robbie and ready to ask him to play," wrote Alexa. That was six years ago. The girls no longer attend the same school as Robbie, but the three of them get together at least three times each year for their birthday parties. Alexa just won an award for an article that she submitted about Robbie. In part, she wrote:

> I believe Robbie taught Meghan and I many lessons about life only he could teach. He taught us to let your imagination run as free as it can and to enjoy life as much as you possibly can. He also taught us how to be better friends to each other, and people we were about to meet in high school. To be unselfish and to care about the ones you love. At our school, he taught everyone to be accepting of people who have disabilities and people who are just different. I also think Meghan and I had a positive impact on Robbie for giving him friends to come to school to, cushioning some of his tantrums and letting his imagination grow. (Fraser, 2008/09, p. 11).

Alexa and Meghan were recently guests for Robbie's 16th birthday dinner. His mother wrote: "with teenagers like these who are caring and compassionate there is hope for people with challenges in our society."

Cultivating friendships is not always easy. Children with PWS, when asked to name their friends, often identify popular students that they would like to have as friends, or others who give them attention, even when it is negative attention. Most teens and adults with PWS, however, are able to name friends and describe activities that they do with them. Friends are usually peers with special needs who they have met through day or leisure programs or residential situations. In some cases they are school friends with whom they have maintained contact. Some enjoy just hanging-out together. They describe spending time watching a movie or playing a game. Peer support is often simply sharing social activities together.

Parents have described a lack of peer friendships and the need to encourage or structure the opportunity for their child or adult with PWS to have a friend. They have pushed participation in school and leisure activities as a way to encourage friendship experiences. When helping to cultivate friendships it is important to consider the question, "Who are his/her real peers?" Some parents, in the quest for normalcy see peers in integrated classrooms, others see peers at the Saturday morning Special Olympics bowling. When encouraging friendships there is a need to take a child-centred perspective and not project parental desires. In many towns it is normal for young adults to leave home and community after high school in order to work or pursue post-secondary education. Those with special needs are left behind. Parents need to consider who the friends will be five or ten years down the road.

At the adult level, participation in Special Olympics and Association for Community Living activities have provided a very meaningful social context for many friendships to develop.

Professional supports

Given that many individuals with PWS receive support from professional care providers it is not surprising that they identify such workers as friends. There is a familiarity that mimics elements of a friendship. Often a trust relationship grows and there is a longevity of service. Indeed, the individual with PWS may value the relationship and consider it a true friendship.

When asked to identify their friends, adults with PWS have cited residential and day program workers. In one case a woman identified a respite worker that she had a decade earlier as one of the two most important people in her life, describing her as her "second mom." She valued their relationship, and despite irregular contact still considered her an important friend. In another situation, a day worker went beyond the call of duty and would invite the woman with PWS to spend a weekend at her home with her family. This gesture was one of friendship, beyond the requirements of the job. In return she was valued as a friend. And Anne, who had been Lindsay's educational assistant for six years through high school now describes having a friendship relationship with both Lindsay and her mother.

One contractor, providing residential supports for several adults with special needs, explained that she wanted her staff to become friends with the clients. She wanted them to have caring relationships and hoped that they would continue to care about them after they leave employment or the residents move on. She hoped that if they met in the street that they would take time to go for coffee. She recognized that trusted professionals who have been open to the role of a friend are in a position to continue to provide support and influence long after their employment role has ended.

Social activities

Social activities require the company or companionship of others. They may be informal, as in just "hanging-out" together, or more formal, as when participating in classes or organized group activities. Often parents and caregivers feel the need to structure social activities in order to encourage socialization. This section discusses some of the more more popular social activities.

Childhood play and social experiences

Developmental play with other children often takes place in the context of the family home. Parents facilitate in-home play sessions by contacting parents of the child's peers. But as one parent lamented, "friends come to our home to play, but she never gets invited to their home." However, parents are extra-cautious about letting a child with

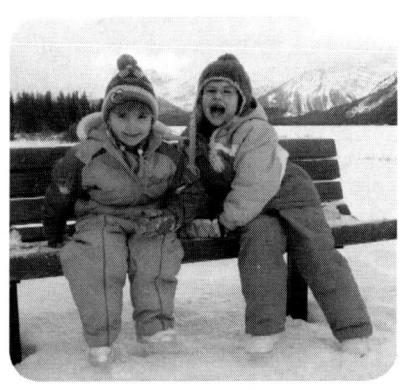

PWS friends -
Madison and Janine

PWS go to anyone else's home. Visiting happens most with close family friends, relatives, or other PWS families. Sometimes families form close friendships and share special occasions together for the benefit of their PWS children.

Recognizing the need for normal social activities and experiences for their children some parents report hiring peers, older teens, and even student teachers to take their child, and at times one or two friends, on outings.

While there are many stories of parents running out of energy or burning out, and thus not providing the extra social activities, there are also stories of parents programming the child with PWS into a year round schedule of enriching community-based social activities. The ability of the family to provide support for such activities is dependent on a number of variables, for example: position of the child in the family, work schedules of parents, ages of siblings, willingness of extended family members, family income, and availability of transportation.

Playing table games

Card games and board games are popular activities which encourage interactions with others. Some with PWS have become highly skilled at crib, a game which requires attentiveness and quick mental arithmetic. Others prefer board games such as Monopoly, which requires planning for the acquisition and upgrading of properties, the handling of money and coping with risk. Of course, not all can play games at high skill levels. Board and card games are available, however, to challenge all ages and levels of intellect. Such games are often a preferred activity because they are sedentary activities which require little output of energy.

Dancing

Dancing is an activity requiring the expenditure of energy which is attractive to many with PWS. The type of dance does not seem to matter, rather it is the beat of the music. Dancing is a highly social activity which permits physical contact and encourages relationships. The dance is a highlight of the PWSA-USA conferences. Here romances begin. Local Community Living Associations also often sponsor dances. Margaret expressed that she liked going to these dances in Calgary. Others enjoy more specific forms of dancing, for example, Kate takes ballet lessons and Angela clogs with a community group.

Group outings

The advantage of group outings is that they are "all-inclusive," that is to say that someone else has made all of the arrangements and provided the transportation. Participants usually know and have a good degree of comfort with one another. Some activities may involve a small group, for example, the residents of a group home doing a common activity together; other activities may involve a large group, for example, attending a bowling tournament or going to a community picnic. Some group activities may even be exotic, like international travel trips. Participating in an activity as a member of a group provides comfort and reassurance when facing new experiences.

Going for coffee

Going for coffee is a favourite and common social activity for adults, whether with workers, friends, or family. In Richmond, Carrie walks a mile to Tim Hortons on her own for a cup of tea. In Selkirk, a man used to have coffee at Tim Hortons but now gets a better deal by buying a senior's coffee at McDonalds. As one mother commented, despite her son's mental age, he functions like an adult when he goes for coffee. Those who might be critical of staff taking individuals with PWS for coffee regularly might need to be reminded of the importance of this activity as an opportunity for social skills training. For example, it encourages: the reading of menus, ordering, handling money, conversing and good manners. Going for coffee is often considered to be an acceptable dating activity. It adds to the individuals's quality of life, and also that of the parent when it can be a positive shared experience.

Solitary activities

Some children with PWS are quite happy to spend time on their own. For some, having their own "space" or "quiet time" is essential as part of their routines. They enjoy time with stuffed animals, pets, television, video games or other solitary activities. Parents recognize that sometimes social activities create too many pressures on children.

Some preferred activities for teens and adults with PWS do not involve social interactions. Doing jigsaw puzzles, word searches, or reading, are basically solitary activities. Watching television or doing crafts, such as knitting, crocheting, or rug-hooking are also usually done alone. Most individuals have a balance between solitary and social activities.

Personal relationships

It is natural for young people with PWS to desire friendships and for some to seek more intimate relationships. There are both subtle and overt pressures to engage in relationships. At school, they see peers flirting with the opposite sex. It is in this environment that they usually experience their own first flirtations. Parents have sometimes been surprised by the sudden announcement of having a girlfriend or boyfriend. In some cases, the modelling of older siblings has seemingly encouraged an interest in the opposite sex. And of course they are bombarded with sexuality on television, on DVDs, and in movies.

Hopes and aspirations

Teens with PWS often express age appropriate hopes and aspirations about future relationships. Like other teens, most say they want a girlfriend or boyfriend, and express a desire to marry and have a family. One mother reported that her son always said that he " wanted to marry, have six kids and live across the street." Influenced by siblings, peers, and media, they may also consider cohabiting or living common-law. In the past some families discouraged relationships and denied sexuality. Today, families more readily acknowledge the normalcy of sexuality, the meaningfulness of relationships, and the possibility of marriage or cohabitation.

PWS conference relationships

PWS teens often form relationships when attending PWS conferences. Families who have attended an American PWS conference will recall the youth program and dance. How young people with PWS love to dance! Relationships are made through the youth activities program and dance. The memories of "boyfriends" and "girlfriends" may last all year, without further contact, but with a memory that may build expectations for the next conference. As one parent expressed, her daughter is still in love with a young man that she met at the PWS (USA) conference about 15 years ago, and hasn't seen since.

Teen crushes

It is not unusual for a PWS teen to have a crush on a guy or girl, or a movie star or teen idol, even without contact. They may become the "boyfriend" or "girlfriend." One mother reported that her PWS daughter had a crush on an older sister's boyfriend, causing her to act shy in his presence. Another had a crush on a friend of her older brother. Others have had crushes on adult workers or professionals in their lives. While most of the crushes are experienced by PWS females, some males do show an interest in the opposite sex. One mother reported that her son began wishing he had a girlfriend when his younger sister began having boyfriends. Another began to reciprocate when girls began to show an interest in him.

Dating and companionship

For most people with PWS the opportunity to find companionship is difficult. The majority find friendships through events sponsored by community living associations, Special Olympics, or through sheltered work environments, day or residential programs. Without

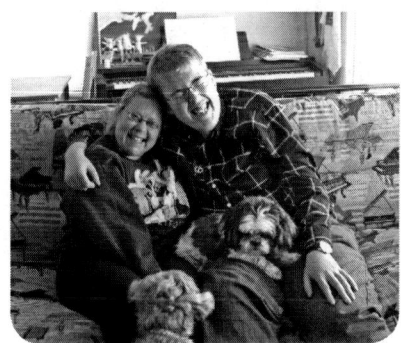

Angela and Joel
enjoy some time together

an independent means of transportation there is usually reliance on group-centred activities or the facilitative support of family members or workers. One young man, living in a rural setting, however, reportedly walked 10 miles and then talked his way onto a bus in order to go to the city to see a girlfriend.

Parents of a 24-year-old who was no longer living at home, explained acceptance of their daughter's dating, saying "if she has an interest, we have no problem." Dating was described as being "good for her." She was described as "more relaxed around boys," and "not so wanting" when in a relationship. After attending a banquet with the young couple, and knowing that diet had been discussed with the young man, they felt "more comfortable now."

One parent described her son with PWS going on a dinner date with a young lady with PWS. The parents facilitated the evening and enjoyed their own meal with her parents, a couple of tables away. Similar dating experiences have taken place, with the support worker chaperoning at a distance. Such facilitative dating can be a life skills lesson, as it presents the opportunity to explain the social importance of such things as taking turns, cooperative decision making, and the social appropriateness of public displays of affection, such as holding hands and kissing.

Dating is a worry for all parents, but as Heinemann (2000) stated "we are probably the only parents who worry more about our kids going into their date's kitchen than into their bedroom" (p. 7). Most dating takes place with individuals with other disabilities. There are two reasons for this according to Heinemann, Wyatt, and Goff (2006). First, "many individuals with PWS do not want to be identified by their disability and establish relationships with people who are not as readily identifiable." Second, "they know that their non-PWS partner will have greater access to food and money" (p. 458). The reasons might be different in Canada. Given the low incidence nature of the disorder and the vast geography of the country, most young people with PWS do not have regular contact with others with PWS, hence there isn't a large PWS dating pool. Most live and participate in programs which are not disability-specific, thus the potential for dates comes from a more generic special needs pool. The present study found only one relationship between two individuals with PWS, and that was short-lived.

While dating fulfils some needs, it can also create some problems. One parent described how supportive intervention was needed in her son's active social life with his girlfriend:

They were seeing each other too much and she was becoming very needy and putting a lot of demands on him. Their relationship was becoming strained, so we helped them to back off on going out together every weekend. Instead of phoning each other every day, they now talk 3 times a week and now they have more to talk about with the space between them.

The issues faced in this relationship are not unlike those that might be faced by parents with any teens or young adults who are dating.

Even when there is an interest in a prospective companion, circumstances may prevent the opportunity to get together. For example, one woman said that she had met a nice guy at a dance, had talked to him on the telephone a couple of times, and had been to a movie with him. While the relationship had potential, she explained that he went home to visit his parents on weekends, and she always went to visit her mother, so they really didn't have much time when they could get together.

Adult intimacy

Relationships do mature. For some young people this includes the desire for intimacy. In another country, parents were upset that their daughter who lived in a group home had the right to have her boyfriend sleep over and share her bed. The desire for intimacy is natural, particularly as part of a long-term relationship. The possibility of an intimate relationship for someone with PWS, however, is often confounded by the chronic level of supervision, and others' views of morality. How does the PWS adult living in someone else's home bring a date home for the night? The answer is: only with permission and support. In one instance, a parent reported that a relationship had been sabotaged by staff, who were uncomfortable with supporting the intimacy.

Of course, the desire for intimacy can create a vulnerability. Parents have expressed fear about males taking advantage of their daughters with PWS. This fear is augmented with the possibility of sexual favours being exchanged for food. Another fear is that of sexually transmitted diseases. One sexually active young woman with PWS contracted chlamydia from relations with her boyfriend.

Some parents admit that they face the challenge of their daughters wanting to be intimate. This is particularly so once they have already enjoyed the pleasures of intimacy. For males with PWS there is less desire for intimacy noted. As John wrote in a letter, "I do not have the feelings of other men." Despite not having a normal sex drive, PWS men may still have feelings of "love." Dating can certainly involve holding hands and kissing. One mother of a young male described her son as a "ladies man." He was attractive with good social skills. As a consequence, he always had a girlfriend. It was the girls, however, who were more intimately aggressive, even to the point of getting him into bed.

Fear of pregnancy

The likelihood of pregnancy is slim. There have been at least two published cases, however, of females with PWS becoming pregnant. The first case was that of a 33-year-old Swedish woman who gave birth to a child who was reported to be developing normally. The second case was that of a 32- year-old Danish woman, who gave birth to a daughter with Angelman syndrome. In reviewing these two cases Schultze (2000) concluded that "it is likely that females with PWS may ovulate and that there is a variable degree of reduced fertility in untreated females with PWS. We suggest therefore that infertility is not a consistent feature in females with the condition" (p. 17).

Some PWS women, if sexually active, are encouraged to take birth control pills. One parent reported a more regular monthly cycle and decreased behavioural concerns while her daughter was on the pill.

Marriage and common-law relationships

A small number of individuals with PWS have entered into marriage or a common-law relationship. Several parents explained that they supported the idea of co-habitation rather than marriage. They did not want to deny their child the opportunity for intimacy but had reservations about his or her ability to commit to a lifelong partnership. Perhaps they were wise. In three out of four cases the live-in relationship ended for reasons of incompatibility, abuse, or declining health. In each case it involved a female with PWS and a male with other identified special needs.

Other parents oppose the idea of sex outside of marriage and believing that the young adult lacks the maturity to be able to handle marriage, discourage any discussion of the topic. Herein lies a troublesome moral/ethical issue: Should the parents' religious/moral viewpoint deny their adult offspring the opportunity for love and intimacy? This is a sensitive question in many homes, particularly when it is the expressed desire of the young adult.

Two individuals over age 40, interviewed in 2007, were both proud of their "engagement" to be married. One woman displayed her ring and spoke fondly of her fiancé. According to the mother it may be an "eternal engagement." In the other instance a male with PWS had given a ring to his fiancée and they were cohabiting with the support of family.

One young woman was married at 23 but the marriage terminated after five years because her husband had a drinking problem. She later lived in a common-law relationship which didn't work out. Now in her forties she expresses no interest in having another relationship.

Love and intimacy are a natural part of adulthood, and can be found and experienced in different ways. Parents and support workers cannot deny a teen or adult with PWS the right to be in love. The main issue is: to what degree do family or workers support their desires and facilitate opportunities? Parents and residential care agencies do not always come from the same perspective on this issue, the former wanting to exercise precaution and control, and the latter needing to support individual rights and expressed desires. While there may be lots of questions about how to support a common-law or marriage relationship, the most pressing issue is still the matter of food supervision.

What parents want

Parents' hopes for their child with PWS are not unlike those that they have for their other children. They include social relationships. The mother of a preschooler hoped that her son would be "the best person he can be." She wanted him to be honest, accountable, to know right from wrong, to be able to cope, and "to have friends." Parents of a young adult said, "We want her to be happy with herself and with others, the same as for the other kids."

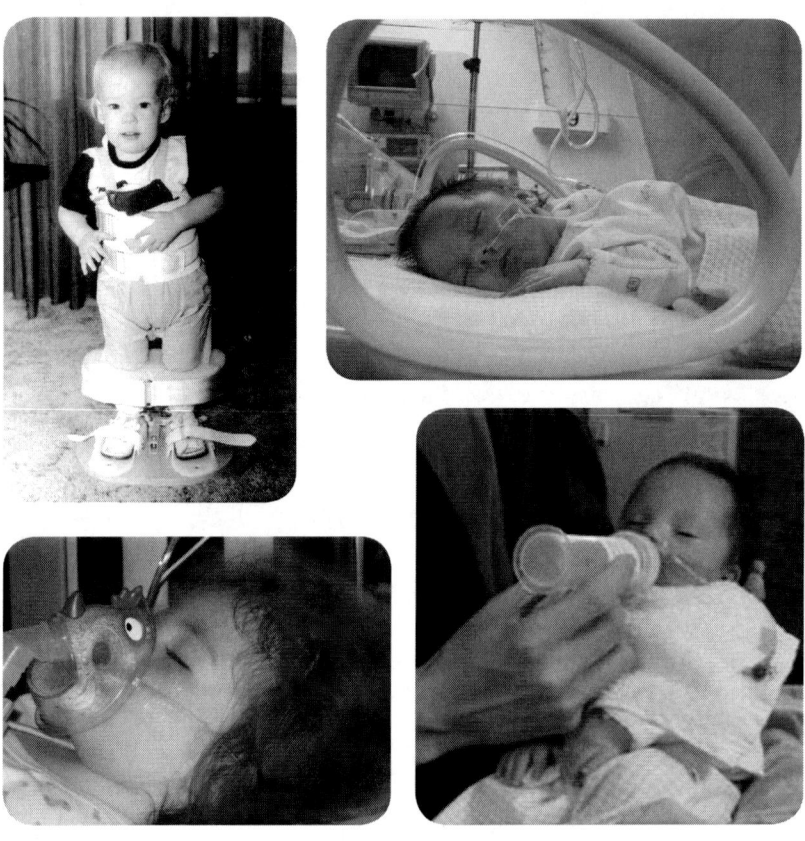

Infants

6

Health and development

Having a syndrome does not mean that the person is sick. Generally, individuals with PWS are quite healthy. There are, however, known health risks associated with the syndrome. Minimizing the health risks is a stressor for many families, particularly where others do not understand or are unwilling to accept the information provided.

Differentiating between what is normal growth and development, and that which can be attributed to the PWS syndrome, is another stressor for most parents

Stages of development

The literature documents two distinct phases which are universally common to all individuals with PWS, the first phase often defined as "failure to thrive" and the second phase which is characterized by an "insatiable appetite" or "thriving too well." While medical assistance is usually required in the first stage, it is less so in the second stage. In fact, because of the high pain tolerance individuals with PWS are less likely to report symptoms requiring medical attention in the second phase. This is a concern addressed by the medical alerts published by the PWS associations. Given the high pain threshold, any complaints of physical ailments should be considered seriously.

Failure to thrive

Failure to thrive is a first stage characteristic of PWS. Immediately after birth mothers are faced with problems associated with feeding, for example: failure to awaken for feeding, weak sucking reflex, inability to swallow, and poor neck and head control. Many parents indicated that

they initially had to resort to "tube-feeding" ("NG" or "nasogastric" tube). The lack of sucking reflex made breastfeeding difficult and often unproductive. Some found success with bottles and large latex nipples with big holes. Some used expressed breast milk; others tried infant formula. In some cases, shorter more frequent feedings were helpful. Some parents found that their infant required stimulation to awaken for feeding.

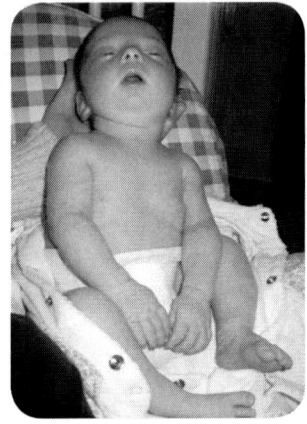

A floppy baby

In some cases there are medical complications which require a period of time in a neonatal intensive care unit. Generally, failure to thrive places the PWS infants at risk for normal development. Insufficient nutrient intake will result in poor weight gain. The time required and the emotion associated with feeding concerns place a physical and emotional drain on the mother. Suddenly the pressures associated with having a baby with special needs become all-consuming. Life revolves around the child. Thoughts of returning to work may have to be put on hold. This may translate into unexpected financial consequences to the pregnancy.

Thankfully, the issues associated with the hypotonia improve, usually after the first year or two. Parents are relieved and encouraged when they finally see the child feeding with ease and thriving. Normalcy seems to follow and there is improved quality of life at meal times.

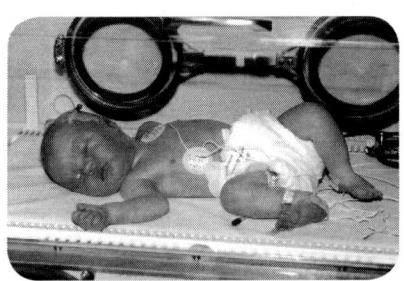

Baby Joel in the incubator

Thriving

The literature describing this second stage indicates that the insatiable appetite is life-long. It is characterized by such descriptors as "chronic hunger," "food preoccupation," "food-seeking," and "thriving too well." If uncontrolled, this stage results in significant weight gain and medical complications.

From a quality of life perspective, this stage is most problematic. Because of the food-related behaviours considerable supervision is required. The volume and rate of food consumption necessitates dietary restrictions. The imposition of diet management and behavioural supervision restricts the freedoms and desires of the individual with PWS, often resulting in confrontation. Parents are torn between wanting to alleviate the chronic hunger and wanting to manage weight (and longevity of life). Combined with the often daily confrontations, they find the emotional stress of parenting draining. As a consequence, their quality of life is below previous expectation.

Aging

While the characteristic appetite is considered to extend throughout life, there is some evidence that behaviour "mellows" with age. Dykens (2004) reported less skin-picking, compulsiveness and non-compliant behaviours amongst 30 to 50-year-olds. Similarly, members of the over-40 group in the present study showed evidence of mellowing. At 55, one woman was said to be more relaxed, less anxious and not as easily upset as in earlier years. At 44, another was described as being more mellow and better able to tolerate crises. And the mother of a woman of 40 years, said that her daughter's anger dissipates easier now. The profiles of others also showed improvements of behaviour in latter years, although the reasons were not clear. Parents suggested that improvements may be due to medications, a change in guardianship, or a move into a supported independent living model. Regardless of the reason, there appears to be a positive change in behaviour as adults transition to their senior years. For the most part, the over-40 group expressed satisfaction with their own quality of life (James, 2010).

Height management

When doctors Prader, Labhart, and Willi published the first article on what was to become known as Prader-Willi syndrome, two of the cardinal features that they described were "short stature" and "obesity." While the management of obesity has been a focus in dealing with PWS from the start, it is only recently that there has been an intervention for short stature.

Short stature

Appearances are important. To be short for one's age, visibly overweight or proportionately different makes one stand out. "Fitting in" is difficult when one "stands out." Height for females with PWS is shorter than for males. For young females with PWS, the 50th centile (i.e., percentile) closely approximates the normal 5th centile, but by 12 years of age the 50th centile falls below the normal 5th centile. For males with PWS, the 50th centile falls below the normal 5th centile by age 14, and then drops off more quickly than for females (Butler & Meaney, 1991).

In an analysis of 315 patients from Germany and the international literature, Wollmann, Schultz, Grauer, and Ranke (1998) found near normal growth during the first year of life, with short stature present in 50% of patients thereafter. Between the ages of 3 and 15 years, the 50th percentile for height in PWS roughly equated to the 3rd percentile in normal controls. Mean adult height was 162 cm for males and 150 cm for females. An earlier study of 232 American cases by Greenswag (1987) reported slightly lower values of 155 cm for males and 147 cm for females (152.4 cm = 5 ft.).

Tall stature

While short stature appeared as one of the cardinal features of PWS in the original work by Prader et al. (1956), it is only a minor criterion in the consensus diagnostic criteria for PWS published in 1993 (Holm et al.). Tall stature can be an atypical characteristic of PWS (Harty, Hollowell, & Sieg, 1993), although relatively rare.

One 22-year-old male from Alberta, with genetic confirmation, was short when compared to sibling height, but measured just over six feet tall. And Bob, a 66-year-old man described as "PWS-like," is also six feet tall (James, 2010). While treated by the house parents for many years as though he had PWS, a diagnosis was never pursued. His tall stature did not fit the stereotype of PWS and may have prevented the possibility of a diagnosis.

Growth hormone treatment

Some parents, in their desire to give their child every available opportunity for normalcy, have energetically pursued growth hormone (GH) treatment. After referral to a specialist some have been dismayed when GH treatment was not prescribed by the doctor because the child was not considered to be growth hormone deficient. On chat lines parents counsel each other on who to see and what to say in order to present the best case to obtain GH. There are an increasing number of papers describing the benefits of GH treatment.

Infants. In 1992 James and Brown reported the unorthodox nature of the crawling experience described by parents. Infants rolled everywhere, wiggling on stomachs or scooting on the buttocks. The latter was creatively described as: sit-crawl, bum-slide, sitting sideways crawl, bum-scoot, and bum-shuffle. In an American study (Carrel et al., 2004), infants and toddlers receiving GH for 12 months showed decreased body fat, increased lean body mass, and increased height velocity. Compared to peers, those who began GH before 18 months showed higher mobility skill acquisition.

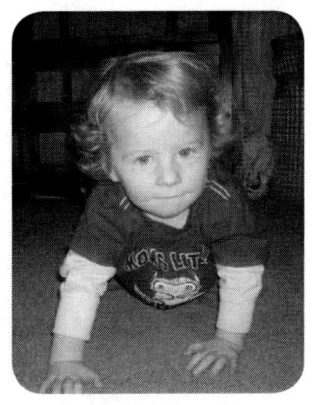

Silas crawling

Children. In a five-year study of 18 prepubertal Swedish children Lindgren and Ritzen (1999) reported that GH treatment had favourable effects on growth (increase in height) and body composition (decrease in body mass index). In a two-year study of 4-16 year old American children with PWS, parents reported more ready participation in prescribed exercises such as physical therapy, occupational therapy, physical education, walking, and swimming. They also noted a decrease in symptoms of depression in their children. In this same study siblings reported that they felt less embarrassed by the physical appearance of their sibling and parents reported fewer "snide remarks" from the public (Whitman, Myers, Carrel, & Allen, 2002).

Adults. In Sweden, Hoybye, Hilding, Jacobsson, and Thoren (2003) studied 17 adults with PWS, aged 17 to 32 years, and reported beneficial effects of GH treatment on body composition (reduction in body fat and an increase in lean body mass) without significant side-effects. Beneficial effects in mental speed and flexibility, and motor performance were documented during GH treatment. However, with the cessation of treatment, impairment was seen in physical and social status as well as overall functioning (Hoybye, Thorren, & Bohm, 2005). In a five-year follow-up Hoybye (2007) also reported that there were sustained and favourable effects on body composition, without significant side effects, with long-term GH treatment.

Fatalities. It should be noted that there have been reports of fatalities in children with PWS after beginning GH treatment. In response to the controversy over the safety of GH treatment in children, Eiholzer

(2005) reviewed the deaths of 13 children under the age of 18 receiving GH treatment and 23 not receiving treatment, and concluded that:

in general, infants with PWS already suffer from hypoventilation. Hypoventilation is probably the consequence of insufficient respiratory muscles, some pharyngeal narrowness and the development of decreased CO_2 sensitivity. Obesity plays an important role in fatal outcomes, possibly enhancing the ventilation disorder, as does kyphoscoliosis. Hypoventilation further leads to a higher susceptibility to infections, which in its own right may aggravate respiratory insufficiency. We consider that in most if not all patients who died during GHT, a combination of extreme obesity and pre-existing ventilation disorder might not have been given the attention it merited. We hypothesize that all of these children had hypoventilation with impaired respiratory regulation even before GHT was begun (p. 38).

Risk factors include: severe obesity, history of upper airway obstruction or sleep apnea, or unidentified respiratory infection. Males may be at greater risk than females. Patients with PWS should be examined for upper airway obstruction and sleep apnea before initiating treatment. (Eli Lilly, 2008).

In an examination of short-term effects of GH on sleep abnormalities in PWS, Miller et al.(2006) reported that most of the patients had improvement after short treatment, but 32% had worsening of sleep disturbance. They noted that "a subset of PWS patients are at risk during this window of vulnerability shortly after initiation of GH."

Scoliosis. Given the high frequency of scoliosis in PWS it is natural to query what effect GH therapy has on it's progression. A Japanese study followed 72 subjects, ages 1 to 49 years. They concluded that "rapid height gain by the use of GH does not increase the risk of scoliosis, and early start of GH administration does not induce scoliosis" (Nagai, Obata, Ogata et al., 2006, p. 1627). In an American study of 25 subjects, ages 4 to 37 months, followed for two years, only one subject experienced progression of scoliosis while under GH therapy (Myers, Whitman, Carrel et al., 2006).

Canadian experiences. There is increasing testimonial evidence in Canada about the beneficial effects of GH on children and teens. The youngest child to receive GH in the current study was 7 months of age. Isabelle, pictured on the next page, began GH at 13 months.

She was at the 50th percentile for weight and not even on the charts for height when GH was begun. At 24 months she was almost at the 75th percentile for weight and the 75th percentile for height. At 3.5 years her mother reported that:

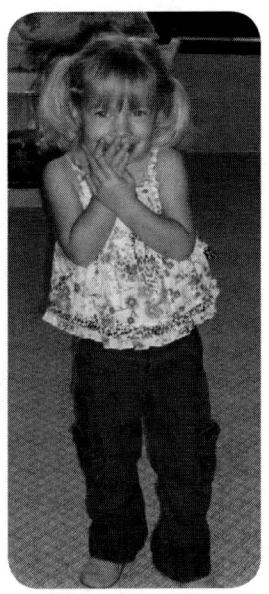

Isabelle at 21 months

> Isabelle keeps up with her peers in the playground, climbs ladders, runs, pulls wagons, pushes pals on a swing, hikes the mountains behind our house, can dress herself (not shirts over her head though), and has the energy to maintain a very active routine. Her hands and feet size have normalized as has her body fat/ muscle composition.

Susan, the mother of a 9-year-old who had been on GH treatment for two years described how her son had grown in height, lost weight, improved coordination, and increased stamina as a result of GH. Today he has a BMI in the normal range and cannot be distinguished from his peers by height. Another mother, whose daughter began GH at age 9, described it as "a very good experience," describing increased muscle strength (e.g., ability to climb stairs and jump) and greater peer acceptance.

From Ontario, Stephen's mother described the benefits that her son received when starting GH at age 16:

> Before GH, he was considered obese with a BMI of 43. Not only has GH increased height and given him a leaner muscle mass, it has enabled him to have an increase in energy and exercise capacity. He has been able to maintain a weight of 140 lbs at 5'6".

In three years, Stephen went from 4'11" to a completed height of 5'6". Along with GH he is maintained on a healthy diet of 1200 calories and 30 minutes of exercise per day. His BMI is now in the normal range and his confidence in social situations has increased.

One common question from parents is "How long does a child have to take GH?" One 14-year-old received GH for a six month period, until his father lost his job and his health plan coverage. The parents did not observe any benefit in this short period of time. In all other cases, the children had not terminated GH treatment.

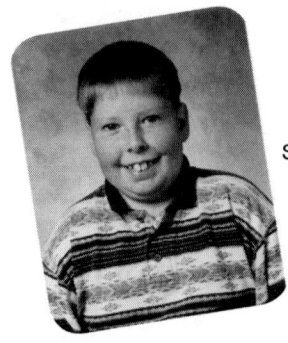

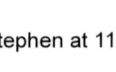
Stephen at 15

Stephen at 11

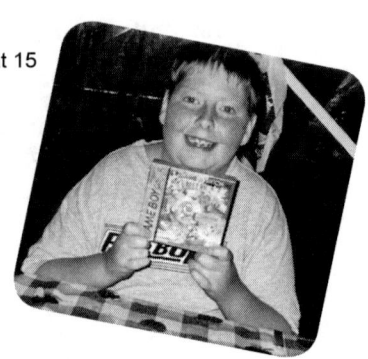

As an adult Stephen continues to receive GH. His mother explained:

> For the last four years after completing growth, we have been able to continue Stephen on GH as an adult due to the fact that he has been proven deficient. He has been able to maintain a healthy weight, an increased exercise and energy capacity, learn muscle mass, good sleep quality and psychological benefits. We hope that other parents and endocrinologists will realize that GH therapy is just as important to the quality of life for adults with PWS as it is for the children, since many will continue to remain deficient throughout their adult years.

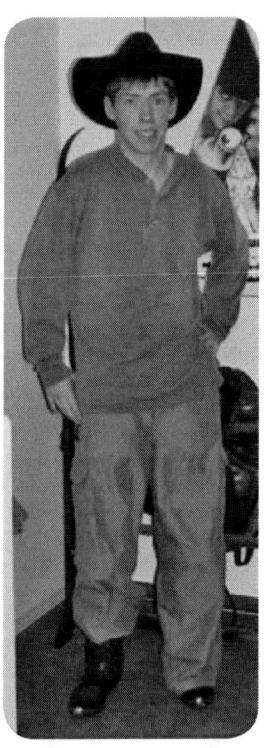

Placebo-controlled randomized clinical trials have shown that GH therapy "improves body composition, lipid profiles, bone density, and quality of life in GH-deficient adults" (Carrel et al., 2006, p. 220).

Getting approval for GH

Growth hormone was first approved by the FDA in the USA for use in children with PWS

Stephen at 21

in the year 2000. In Canada parents have been frustrated in their struggle to get GH treatment. Because there does not seem to be a uniform approach across the country, parents are left to shop for the treatment that they want. Generally, they require a referral to an endocrinologist and ear, nose, and throat specialist. Children must undergo a sleep study to rule out sleep apnea or other respiratory problems, as well as being checked for growth hormone deficiency.

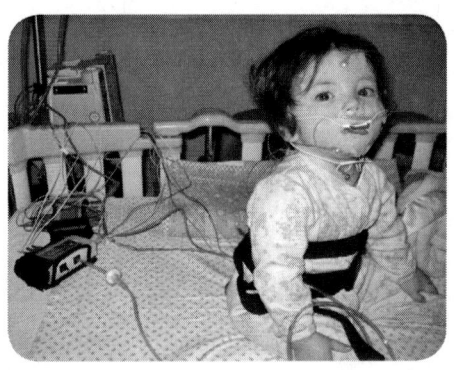

Amaia undergoing a sleep study

The option of GH therapy is not routinely presented by doctors. Parents describe having to "push" or "do battle with" their doctors, particularly the endocrinologists, who are commonly perceived as dragging their feet on the GH issue.

Parent networking is educating parents on how to seek out this treatment. The mother of a two-year-old described how the topic of GH was handled by the endocrinologist. After waiting six months for an appointment, she raised the topic with him. He was not very encouraging, saying it was expensive and some insurance companies wouldn't pay for it. He also said that he would not give it before age 2. Having already done her research on the Internet, she pushed for it.

> I wanted the sleep study moved up. I had to push for it because they didn't see a need. When we had the sleep study it took another six weeks until the doctor interpreted it. It was very frustrating.

Ultimately, her son began GH treatment at 18 months. She offers this advice to other parents:

> You need to push the Endo. Go to the national group. Stay current. Come armed with data. They seem to respect that. Ask what steps need to be taken and make sure they follow through. If the costs are not doable be aware that drug companies may provide it for a year on compassionate grounds.

GH therapy - the funding issue

Funding for GH therapy is a big issue with parents. There are great inequities. As one parent crassly stated, "it is a crap-shoot for every family to try to get coverage."

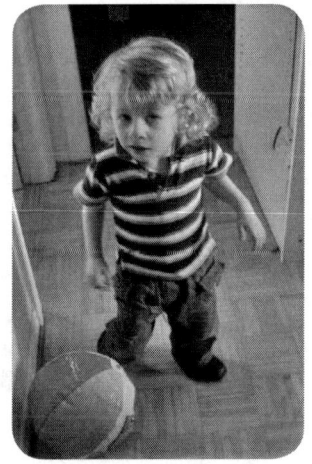

Silas began GH at
18 months

Where will the money for GH come from? At the time of writing parents report paying from $600 to $2,300 per month. Once growth hormone deficiency has been established, some Canadian parents have been successful in obtaining funding from their private health insurance programs, or through participation in research studies. In one case, where husband and wife both have extended health care coverage the two companies cover the costs. In another case the husband's insurance covers 80 % of the cost and social services covers the remainder. Others, however, have been rejected.

After rejection by the insurance company some have been provided GH on compassionate grounds by a pharmaceutical company. This offer, which covers one year, provides time to work on alternative funding - but also creates pressure on the parents. Who would want to terminate something after a year when it was producing results? According to one company representative, an extension may be possible as each compassionate case is decided on its own merits and is reviewed annually.

Each family circumstance is different. One father, after having discussed the need for GH with his employer, pointed out that if the employer facilitates obtaining GH then the employee may feel indentured to the company. Another parent described the dilemma of discontinuing GH treatment for the child after losing employment and health coverage. Other parents described the economic pressures for those who are self-employed with no third party assistance.

Future hope

Butler, Hanchett, and Thompson (2006) state that it is "reasonable" to believe that improvements noted with GH therapy "should lower the risk for co-morbid diseases (e.g., diabetes, high blood pressure, cardioivascular disease)." They also believe that a longer life span and better quality of life can be anticipated. Certainly the early testimonial evidence from young Canadian families is suggestive of improvements to quality of life.

Weight management

The management of weight (i.e., the control of obesity) is the primary task for all parents of children with PWS, or caregivers of adults with PWS. There are three important aspects to weight management:
- diet and nutrition
- food access controls
- exercise.

Best practice requires significant effort in each of these areas. Parents who have been most successful at maintaining their child's weight within normal limits have approached each requirement with diligence, researching and learning all that they can in order to establish good structures and routines. For both males and females with PWS, the 50th centile approximates the normal 95th centile for weight (Butler & Meaney, 1991).

Effective weight management affects the health, self concept, and social life of the child or adult with PWS. The structure and routines of the home, while perhaps limiting some aspects of home life, generally provide for more stability, an important aspect of quality of life for parents and siblings.

Body mass index

The calculation of body mass index (BMI) has been useful for some parents and caregivers in order to monitor weight. BMI is calculated by taking weight (in kilograms) and dividing by height (in metres squared). There are a number of websites providing this calculation free of charge. The BMI number indicates whether or not weight falls within a healthy range.

Table 6 Body Mass Index	
BMI	Classification
under 18.5	underweight
18.5 to 24.9	normal
25.0 to 29.9	overweight
30 to 34.9	obese Class I
35 to 39.9	obese Class II
over 40	obese Class III

Table 6 shows the BMI ranges used by Health Canada (2003). The use of BMI calculation is not intended for those under the age of 18.

One man, now in his forties, has been able to maintain his body weight in the normal range throughout his adult years. His regimen requires him to weigh in daily. Staff report the information to his parents who monitor the weight closely. Staying within his normal target range allows him rewards and treats.

Obesity and risk

Obesity will result from poor weight management. Obesity increases the risk for: heart disease, diabetes (type II), high blood pressure, stroke, orthopaedic problems, sleep apnea, and mortality from cancer (Christensen & Hainline, 2001). Individuals in the present study have given testimony to all of these conditions except stroke.

In an international review of 27 cases, researchers in the Netherlands found that obesity and its complications, leading to death, were pronounced in the adult group (Schrander-Stumpel et al., 2004).

Hypotonia with hypoventilation were noted in babies, and acute respiratory illness, with unexpected sudden death, was reported for young children.

A review of 20 PWS deaths (age range 17 to 54 years) in the author's files indicated only one BMI in the normal range, and 13 (65%) considered obese (i.e., BMI > 30). One additional individual was described as "overweight" at the time of death. The weight in the last year of life was undetermined for six people. Known causes of death included: heart attack, pneumonia, embolism, cancer, kidney failure. Only one individual died "peacefully in his sleep."

In a related study of individuals over the age of 40 (James, 2010), 10 out of 13 of those profiled had BMIs in excess of 40 at some point during their twenties and thirties. The highest BMIs were 74.3, 64.6 and 62.8. The weight histories were equal to, or more serious than, those of peers who died; yet 3 (including 2 who were previous obese) were not considered to be obese in their senior years.

Heinemann (2008) reported that morbid obesity (i.e., BMI>40) declines with advancing age. She speculated two reasons for the decline: those who were morbidly obese as younger adults may not have survived beyond age 35, and those who were over the age of 35 were more likely to be in a care facility where they would get better nutritional management. The BMI data for the over-40 group studied by James challenges these assumptions. Almost all were morbidly obese as young adults and survived. And while better nutritional management might well be a factor, it is not necessarily because of placement in a care facility. Four individuals lived with family, seven in supported independent living, one in a private residence with caregivers, and only one in a PWS group home.

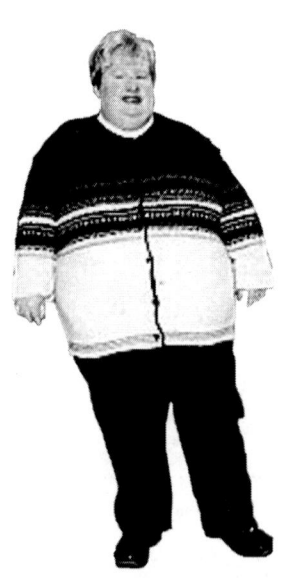

Carrie at age 30
and 259 pounds

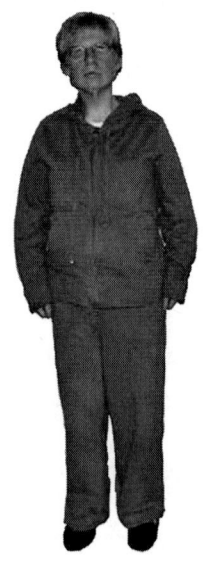

Carrie at age 34 and
90 pounds

The before and after pictures of Carrie on the previous page illustrate the type of weight loss which is possible. At age 30 Carrie weighed 259 pounds; at age 34 she has been maintaining her weight at her target of 90 pounds. She is 4 feet 8 inches tall. She attributes her success to a change of residence, a low-carb diet and Xenical. She says that her feet used to hurt from walking and she had breathing difficulties. Today she says that she is "happier than I've ever been" and particularly enjoys shopping for clothes. Others, too, have shed in excess of 150 pounds. In every case there are descriptors of better health and a healthier lifestyle, for example: no longer requiring oxygen, able to participate in sports, commitment to a daily exercise regimen, greater enjoyment of social and physical activities, and enjoyment of healthier food choices.

Individualized concerns

While the hyperphagia (excessive eating) is a cardinal characteristic of the syndrome, the degree of weight gain is dependent on a number of individual variables. Heinemann (2000) poses the following questions for professionals to consider:

- How much of a food forager is the child?
- How many calories does it take for this child to gain weight?
- Should food be locked up?
- Who else in the extended family and community needs to be educated?
- Who and what makes up the parents' support system?

The questions incorporate personal as well as family variables, and while asked in relation to children can apply equally to teens and adults. While there are commonalities associated with PWS each situation is different. Environmental factors contribute to the uniqueness and must be examined from a weight management perspective. For example, parents should consider the lay-out of the home (e.g., the location of the bedrooms, the traffic lanes to the kitchen), the ability to secure food (e.g., location of food storage, lockable areas), and the temptations of the neighbourhood (e.g., access to vegetable gardens, community garbage disposal). It is generally easier to control environmental variables than personal or family variables.

Heinemann (2000) points out that before the final year of life for Christina Corrigan, the young American teen had seen a doctor and nutritionist 90 times, resulting in placement on the typical diet. She emphasizes that it takes far more than a diet to get PWS weight under control. Christina unfortunately passed away at age 13 at 672 pounds (BBC, 1998). By contrast, there are many families that are managing diets well, with or without the assistance of professionals. However, they may have difficulties with environmental controls or incorporating exercise into the daily regimen. Each family circumstance is unique.

Nutrition

Diet and nutrition are central to the management of PWS throughout life. The primary concern is obesity prevention. Diet management is difficult because the individual with PWS almost always feels hungry. From the parents' perspective, it is natural to want a child, or adult, to have their hunger satisfied. However, a person with PWS has a large appetite that is not easily satiated. The challenge is to limit calories while satisfying hunger. At the same time, it is essential to provide the vitamins and minerals required for normal growth and development in children or health maintenance in adults.

Calorie needs. Stadler (1995) suggests that daily caloric intake "may range from 600 to 800 kcal among young children and from 800 to 1300 kcal among older children and adults" (p. 99). Balko (2006) explains that "an individual with PWS needs only about 60% of normal energy requirements" (p. 1). She then gives the example of a 20-year-old non-PWS female requiring 2200 calories daily, and a 20-year-old female with PWS needing only 1300 calories for weight maintenance (and 1000-1200 for weight loss). An extra 500 calories per day can result in a weight gain of 48 pounds per year for an individual with PWS.

Supplements. Because meals for those with PWS must be lower in calories, they may not have all of the nutrients required for growth and development. Stadler (1995) maintains that a multiple vitamin and mineral supplement is essential for individuals with PWS, "because prolonged and severe energy restriction predisposes an individual to insufficient intake of many vitamins and minerals" (p. 99). Balko (2005) recommends a multivitamin with iron as a standard after the age of 3. Given that "children with PWS are at higher risk of osteo-porosis or low bone density, due to hormonal abnormalities," she also points out that calcium and vitamin D supplements may be required for children, adolescents, and adults with PWS in order to meet the recommended minimum daily intakes.

While data was not solicited specifically on the use of supple-ments, descriptions of diet did include reference to supplements on occasion. In some cases supplements have been recommended by physicians, in other cases parents have taken the initiative to include them in the diet.

Dietitians. In 1992, a Whitehorse mother went to a dietitian to try to get a detailed menu for her three-year-old son with PWS who also had food allergies. "The second thing on the list was enriched white macaroni and cheese, with frankfurters, and he can't eat that kind of food," said the mother. Her frustration was not just with the recommended menu, but also with the amount of food. Her son gained weight on 850 calories, but the dietitian and the doctor said that 850 calories was not enough, and that he required at least 1,400 calories. But at 1,400 calories he could gain a pound a week (Stewart, 1992). This is not an isolated story. Have things changed over the years?

A father of a young man from Alberta recently related the following story involving a dietitian:

> At one point our son was seeing a dietitian regularly. However, she refused to adjust his diet in accordance with his PWS. She did not compensate for his low metabolic rate. I pleaded with her to contact the Prader-Willi Association in the United States and to speak to a specialized dietitian there so that she could have a greater understanding. At first she was somewhat angry with me, but in the end she did take up my suggestion. However, she continued to be ignorant about his special needs. This became painfully clear later when my son went to see her during the time that he was still on insulin. He informed her that he would have an occasional low. Her solution was to give him some energy bars (which are full of sugar) which he could consume during the time of the low. As you can well imagine, before he even reached the door of the elevator of the clinic, those energy bars had been consumed.

Despite contact with the PWSA-USA, this professional did not have a fundamental understanding of PWS. Of critical importance is any dietitian's attitude to researching and learning about this syndrome.

Diets

Families are usually encouraged by professionals to either count calories or follow a food exchange system. Some, however, choose to maintain established eating habits and simply provide a child with smaller portions. Yet others adapt an eclectic approach with organic foods, balanced diet, and exercise components. Given the tensions associated with mealtimes, following a consistent dietary approach provides structure. Each system has its merits. Exchange systems seem easier because they are balanced, easy to follow, and easily modifiable. Calorie counting, on the other hand, seems more precise, but requires more attention to meal planning to ensure the inclusion of all of the food groups and nutritional balance. The eclectic approach generally requires the commitment of all family members.

Calorie counting.   Counting calories is a way of life in many PWS homes. Trying to find innovative ways to come up with low sugar and low fat meals, however, can be a challenge. Unterberger (2003), a PWS parent and resident of Alberta, has compiled a comprehensive cookbook with low-fat, low-sugar and low-calorie recipes. This book also shares tidbits of information on PWS, and managing the syndrome.

Counting calories can be a way to keep a person with PWS occupied during meal preparation time (it also improves math skills!). PWS parent organizations, and their websites, are good sources for low-cal recipes and food ideas.

Food exchange systems. Food exchange systems are preferred by some families because they are easier to implement. They offer a well-balanced diet which includes all of the food groups and takes into consideration calories and nutrient values. The systems are flexible and can be modified as the child ages. The "exchange" allows for the exercise of food choices from established lists. The two most popular systems are:

- *The Canadian Diabetes Association (CDA) Food Choice System.*   This method of meal planning is based on the needs of people with diabetes. In order to control the amount of glucose (sugar) in their system, a certain amount of carbohydrate, protein, and fat must be eaten at each meal. Food is classified into groups and is interchangeable with other food in the same food group. This system empowers an individual to have some control over diet by making choices.
- *Red Yellow Green (RYG) System for Weight Management.* The Ontario PWSA (2006) has adopted a new version of the RYG system based on the 1970s "Stoplight diet" developed by Dr. Leonard Epstein, University of Buffalo, and the RYG diet from the The Children's Rehabilitation Program in Pittsburgh. The RYG system is based on the metaphor of a stoplight. There are red "stop" (high calorie) foods, yellow "caution" (moderate

calorie) foods, and green "go" (low calorie) foods. Colour charts are attractively presented for non-readers. Serving sizes are identified in each of the food categories. This system also empowers an individual to have some control over diet by making choices within the exchange system.

Balko (2006) maintains that the obesity of PWS can be reversed, reduced, and prevented. Her practice-based research indicates that the RYG system is an effective tool for the prevention and treatment of obesity in PWS. This system has been used successfully with more than 100 patients with PWS at the Prader-Willi Clinic at North York General Hospital. The revised Canadian RYG system is a collaborative effort of the Prader-Willi Clinic, the Ontario Prader-Willi Syndrome Association, the Vita Community Living Services Prader-Willi group home staff, families, and patients (Balko, 2005).

Just smaller portions. While children are younger the "just smaller portions" approach has some logic. After all, adults get to eat more than children. There are additional tricks, however, which must be used with this approach in order to give the illusion of a full portion, for example: choosing smaller size dinner plates, spreading food out (rather than piling it up), and using low-cal garnishes to cover open plate space.

Susan says she doesn't follow any particular diet and does not count calories. Evan is nine years old and has little variation in his meals, except at suppertime. Meals have routines and patterns. He gets smaller portions, but is allowed seconds. He always gets a dessert (90% fruit). If he obtains food between meals, he gets less at the next meal. He is on GH and his BMI is within the normal range.

Others have found that as the child grows older, the size of portions may be challenged. When compared to calorie counting or a food exchange system there is an element of arbitrariness by the person apportioning the food. The previous two approaches are more objective as there are measurable standards.

Eclectic approaches. A small number of families described an approach to weight management based on a better than average understanding of nutrition, a strong emphasis on avoiding additives and eating naturally, and combining exercise as an integral family activity. This approach may have elements of calorie counting and food exchange systems but is more creative and less rigourous in its approach.

In Sooke, Marion keeps a large organic garden. Her son's diet is low-cal and strictly organic. There are no sugars, chemicals, or additives. David has learned to read labels well. He grinds his own organic oatmeal for breakfast. David expects desserts. Typically he gets plain yogurt or gelatin with organic fruit or frozen sorbet. When he comes home from his day program he enjoys smoothies made from organic fruits and vegetables (e.g., raspberries and kale). Marion loves her Vitamix machine which she uses daily to prepare fruits and veggies, often added to green tea. She uses herbs and spices generously to make meals interesting.

In Cumberland, Rosemary uses natural products, makes everything from scratch, and never counts calories. She grew up with gardening and canning and has never wavered from it. She maintains that "food is not the enemy, the syndrome is." She believes that everyone has an optimal body weight that can be found with a more natural diet. If Lindsay transgresses, she is never punished with a food reduction. Her BMI has dropped from the "extremely obese" category to within the "normal" range with this approach (losing over 100 pounds). When asked about her diet, Lindsay said that the food is "excellent" and then added that "organic food is more satisfying."

Another mother described how a vegan diet worked for her daughter while she was at home. This included lots of veggies, high fibre, tofu, and beans. However, when she went to live in a care home and went on a meat diet her weight increased.

Self-regulatory behaviours

There is ample testimonial evidence that many teens and adults with PWS are capable of:
  • understanding the concepts of calorie counting and/or food exchange, and
  • understanding logical consequences (if you eat more now you get less later).
The difficulty, however, is in applying these concepts. While some might demonstrate some self-regulation (e.g., low-cal choices, leaving food on the plate, resisting temptation in the presence of food, sharing food with others), this is most likely to occur when there is an audience.

There are examples of self-regulatory decisions that hold over a span of time. Evan decided to give up his lunch cookie for the duration of a Healthy Living Study Unit in grade 4. In high school Jill worked in the canteen without giving in to temptation in the presence of junk food. And Lindsay chose not to take a mid-morning snack to her day program, even though she knew that co-workers would be eating. These examples suggest a strong degree of self-control and are in contrast to the stories of poor impulse control and instant gratification.

Angela, age 40, describes having a "shut-off point" with respect to food:

> When I am at a restaurant and someone tells me what and how much to order, or tells me that I cannot have a glass of wine with my meal (because it is alcohol, even though I am an adult), the control makes me so angry that I choose not to eat at all (Kinash, 2007c).

Despite her anger, Angela says that she is able to make a decision not to eat. And one mother reported that her daughter will say "I am full." These are expressions of self-regulation. Others, too, are able to stop eating. Whether they actually reach a point of satiety, or simply respond to a social cue to stop, is perhaps not important. The fact that they can make a decision to stop means that they have a degree of self-control.

One mother explained how self-regulation was instilled from day one. She introduced the diagnosis of PWS to her son at age 4, explaining to him that he had a condition that would make him hungry and wanting more food. She emphasized that mommy and daddy would give food, but that he had to ask them for it. They have never locked food up. As a young adult her son gets three meals and two snacks per day and reportedly "would never take anyone else's food."

Food access controls

There are two primary food access controls, supervision and modifications to the environment. Both can have a substantial impact on quality of life for parents and child.

Supervision. The need for supervision begins in toddlerhood when the child begins to explore the environment. This level of supervision is primarily safety oriented, is normal and can be expected for all children. As a child with PWS begins to seek out food, however supervision is required to prevent access to food and reduce caloric intake. As children grow, some become skilled in "hovering" around potential food sources, "stealing" food from unsuspecting parties, and "gorging" themselves for fear of being caught. Sometimes they acquire food with clandestine skill, that is to say with insight, patience, and in an inappropriate manner. The premeditated thought required to circumvent schedules, personnel, and lock systems suggests a level of problem solving ability unmeasured on standard intelligence tests. Parents often describe having to "stay one step ahead of them" in securing food. It always brings a smile to hear how physically over-weight children and teens can adroitly manoeuvre through trip lines, alarm systems, creaking floor boards, and still manage to gain access to food unnoticed.

Most parents maintain that supervision is required in all environ-ments. The lack of supervision for food access control has often been cited as a reason for curtailing visits to grandparents or for not using certain individuals for respite or babysitting. Lax supervision results in food access, which complicates things for parents. Most often parents invoke a response cost, trying to reduce the calories consumed in snacks or at the next meal by making the child forfeit some food. This approach often results in behavioural issues, diminishing the qual-ity of life for parents and child. Thus it is often easier not to entrust supervision to others, particularly when the child is younger. Parents often choose stability and the status quo over an evening out.

Parents have high expectations around supervision. When the su-pervisor is an employee of the education system or some social service agency the assumption is that the person is trained and is being paid to provide a level of supervision commensurate with what the parents could provide. Anything less usually results in complaints.

Like most children, those with PWS will test new staff to see what they can get away with. They may tell fibs or play both ends against the middle in order to manipulate the situation to their advantage. Recognizing that their goal is to get food should help staff to focus supervision efforts and prevent becoming side-tracked.

Environmental modifications. Parents have found many creative ways to secure food and limit access. Denying access to the kitchen, particularly during meal preparation time, has been successful for mothers strong in organizational skills and strict with enforcement. In some cases, food has been secured in a lockable pantry area. In one home a spare bedroom became the pantry, and also housed the freezer. Families with the luxury of creating their own floor plans for new construction are recognizing the value of the old-fashioned pantry (because it is easily locked).

Most often parents simply lock food cupboards and the refrigera-tor. For young children, any of a number of commercially available cupboard door locking devices will do the trick. As a child grows, however, something more sophisticated is needed. For example, magnetic locks or keyless, digital code locks which can be re-programmed from time to time.

In the past, refrigerators were made secure with a bicycle chain and lock or similar piece of chain and padlock. However, the appearance was not attractive and the chain marred the paint. There are, however, creative ways to use existing pre-drilled hinge holes to add a hasp and lock to newer refrigerators. This is possible, because most fridges are now pre-drilled to allow for either a right or left hand door opening.

Freezers should not be overlooked. Frozen food can always be thawed, or consumed in a frozen state. The freezer may contain the most easily accessible food in a neighbour's home. When located in a basement, carport, or porch area it may be easier to access than a fridge in a high-traffic kitchen.

At school, access to other children's lunch bags is a major concern. Selecting a desk close to the entry/exit door, and not requiring the child to go through the coat room area might help, but vigilance is needed. Teachers should be cautioned to put their purse and lunch in a lockable desk or filing cabinet drawer. For secondary students, the strategic location of the locker is important. It should be away from the cafeteria, foods lab, and vending machines. Janitors should be asked to make the removal of waste food from garbage containers a priority right after recess and lunch.

Most parents and caregivers find it necessary to modify the environment. Whenever possible, they prefer to choose environments where, as Kinash (2007c) suggests, food does not have a salient presence. Being in an environment free from the sight, smell, or sound of food minimizes distraction and allows the individual to focus on the activity at hand.

Exercise

Exercise is the third of the three cornerstones of a good weight management program. Exercise burns calories, tones muscles, builds strength, increases stamina, and improves flexibility and balance. As can be seen in Chapter 8 (Leisure), individuals with PWS engage in a wide range of physical activities.

Children's fitness tax credit program. Effective January 1, 2007, the Government of Canada implemented the Children's Fitness Tax Credit. The guidelines support children's participation in all programs that contribute significantly to their fitness with substantial additional support provided to children eligible for the disability tax credit. The age limit for the disability tax credit was raised from under 16 to under 18 years of age. Also, for eligible children, a $500 non-refundable amount was introduced, subject to spending a minimum of $100 on registration fees. This amount recognizes the extra costs associated with specialized equipment, transportation, and attendant care for children with disabilities.

Motivation. Not all parents are motivated to exercise - they need encouragement. Similarly, most children and adults with PWS must be motivated to exercise. Introducing new activities is often difficult. When children are young parents can challenge them to exercise by taking them to the beach to walk on logs or to a children's park to use the climbing apparatus. Toys can be provided which promote safe physical activity, such as push toys, tricycles, and balls. It is important for parents to both promote and participate in physical activity with their PWS child.

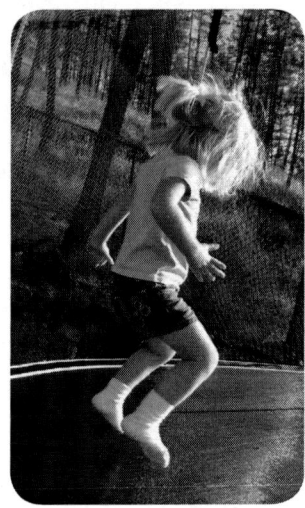

Isabelle on her back yard trampoline ·

Some families exercise together. Carrie, a young B.C. woman with PWS who has represented Canada at the Special Olympics World Games, was introduced to exercise as a family activity. The role modelling of parents and siblings, the enjoyment of shared time learning and recreating together, and the routines of a lifestyle commitment are obvious when families are physically active together.

Companionship while exercising is helpful. Lindsay and Madeline each go for walks with their caregivers in the evenings. Some individuals enjoy the encouragement and company of their educational assistant or program worker while they exercise.

Individualized program plans usually have an exercise component. Paul gets lots of exercise during his individualized day program, whether he is cleaning floors or swimming with his worker. At 56, Anne

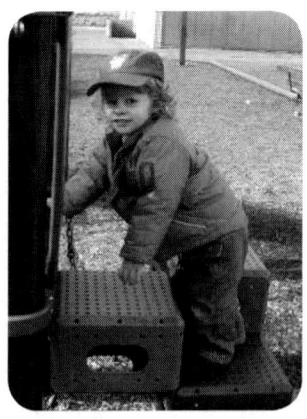

Silas climbing at the park

Marie has an exercise component to her daily routines, including lots of walking and twice weekly trips to the gym.

The Special Olympics Organization fosters personal growth and motivates individuals to exercise in order to compete in sports. It provides skill development, the camaraderie of peers, new social experiences, opportunities to travel, and tangible incentives such as ribbons and trophies.

Sometimes motivation has been increased by offering rewards for exercise achievement. Parents and caregivers have offered material incentives such as new clothes, tickets for concerts, or special holidays.

A cognitive approach is used by some parents to increase exercise motivation. This involves reasoning with the individual that the benefits of exercise are worth the effort. For example, exercise will mean greater choice in clothes, more opportunity to participate in sports and recreation, less breathlessness, more strength and balance. This approach requires good timing. It is hard to reason things out just before a meal or snack time, when behaviour is a topic of concern, or when the child is tired and unable to focus attention.

Some individuals are definitely self-motivated to exercise and do not require supervision to do so. Carrie maintains a rigourous athletic training program that has allowed her to compete internationally in swimming and snowshoeing. Bill enjoys competitive curling with Special Olympics and has competed at the national level. He enjoys walking six kilometres round trip to his program daily. Erin competed in a public challenge to swim 40 km over a period of weeks. Others, like Robbie, are faithfully committed to their responsibility for dog-walking.

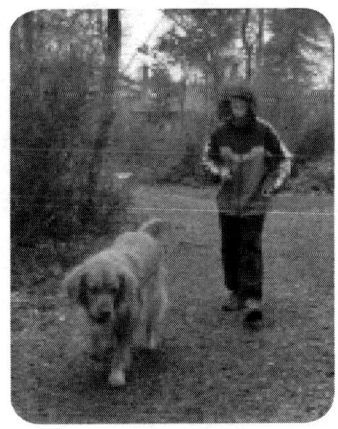

Unless there is some self-motivation change will be hard to achieve. Exercise is a necessary component for significant weight loss. One 22-year-old man reduced his weight from 355 to 175 pounds. His motivation began when he went to a PWS-USA conference in Minneapolis, where he had the opportunity to talk with others who had lost a lot of weight. He decided that he wanted to lose weight too. According

Robbie on a daily walk
with Dublin

to his father:

> once he decided he wanted to lose the weight it was much easier to get him to agree to a reduction in food as well as an increase in exercise. This did not always meet with his approval, but he knew he wanted to lose the weight. If it wasn't for his cooperation the weight loss would not have happened.

He understood that his parents were trying to help him reach *his* goals.

It is important that exercise not be beyond the capability of the individual. A bad experience will result in future resistance and could possibly cause physical harm.

Physio and other therapies

Because of the hypotonia, many infants and children with PWS receive physio and/or occupational therapy. These help with gross and fine motor development and the support of physical activities that encourage weight management and good health practices. For teens and adults these therapies often support activities of daily living and work tasks. At times these therapies focus on rehabilitation after surgical interventions.

In some cases the hypotonia affects speech production and communication difficulties result. These can be compounded by the degree of cognitive ability. The services of a speech and language pathologist can be helpful in identifying structural, oral, and language development problems.

Some children and adults with PWS participate in "hippotherapy" or "therapeutic riding." Hippotherapy is a rehabilitation strategy which uses a horse to stimulate postural and muscular reactions in the rider. Participants also learn protocols, provide care, and develop bonds with a horse which may help to address goals of a cognitive, behavioural, or social nature (for more information visit the Canadian Therapeutic Riding Association at www. cantra.ca).

An article in The Sudbury Star (Bradley, 2009) gives testimony to the value of the therapeutic riding program. Jason, a 24-year-old

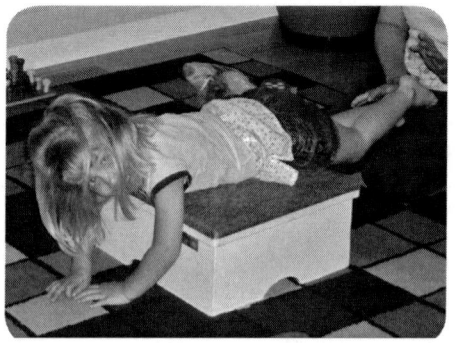

Isabelle doing physio exercises

with PWS, who has been riding for eight years described therapuetic riding as "an amazing experience":

> Because I have Prader-Willi syndrome, gastroparesis, osteoperosis and arthritis, I cannot take part in many activities in my community....they have helped me feel like part of my community,

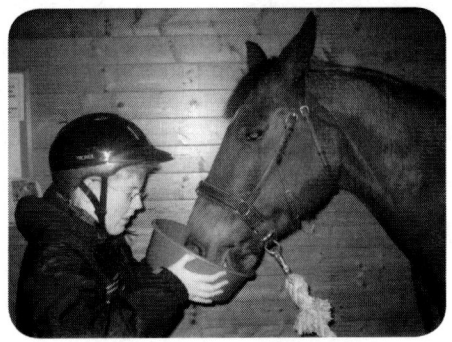

Robbie enjoys hippotherapy

> improved my balance and muscle tone, helped loosen my joints and, not to mention, I love riding with the horses. When I'm with the horses I forget all about having any disabilities. I feel like I belong and make many new friends.

The importance of choice again

Permitting individuals with PWS to make choices is important, particularly in the area of food and exercise. It is possible to present choices and thus empower the individual. The testimony of 20-year-old Grace (1998) emphasizes the importance of choices. Her weight was out of control in high school, and she went up to 214 pounds. She said, "I could hardly walk, my blood pressure was so high, and I had a hard time breathing properly." After exhausting a number of foster homes, she was placed with Barb. In her own words:

> Barb said I have a choice... to have a good life and feel great, or..... to have an unhappy life and die! I chose to have a good life and let Barb help me!

> We started with walking the dogs and controlled meals of low fat and sugar, high in fibre (whole grains) lots of fruit and veggies. We tried lots of different things such as Barb gave me all my food for the whole day.....I liked that but sometimes I couldn't help eating it all at once....so I asked Barb to monitor it for me.

> I'm given lots of choices on snacks and if there is any sneaking or stealing of food I lose out big time on those choices.

After a year and a half Grace was down to 105 pounds. She was eating 1500 calories a day, taking vitamins and mineral supplements, and biking three miles daily (adult three wheeler) or jogging two miles. Choices were an important part of Grace's day. She went off Prozac and said "my blood pressure is excellent and I feel great!"

Health support

Generally, individuals with PWS experience good health. Because of their high pain threshold, however, any health complaints should be taken seriously.

Parent support networks

The need for more information on PWS is a priority for most PWS parents. One of the main criticisms by the pioneer parents was the lack of information available to them. The highly technical papers provided by medical personnel provided little insight for coping with PWS.

In response, parents banded together to share their experiences, knowledge, and resources. They joined local associations supporting children with special needs and formed regional and provincial PWS parent associations. Many took out membership with the PWSA-USA group and enjoyed receiving *The Gathered View* with its research updates and practical helps. They began to network through conferences and email. More recently they have enjoyed the expanding social media networking capabilities. Parents can now get an almost immediate response from another PWS parent somewhere in the world. Frequently, parents are seeking information relating to health issues.

The Internet as a source of medical information

Younger parents are quick to use the Internet as a source of information. This was not available to the pioneer parents, although some have now embraced the new technology as a source of help. In the words of Driscoll and Butler (2002), "the Web can be a good starting point to gather information, but don't let it be your last point." They caution parents to check the source and reliability of the medical information found on-line. They suggest asking, for example:

- Have clinical trials been done and published?
- Was their publication in a respectable medical journal?
- Were the results significant?
- Did other groups get similar results?
- What are the possible side effects?
- Are the suggested medications approved by the FDA?

It must be recognized that anyone can post anything they want on the Internet without the information being verified. Unsubstantiated claims of success need to be further investigated. Basically, contributors to the Internet fall into three groups:

- professionals sharing research or clinical experience
- parents seeking support and/or sharing their experiences as support for others
- promoters selling products and services.

It is important that parents understand the source, and the credibility, of the information that they are reading.

Medical alerts

The PWSA(USA) publishes Medical Alerts for routine and emergency treatment of PWS. Table 7 summarizes the topics covered by these alerts. In emergency situations, the organization can provide information to emergency departments and hospitals upon request.

An article in a 2004 edition of *The Gathered View* illustrates the value of the Medical Alert in an emergency situation. Heinemann describes receiving a call from a physician who had treated a 15-year-old girl with PWS in the emergency ward. In the doctor's words, "If she had not brought the articles and insisted that I go to your website, this child would have died" (p. 6). After an episode with binge eating the girl had been brought in with vomiting and belly pains. Typically the symptoms would have been treated like the flu for a couple of days. However, due to the Medical Alerts the doctor pursued it further. The girl had such a bad hernia that "her spleen, stomach and duodenum were in her chest."

Wharton (2004, September-October) emphasized that individuals with the following symptoms should receive *immediate* medical attention:

Table 7 Medical alerts
• anesthesia, medications reactions
• adverse reactions to some medications
• high pain threshold
• respiratory concerns
• lack of vomiting
• severe gastric illness
• body temperature abnormalities
• skin lesions and bruises
• hyperphagia (excessive appetite)
• surgical and orthopedic concerns
• central adrenal insufficiency
• osteoporosis evaluation and therapy
• pediatric postoperative monitoring
• inpatient care
Source: www.pwsausa.org

- abdominal pain
- bloating, or distention, and/or
- vomiting.

The PWSA(USA) encourages all families to keep a copy of the Medical Alerts and significant medical articles in their car and to give copies to all care providers. All of the recommended articles are available on their website under the Medical Alert button (www.pwsausa.org).

Parents have reported extreme frustration and anger over the manner in which their child has been treated by the emergency department of their local hospital. Given the nature of the emergencies the doctors are required to handle it is perhaps understandable when they do not take time to read up on PWS. Of greatest concern, however, is that they listen to the in-put from the parent and avoid mis-diagnosing or mis-prescribing medications. For example, vomiting and abdominal pain are rare in PWS and require emergent evaluation for gastric rupture and necrosis. In a review of 152 American PWS deaths, Stevenson et al. (2007) found that gastric rupture and necrosis accounted for 3% of the causes of mortality, with another 3% suspected to have gastric rupture. The PWSA(USA) has put out a medical alert for severe gastric illness.

For hospitals that are now "paperless" it should not be difficult to flag the individual with PWS on the computer so that any attending physician could be aware of the medical alerts. After a bad episode, one parent and physician made arrangement with the emergency department to have the child immediately sent to pediatrics rather than be treated by the emergency department personnel in the future. Parents can be proactive in discussing this with their child's physician before an emergency occurs.

Medical histories

Many parents related that their child was hardly ever sick. Anecdotal information provided on medical histories of adults underscored the importance of responding to any complaints of physical ailments, as covered in the medical alerts. For example:

- a 22-year-old woman, weighing 247 pounds, was having difficulty breathing and was falling asleep at work. She could only walk a block or so before getting *a stitch in her side*. She was admitted to hospital suffering from heart failure.
- a 24-year-old man with a morbid level of obesity went into a pharmacy to get a prescription filled. A clerk came out to get the mother who had remained in the car. The man was

complaining of *back pain* while sitting in a chair waiting for the prescription to be filled. He was having a heart attack and died on the spot.

- a 25-year-old young woman twice complained of a *back ache* while on an outing. She collapsed after mentioning it a second time, was hospitalized and had her gall bladder removed.
- a 27-year-old young man was *feeling unwell* for a week. He had an unsteady gait, slurred speech and excessive thirst. He was hospitalized, started on IV antibiotics and insulin. Three days after admission, he collapsed suddenly following a return from the bathroom. He deteriorated quickly and died. The autopsy concluded death was due to pulmonary thromboemboli (blood clot) originating from the deep leg veins.
- a 45-year-old man on a well-maintained diet attended a house party where binge eating took place. Later he *vomited all night* and the next morning. This was the first time he had ever vomited. He appeared "blown up." He was hospitalized with necrosis of the stomach.
- a 45- year-old woman was taken to Emergency because she had *no standing nor sitting blood pressure and her heart rate dropped below 50.* Her whole personality seemed to change. She was very confused, withdrawn, lethargic and lost interest in food. The diagnosis was that she was over medicated. Medications were changed and within five days she was back to normal.

The high pain tolerance and the lack of vomiting are misleading to those unfamiliar with PWS. With the high pain threshold there is a risk of undetected infections and broken bones. Families have provided reports of lack of pain under circumstances which would cause persons without PWS great pain, for example: impacted bowel, appendicitis, and broken arms.

Cassidy, Devi, and Mukaida (1995) identified hypertension and diabetes as the major health problems of adulthood, with obesity, osteoporosis, and restrictive lung disease also problematic. According to Eiholzer and Lee (2006), respiratory muscle weakness and the inability to compensate during acute lung disease may account for a "relatively high occurrence of pneumonia and fever-related mortality" (p. 122).

At the time of interviews, those over age 40 were in stable health, although there was one death before the printing of this book. Almost everyone had a history of earlier hospitalizations. Surgeries were required for: hernia repair, gall bladder removal, intestinal by-pass, insertion of rods in the back, knee repair, hysterectomy, and correction of pulmonary embolism. Other hospital stays were required for heart failure, skin lesions, and psychiatric care. There were multiple occurrences of diabetes, arthritis, and scoliosis.

Medications

Not all children and adults with PWS require medication. As stated earlier, most are very healthy. Yet medications may be suggested to help manage problematic aspects of the syndrome - chiefly to address the hyperphagia and resulting obesity, and to moderate emotional and behavioural aspects of the syndrome. Reports on the use of medications vary, emphasizing the individuality of the syndrome.

Hyperphagia and obesity. The question is often asked, "Isn't there some medication that can be taken to curb the appetite?" According to Driscoll and McCune (1998), appetite suppressants, thermogenic agents, and digestive inhibitors all have their strengths, weaknesses, and side effects. Whitman (1999), however, points out that "all medications have been ineffective in addressing the brain signals that drive the person with PWS to seek food and overeat." She cautions:

> Until such a medication is discovered, good management depends on environmental protection against overeating, as well as an understanding caregiver who recognizes that a constant feeling of being hungry is a natural stimulus for being irritable and occasionally hard to get along with (p. 18).

An article about Bill, one of the participants in the 1987 study by the author (James, 1987), attributed weight loss to the use of Bupropion (Wellbutrin), a drug used to switch off nicotine cravings. At 40, Bill weighed 265 pounds. After only two weeks of Bupropion his eating habits became more appropriate. Thereafter, his weight dropped steadily. Two years later, he weighed between 130 and 135 pounds (Pound, 2002). A follow up visit by the author in 2007 verified that Bill has maintained his weight in the 134 to 140 range over the last five years. He has continued with the Bupropion. When the question of the effectiveness of Wellbutrin/Bupropion with PWS was asked of the PWSA(USA) medical board members the responses were varied. In short, it might help some individuals and not others (PWSA-USA, 2004).

Emotions and behaviour. Emotional lability (the "mood swings") often associated with PWS may cause parents to seek medical assistance for their child. Similarly, behaviours too difficult to manage with behavioural interventions may go the route of the family physician or psychiatrist, resulting in a prescription for medication. Whitman (1999) asserted that "almost every behaviour change medication 'known to man' had been tried both singly and in multiple combinations in an effort to help alter severe behaviour problems in persons with PWS." She went on to describe as "startling" the " range from ineffectiveness to absolute toxicity of most of those medications" (p. 19).

Certainly many individuals with PWS are taking medications for behavioural reasons. There is great variability in response to these medications. For example, one man takes 20 mg of Prozac and is less agitated and has no more tantrums. This amount is ineffective for another - she requires 30 mg to effect change in her behaviours. And while Wellbutrin helped Bill with anxiety reduction, weight loss, and more appropriate eating behaviours, a female went on the same drug and lasted only three months because she became an "unbelievably impossible person." One woman, who has taken Haldol for more than 20 years, has tried alternative drugs many times, all with negative consequences. These examples illustrate unique dosage needs and individual reactions to specific medications. The literature emphasizes that there are no universal drug solutions with PWS. It must also be pointed out that medication is not always needed, and if prescribed may only be needed for a period of time.

Adverse drug reactions. Finding the right medication may take some experimentation. In some cases there will be adverse reactions to drugs. For example, while in hospital one young woman was prescribed Valium. According to her mother, "this sent her wild - we went in to find her talking nonsense and heard that she had been standing on the window ledge on the tenth floor." When taken off the Valium her behaviour stabilized. In another hospitalization she was put on Prozac. Her mother's diary described her as "hyper and saying and doing senseless things. She is not eating her meals. Everyone is concerned at her lack of sleep. She is spaced out." A week later she was on Haldol and her mother noted "she was sitting on a chair, head down, drooling, and making no sense at all when she spoke. She certainly needed the sleep but this deterioration is frightening to see." She was taken off the Haldol and the next day the mother recorded that "she seemed a bit more alert, but still far from being herself." Eventually Bupropion became the medication of choice.

Self-medication. Self medication can be an issue with older teens and adults, particularly amongst those who are higher functioning.

They may respond to commercial advertising, and be able to get assistance to locate the product. The following case illustrates the difficulties associated with self-medication.

A high functioning young woman of 19 years was living at home and attending a day program. She was normally cooperative in both environments. Suddenly, she presented as angry and argumentative, with frequent blow-ups. She became confrontational and loud. She complained about dizziness, couldn't focus, was unable to make decisions, and presented as tired and sleepy. She was agitated, delusional, repetitive, demanding, unable to organize herself, or play favourite games.

During the month she was seen by her GP, referred to a psychiatrist, observed by mental health team members and a private PWS consultant. In order to rule out the possibility of side effects, all medications were stopped. It took a month for her behaviours to normalize. At a team meeting the psychiatrist explained that the sudden on-set behavioural change coincided with the young woman, who was already taking over-the-counter medication for cat and dust allergies, independently adding an extra strength cold medication. As there were no medical concerns as a result of all of the medical assessments, the psychiatrist explained that there were two possibilities for the behavioural changes: either interaction effects or high dosage effect of self-administered over-the-counter medications.

Skin-picking

Skin-picking is listed as one of the minor criteria to be considered when diagnosing PWS (Holm et al., 1993). In a retrospective study of patients with genetically confirmed PWS, Gunay-Aygun et al. (2001) found documented skin-picking in 81% of the cases.

Social implications. Open sores on exposed parts of the body are not attractive. Sores on the face and hands are problematic because they are most easily seen; sores elsewhere are problematic because they cannot easily be detected. Apart from the health risks associated with infection from skin-picking, the resulting appearance of open sores, scabs, and scars can be a deterrent to social interactions and contribute to a negative self-concept.

When and where? According to Kellerman (2002), an American parent writing for *The Gathered View*, "skin-picking is more likely to occur during periods of boredom or stress, and occurs most often at bedtime, in the bathroom, in class and in the car" (p. 5). There are anecdotal reports from Canadian families suggesting that it does not just occur at times of boredom or stress. Some parents report that skin-picking occurs "at times of idle activity" when otherwise engaged, for example, when watching television, or visiting.

Skin-picking which does not appear on exposed skin is most problematic. How can privacy be respected in the washroom cubicle at school when skin-picking is taking place? In some school settings the child must be accompanied to the washroom by an educational assistant and the cubicle door left open. Because an individual with PWS may be self-conscious about others seeing him or her dress or undress there may be little incidental opportunity for parents and caregivers to see the condition of the skin. This is particularly so during the adolescent years. In some cases it has been the educational assistant, helping in the washroom or changing room at the swimming pool, who has been first alerted to open sores or bruising.

Some parents are embarrassed by their child's skin-picking, as though it is a reflection on their parenting ability. As a result they feel less interested in being out in public with their child on display.

Interventions. So what has been tried to combat skin-picking? Table 8 illustrates the range of interventions parents have reported. Most have some degree of effectiveness. Recommendations for intervention have come from medical practitioners, behavioural specialists, and non-professionals such as other PWS parents and friends.

Interventions are not necessarily agreeable to the individual. Having to wear gloves secured to clothing when in class or in public draws attention and makes the individual stand out as being different. In mild cases, the threat of gloves can be a deterrent. One parent described putting socks on her young daughter's arms and taping them to the pyjama sleeve so that they were hard to remove. In one school situation long evening gloves were worn and pinned under a long-sleeved blouse. One adult daily wears gloves, secured with duct tape at the wrist.

For one teenage boy, Nexcare waterproof bandages "worked wonders" according to his mother. For another young man Duotherm became the application of choice. And another young man applied an imported European udder salve to his skin every day.

One teenager was not permitted to participate in the weekly special needs swim program because of the open sores. Given that she enjoyed the swim program it was hoped that the temporary exclusion would be a social motivation to allow her sores to heal. Others were

Table 8
Skin-picking interventions

- supervision (washroom cubicle, bathing)
- topical skin applications (salves, creams, lotions)
- behavioural contracting (reinforcement, incentives and rewards)
- adjustments to clothing (long sleeves, secured gloves, legs covered)
- redirection (to high interest activity, alternative manipulative activities)
- cosmetic cover-ups (Band-Aids, bandages, Duotherm)
- cognitive strategies (reasoning, motivating)

offered rewards, such as social outings and holidays, for improvement of their skin.

Adults with PWS described various things that they like to do to keep their hands occupied. For example, while watching television they knit, crochet, or do crafts of some type. Some simply keep their hands active playing with string or wool. Several described carrying their word search book with them wherever they go, to prevent boredom.

Health risks. Open sores resulting from skin-picking can lead to infection. They often begin with picking at pimples, scabs, bites, acne, or other skin blemishes. Picking can introduce new bacteria or cause existing bacteria to spread. For example: the parent of a teen reported that picking near the rectum raised a concern for cleanliness and repeated infections, a caregiver for a woman in her twenties expressed concern for repeated staph infections, the mother of a 9-year-old described chronic open sores that needed to be treated with antibiotic ointment, and one older woman required weekly visits to a wound clinic for medical attention to chronic leg sores due to severe picking.

Joint problems

Obesity affects joint wear. "Obese people have a nine-fold greater risk of osteoarthritis - the leading cause of joint degeneration" (Alberta Bone & Joint Institute, 2007). Weight bearing knee and hip joints are most at risk although spine and neck problems can also be anticipated.

In their forties, several individuals have joint problems which limit their physical activity. One woman with arthritis in her ankle and a "gimpy" knee has fallen in the streets and now must use a walking cane and is cautious about walking outdoors. Another explained how she has had three knee surgeries and at 44 needs a knee replacement, which the doctor says she is not eligible for until after age 50. Her mother confirmed their understanding that the age requirement was due to the expected length of service of the artificial knee joint (10 to 15 years) before it would need to be replaced. One older male fell on a hardwood floor and tore ligaments in his leg and was required to wear a leg brace. Another woman in this age group uses leg braces and crutches.

The observance of joint problems in those aging with PWS has important implications for services. A loss of mobility may require adaptations to home and work environments. A more sedentary lifestyle has implications for diet, energy expenditure, and exercise. Almost all joint problems will have requirements for rehabilitation services, thus requiring transportation to scheduled appointments. Joint problems can impinge on individual and family quality of life.

Scoliosis

Scoliosis is a lateral curvature of the spine. In 1987 James reported scoliosis in 35% of the western Canadian population studied, but suggested that this might represent under-reporting. Other published reports of the day ranged as high as 87% for curvature greater than ten degrees (Laurnen, 1981). A recent Japanese study (Nagai et al., 2006), found a rate of 45.8% in a population of 72 patients ranging in age from 1 to 49 years. They found a higher frequency of scoliosis amongst females (57.7%) than males (39.1%). For those under age 5, the rate was 21.7%; for the 6-11 year group it was 25%. For the population over age 12 the rate was 67.6%. "The increased frequency of scoliosis with increased age was evident, irrespective of the use of GH" (p. 1624).

The present study did not gather specific data on scoliosis, although it was identified in some cases in open-ended conversation in the context of lifestyle discussion. One young woman had rods placed in her back at age 18 and was living an active, semi-independent lifestyle. Amongst the over-40 PWS population, only 3 out of 13 individuals (23%) identified scoliosis as an issue. All are females. One woman had required two surgeries to place rods in her back, at age 30. Another had to give up bowling because of increasing back problems. The third now leads a very sedentary lifestyle.

Sexual development

Hypogonadism refers to incomplete sexual development and occurs in more than 80% of teens and adults with PWS (Holm, Cassidy, & Butler, 1993). The extent to which this may impact their concept of self is unclear. Some individuals acknowledge that they can't become mothers or fathers in a matter-of-fact way. More problematic are the feelings and emotions associated with immature physical development and the lack of, or tardiness of, secondary sexual characteristics (i.e., pubic, axillary, and facial hair, voice change) as peers go through puberty.

Cryptorchidism. Cryptorchidism (lack of testes descending into the scrotum) is common in male infants with PWS. In an Italian study examining 42 males, all showed cryptorchidism. This was bilateral in 86% of the cases (Crino, Schiaffini, Ciampalini et al., 2003). Ninety percent of them underwent orchidopexy (operation to bring the testicles into the scrotum). The authors reported that for 22 out of 29 males over the age of 9 years the onset of puberty was spontaneously achieved, however it was incomplete in all cases. One Canadian parent described this surgery on her two-year-old as "relatively minor surgery."

Testosterone therapy. According to Eizholzer (2005), whether missing sex hormones should be replaced is "still a controversial question" (p. 103). There are examples of older males in the present study receiving testosterone treatment. A young man who began treatment at age 18 experienced penis and scrotum growth. His voice deepened and he began to shave every other day. He experienced spontaneous erections that were embarrassing, but a switch from injections to pills corrected this and moderated his mood swings as well. The only downside was acne. The parents of a young man in his early twenties report that testosterone injections, begun at age 19, put their son through a normal puberty development. He gained muscle size and endurance as well, increasing his ability to do physical activities. The oldest male to begin testosterone in the current study was 33 years of age; he now has to shave regularly.

Menarche. Amenorrhea (absence of the menses) or oligomenorrhea (infrequent or scanty menstruation) beyond age 16 are frequently reported with PWS. For example, Crino et al. (2003) reported spontaneous menarche in 44% of females over the age of 15 (36% experienced oligomenorrhea afterwards) and amenorrhea in 56%. In the present study, parents reported precocious pubic hair and an occasional and scanty period as early as age eight, ranging to spontaneous menses beginning at age 32.

Breast development. "Significant breast development, even to full maturation, can occur in girls with PWS" (Lee, 1995, p. 35). Crino et al. (2003) point out that breast development is sometimes difficult to recognize because of excessive accumulation of fat in the body.

In her late teens, one young woman, requiring a size 48G brassiere, expressed an interest in breast reduction surgery. She was referred to a specialist who explained that it was not just a cosmetic issue, but rather it had become a health issue as the breasts were separating from the chest. She was in hospital overnight and took two weeks to recover. With subsequent weight loss she is delighted to wear a 34B bra and enjoys shopping for new clothes.

Bruising

Many individuals with PWS bruise easily. Bruises vary in their size and colouration and might result from a specific accident or from an on-going unhealthy relationship. While falling or bumping into furniture is a common cause of bruises, they have also been the result of poking by peers or manhandling by adults. Some children may seem to be clumsy and accident prone; others may be victimized. Bruising can be a more subtle indicator of quality of life concerns.

Reality of bruising. "Bruising easily" means that skin discolouration will occur more quickly than for a person without PWS. It means that even slight, inadvertent bumps that occur may result in discolouration, while a person without PWS would show no colour. A hit or hold will require less force or pressure to result in a bruise.

Bruising should always be taken seriously. Easy bruising, when combined with a lack of pain, may contribute to a mis-diagnosis. Bruising can be a sign of fractured or broken bones that might otherwise be missed. Unsightly bruising sometimes attracts attention, becomes a topic of conversation, and contributes to gossip.

The reality of easy bruising should not imply avoidance of all activities that have inherent risk of bruising. Rather, this awareness should lead to better understanding of medical and social situations which require additional intervention.

Lack of explanation. The first questions that parents usually ask are: "How did you get this bruise?" "Where did you get the bruise?" "Who gave you the bruise?" "Why do you have this bruise?" Often the response is "I don't know." This may in fact be a very honest response. Considering the high pain threshold, the individual may not have registered pain with an assault to the body which could have resulted in bruising. Hence there could legitimately be no awareness. For example, the bruise might be the result of one of many inadvertent bumps that occur in a crowded bus, hallway, or classroom that go unnoticed during the bustle of activity.

Of concern, however, is when "I don't know" is a cover up to protect the truth from coming out. For example, it is not uncommon for children to poke and prod to get each other's attention, or in more sinister moods to torment each other. Children with and without PWS, have been known to endure bruising in order to protect their "friends." The sharing of bruise information with other members of the school team is one way to monitor school social situations and discover the cause or the culprit.

Bruising and needles. The drawing of blood and the injection of growth hormone both require the use of a needle. Blood tests are a normal experience for most who have PWS. Parents have reported that nurses and laboratory technicians have had difficulty with drawing blood. One parent described her child having to suffer up to 11 pokes in order to get a needle into a vein. Of course bruising usually results.

Suspicion of abuse. Bruising may lead to suspicions of abuse. Professionals who are in the position to observe a child in various stages of undress, and who observe bruising, have to exercise professional judgment about the possibility of physical abuse having taken place. This certainly applies to teachers, educational assistants, childcare workers, and others in the educational setting who may have the opportunity to see discolouration while assisting with personal care, physical education, or recreational activities. Once trained to recognize child abuse, these professionals and paraprofessionals will likely err on the side of caution in order to protect the child and fulfill their obligations under the law. The obligation to report includes not only "abuse," but also "suspicions of abuse." One family's story follows. According to the mother:

> School, on more than one occasion, called about possible abuse due to bruises on his arm. Our son bruised very easily, and if I held him tightly, just to ensure safety or keep him away from food, he'd have a very noticeable bruise. Fortunately I knew the Principal well, and he would understand and accept my explanation, although I know he was bound by law to inquire (I am glad that it is necessary). This however is embarrassing to say the least.

On one occasion, however, a charge did result. When the child was about 10 years old, the mother was in hospital and the father was having difficulty coping with his son's mouthiness and stubbornness (which were probably worse, because mother was away). A tantrum resulted with the boy accidentally banging his head against a light switch, which cut his head. When the school heard the boy's description of the situation, they called the RCMP and Social Services apprehended the boy until his mother got home. The father was charged with child abuse, although the judge ultimately did not agree and the case was dismissed. In the mother's words, "it was upsetting for the family and the cost of a lawyer was significant."

In defence of the professionals, there may be little choice on the matter of reporting. School jurisdictions usually have a protocol agreement signed with police and the social services ministry which defines responsibilities. Investigations of abuse will typically be handled by the police unless there is immediate need for child protection involving social services. Once the report has been made, the one making the report is out of the picture and will not likely know the outcome unless it becomes a matter of public record.

Some websites suggest that it is important to document and report any bruises occurring from a school-related incident. On the one hand, this is self-protective against any mis-directed accusations of abuse; on the other, it can be proactive and can cause school officials to investigate a possibly abusive situation, whether involving students or staff. Good documentation particularly helps when establishing long-term patterns, for example bruises occurring in certain instructional blocks, on certain days of the week or during specific activities.

Bruising should be explainable, regardless of the environment. Vigilance is needed across environments. It should not be assumed that all bruises, or at least the potentially problematic ones, only originate in school environments.

Mental Health

Behavioural difficulties are common with PWS. It must be recognized, however, that like others with developmental disabilities, individuals with PWS are vulnerable to the full range of mental health and psychiatric disorders. One parent explained that her son had "gone through hell and back" resulting in the need for medication to assist with his adjustment. It was difficult to determine the number of people with PWS who had previously seen, or were under the care of a psychiatrist at the time of this study. Caregiver reports were often incomplete. While there were reports of psychiatric ward admissions, psychotropic medications and psychiatrists, the numbers were low. While parents were very open to discussing PWS, it was harder for them to talk about mental health issues.

Critical periods

A German-Swiss study (Steinhausen, Eihozer, Hauffa, & Matlin, 2004) found heightened psychiatric vulnerability for adolescents and young adults with PWS. They found a strong association between high BMI scores and high levels of behavioural and emotional disturbances. A Japanese study found that "adolescents and young adults with PWS showed symptoms of psychiatric illness and that the prevalence rate increased with age" (Hiraiwa, Maegaki, Oka & Ohno, 2007, p. 539). They suggested a prevalence rate of 27.6% for psychotic symptoms amongst young adults with PWS. In a U.K. report, Clarke et al. (1998) described six adults with PWS (ages 20-46) who had developed psychoses. They suggested that "PWS is associated with a vulnerability to psychotic symptoms in adult life" (p. 449). In a study of people with PWS over age 16, Clarke (1998) gave a "crude estimate" rate of 6.3% for possible psychotic disorders amongst adults with PWS.

Genetic sub-types

Of particular interest is a British study, which explored the prevalence of physical and psychiatric morbidity, comparing genetic sub-types (Boer et al., 2002a). The rate of serious psychiatric illness in this study was 28%. However, they found that only 8% of adults with deletions had psychotic illness, compared to 62% for those with disomy. All of the subjects over the age of 28 with disomy had psychotic illness. Boer et al. (2002b) query whether psychotic illness may be inevitable in early adult life for those with UPD.

Dual diagnosis

Dual diagnosis refers to coexisting diagnoses of "mental handicap" and "mental illness." Terms will vary and may include "developmental disability/intellectual disability" and "emotional disorder/psychiatric disorder," amongst others. There is a considerable range in the literature for dual diagnosis prevalence rates. The province of Ontario uses an estimate of 38% (Morris, 2003). Horvath (2006), in a PWS survey in the Central West Region of Ontario, found 8 out of 47 clients to be dually diagnosed. Clients, families, and service providers report that those with dual diagnoses have frequent contact with numerous service providers, health disorders that often remain undiagnosed, and uncoordinated services (Bradley and Morris, 2001). To illustrate this, the authors give the examples of common health disorders, such as an earache or abscessed tooth, being attributed to a behaviour disturbance (e.g., self-injurious behaviour), or mistakenly being associated with developmental disability, and therefore being left undiagnosed. Conversely, psychosis is often over-diagnosed and as a consequence people with developmental disabilities may be over medicated.

The presence of significant behavioural difficulties associated with PWS does not necessarily mean that there will be a dual diagnosis. Only a psychiatrist will be able to provide the dual diagnosis.

Psychiatrist or psychologist?

It is important for parents to understand the primary distinction between "psychiatrist" and "psychologist." Psychiatrists are medical doctors who have pursued specialty training. Psychiatrists usually administer medications, while psychologists employ some form of psychotherapy. Like medicine, the practice of psychology is regulated provincially in Canada. Licensure may or may not require a doctoral degree in psychology.

Psychopharmacological treatment (i.e., medications) may play a crucial role in the management of psychopathology for individuals with a dual diagnosis (Antochi et al., 2002). These include antianxiety, antidepressant, and antipsychotic medications, mood stabilizers and stimulants, among others. Psychotherapeutic techniques, on the other hand, include such options as: individual and group counselling, applied behavioural analysis, play therapy, family therapy, cognitive strategies, and stress reduction. Parents should have some understanding of the possible treatment routes before seeking intervention. Parent to parent communication is most helpful in order to understand the options.

There is no guarantee that either a psychiatrist or a psychologist will have had experience working with PWS. While an inexperienced professional with the right attitude might be helpful, in times of crisis most parents want an experienced professional on their team. Even an experienced and knowledgeable medical doctor, however, might not have the right "bedside manner." General practitioners unfamiliar with PWS are at risk for mis-diagnosis and consequent mis-prescribing of medications. Psychiatrists are more likely to be of assistance for severe behavioural concerns requiring medication.

School districts employ school or educational psychologists who conduct psycho-educational assessments and provide behavioural support in the educational setting. Some adult agencies have the services of a behavioural psychologist. When provided by the school or agency the service is free.

Coping with a dual diagnosis

A parent, suspecting the possibility of a mental health diagnosis, will need a referral to a psychiatrist from a general practitioner. It is important to go to the appointment armed with data on the problem behaviour, for example:

- date and time of onset
- circumstances precipitating onset (e.g., health issues, social or family trauma, head injury)
- frequency, timing, and intensity of the behaviour
- impact of the behaviour on self and family.

If medications are prescribed it is important to monitor the effectiveness of the medications, even if not specifically asked to do so. Parents should query what side effects might appear and report any observations immediately. This is particularly important to assist the doctor in adjusting the dosage. As a general principle, doctors try to maintain the minimum dosage required to address the problem behaviour, but thresholds can be hard to determine sometimes.

It is also important to review the administration of medications. Because the behaviour stabilizes should not mean that the medication will be automatically renewed forever. Sometimes changes in other circumstances (e.g., health condition, living environment, social relationships) can change the need for medications.

Advocates should be vigilant in monitoring medications for another important reason. Over-medication for the purpose of behavioural compliance can occur. Indeed, someone should be asking why medications are necessary in the first place. Are they in the best interest of the child or adult with PWS or are they to aid the caregiver in behavioural management? The same individual managed by someone else or in another environment might not require any medications. So whose quality of life do the meds really address?

Dental health

Poor oral hygiene and dental concerns may interfere with the social acceptance of any one. For a child or adult with special needs these can be unnecessary distractions affecting self-concept. In the U.K., Waters et al. (2007) found a 41.7% presence of dental problems amongst adults with PWS.

Dental caries have been reported by some families. Commonly these are accompanied by thick, sticky saliva. Poor oral hygiene can also lead to gum problems (gingivitis). In a small study of 14 individuals, Nowak (1995) reported the most common oral finding to be generalized marginal gingivitis secondary to poor oral hygiene.

Oral hygiene

It is important to consult a dentist regularly to monitor the condition of teeth and gums. Nowak (1995) explains the reason to be concerned about good oral hygiene:

> The characteristic constant eating by PWS patients greatly increases the availability of fermentable carbohydrates necessary to the development of dental caries. Increased dietary intake coupled with crowded dental arches results in food retention and increased plaque formation, leading to gingival irritation and inflammation (p. 82).

For some individuals thick, sticky saliva is evident at the corners of the mouth, and may even appear string-like when chewing food. Such saliva may contribute to dental caries. If not removed, it may form as a crust around the corners of the mouth.

Teaching children to brush effectively takes time and patience. Some children have difficulty with the physical actions required to floss or brush teeth adequately and require the help of an adult. Parents have reported the need to assist with teeth brushing even at older ages when independence with this task would normally be expected. In one case a young man continued to have parental help with teeth brushing into his adult years until he moved away from home.

Commonly parents have had to give reminders to brush teeth. This is another area which creates a dilemma - to permit independence, may lead to inadequate dental hygiene practice, which may result in dental issues; to ensure good oral hygiene practice often requires being personally invasive, and actually doing the brushing. While this is not a comfortable practice for parents, it is done with the feeling that it is absolutely necessary.

Finding a dentist

In most jurisdictions dental screening occurs when the child enters the public education system. Screening is meant to identify those children in need of urgent dental care. After identification, children are referred for professional dental care and then monitored for action taken. For some this might be the first indication that the child needs to see a dentist. Most, however, have been to a dentist before they enter school. Children should start brushing their teeth as toddlers.

There are special tooth brushes for toddlers and tooth paste that is not harmful if swallowed.

Back in the eighties parents reported difficulty obtaining an effective dentist. Nothing has really changed in this regard. The best advice is still to get the recommendation of another satisfied parent. Networking through the closest PWS association can be helpful in this regard. Posting a query on a PWS chat line might also get a response. Alternatively, parents might want to consider placing a call to the provincial office of the dentists' professional association or to other disability advocacy groups. The primary issue is whether or not the dentist has experience with, and is comfortable with, working with children or adults with developmental delays. If not, there may be difficulties with communication and comprehension, which can compromise dental treatment.

7

Education

A school system, whether public or private, is responsible for children for more time annually than any other agency. For 13 years parents have a close relationship with an education system, albeit with various schools and representatives. Where the child and the parents have a good relationship with the school their quality of life is enhanced; where there is a poor relationship, the quality of life is diminished.

Unfortunately, all parents do not have a positive experience with the school system. In a recent DVD produced in Alberta, (Kinash, 2007a), parents complain about a number of issues with their child's education. In the words of one parent, "working with teachers has been the most challenging part of dealing with PWS." In B.C. a parent went so far as to withdraw her son from going to school after grade 8 due to her frustrations with the system.

It is important that parents understand how their education system works and be able to differentiate between individual and system variables.

Education systems

Education systems aspire to seamless and continuous services. "Seamless" implies the ability to move between systems without any blockages; "continuous" suggests that services are available at all levels within the system. For example, public and private education systems work with preschool systems to make school entry smoother; they work with colleges to make the transition to post-secondary easier.

They also provide special education supports from school entry until graduation.

Parents must be aware that while the service may be continuous, the models may vary. For example, physiotherapy is often a one-on-one hands-on service at the preschool level. In the public education system, however, physiotherapy may be consultative, with the physiotherapist participating in team meetings and in training the educational assistant how to conduct the required physical activities. Similarly, speech and language therapy offered individually at the preschool level may become a group activity or scheduled for only a part of the year in the public school system. In both of these examples, the model reflects the available staffing level. Whereas the preschool system works with a small number and range of students (ages 4 to 5), the public or private school system accommodates a much greater number (ages 5 to 19). Parents are often dismayed at what they consider to be a "lack of service" when they enter the school system. Obviously, education systems are not rich enough to be able to afford the type of one-on-one assistance that parents would like to have. Rather than viewing it as a *lack* of service it should be viewed as a different *model* of service.

It should be noted that there are important differences between the American and Canadian education systems. Education is a provincial responsibility in Canada, whereas in the U.S. special needs legislation is federal. Children in Canada can generally participate in public system special education programs until the age of 19, while in the U.S. the Individual with Disabilities Education Improvement Act of 2004 serves children from ages 3 through 21 (Whitman, 2006). After leaving secondary school in Canada, adults with special needs are eligible for adult special education through the college system.

Regular or special education?

When a child is identified with special needs in infancy a number of specialized support services are usually made available, for example: infant development program, physiotherapy, occupational therapy, speech and language therapy. These are special services that young children receive based on their identified special needs. As they transition to the larger public or private education systems the same services are usually available although, as indicated above, the service model may change. Education systems, however, have additional supports for children with special needs, for example: special classes, learning assistance, and counselling.

Parents are often polarized on whether they want "regular" or "special" education services for their child. Proponents of normalization often want their child in a regular classroom. They see this as the least restrictive environment. At the elementary level parents' arguments are often based on principles of equity, non-discrimination and child rights. By the secondary years, however, commitment to such principles often give way to more practical concerns such as the need for life skills, socialization, and work training. Somewhere along the way, idealism usually subsides and pragmatism grows. Idealism requires more parent energy in monitoring, advocating, and educating in order to keep a child with special needs in regular education. Pragmatism, on the other hand, is much easier as special education systems are usually well-equipped to make education relevant to special needs.

Some parents fear that the use of the word "special" will forever label a child within the system, predisposing teachers to embrace the "self-fulfilling prophesy." They prefer to give the child the full benefits of the regular education experience, knowing that placement in special education is always there as a back-up. While neither decision is irreversible, it is certainly easier to move from regular to special education, than from special education to regular education. In this latter case there will be academic gaps that will be hard to overcome, placing additional stress on the child.

Most PWS parents recognize and value the additional specialized services which can be available under the special education umbrella. In some jurisdictions, students with special needs can be in regular classes and still receive the benefits of some specialized services. It is important to understand that models and service levels vary across school jurisdictions within provinces. Learning is faster-paced, with higher expectations and a sense of competitiveness or comparison in a regular class. Special education classes offer a slower pace and more individualized learning.

In the past, students with PWS were usually recommended for special education placement. It was not always a pleasant experience. Thirty years ago, one mother had to send her daughter to a new school on "the retarded bus - that's what the kids all called it." It was a hard move, for mother and daughter:

> It was a whole month of her crying every morning. 'Mum, I don't want to go on the retarded bus. Don't make me go. Mum I'm not retarded. Why do you keep doing this?' It was very heartbreaking. I was always concerned about the damage it was doing to her emotionally (Kinash, 2007a).

Busses for students with special needs were often smaller capacity vehicles provided by service organizations. They were visibly different with different colour, prominent advertising , and wheelchair lifts. Today, while still being smaller vehicles, they are more likely to look like other school busses.

Reflecting on her daughter's special education experience, the mother went on to say that her daughter "got away with more stuff because she was special needs. No one seemed to be monitoring what the teachers were doing." In the past few decades special education services have evolved. Today, the options of integrated placements, individualized programs, and educational assistant (EA[1]*) support in the neighbourhood school make the special education experience more positive. The accountability mechanisms are more rigourous and parents are integral members of the team. Still, it is not an easy decision and parents must weigh the educators' recommendations with what they believe will be the best for their child.

Eligibility for services

To work effectively within a system, parents must understand how the system functions. The issue of "eligibility" is important to understand. Many parents enter the public education system believing there is an "entitlement" based on their child's medical diagnosis. However, almost universally special education systems provide services based on meeting eligibility criteria, not entitlement based on a medical diagnosis.

Most often children with PWS are eligible for special education services because of their level of cognitive functioning. Generally, they meet the criteria for a moderate or severe to profound level of intellectual disability, as assessed by a psychologist. However, some children with PWS are within the normal range on standard intelligence tests (cognitive and adaptive behaviour measures) and will not meet eligibility criteria due to intellectual disability. They may, however, meet criteria by virtue of a physical disability or chronic health needs, as assessed by medical doctors.

Eligibility requires that comprehensive assessment data be available for the child. A parent unwilling to allow their child to be

---

* Paraprofessionals in the classroom have a range of job titles. While "education assistant" (EA) has been used in this text, it should be understood to mean any paraprofessional role in the classroom, e.g., teacher aide, teacher assistant, classroom aide, instructional assistant, etc.

assessed by a psychologist, or to share their child's medical history, for example, may prejudice a child's eligibility for service. Eligibility criteria vary across categories. Likewise, the source of required documentation differs. It follows that there must be an individualized education or program plan in place for students who meet eligibility. The plan is determined by educational needs and not a medical label.

For most parents, eligibility is synonymous with getting sufficient paraprofessional support time. While time from an EA is always assigned based on need, the perception of need often varies between the parents and the special education administrators who have to comply with system-wide requirements and financial constraints.

One parent from Manitoba related that her son was the first child with PWS in the school district and she had to advocate for services. There was a new special education coordinator, who didn't know her son. The boy had been seen three times by the school psychologist, "to validate the school's point of view." The result was a 50 percent cut in the allocation of EA hours. Meanwhile, her son gained 20 pounds, was stealing money, was functioning academically at a grade two level, and the grade 5 educational planning meeting had been conducted without the parent present. It is easy to understand a parent's frustrations with a school system when listening to such stories.

While some jurisdictions utilize special education funding categories, others use a block funding approach. In the former the requirements are centrally administered and are more stringent, in the latter the local school has more flexibility to determine priorities.

Low incidence versus high incidence

Incidence refers to the frequency or occurrence within a population. PWS is a low incidence condition, that is to say that there are not many students with this condition. High incidence means that there are considerably more students with a condition on a per capita basis. For example, there are considerably more students with a mild mental handicap or a learning disability. Remember that funding is not provided for the diagnostic label of PWS. Rather, the need for service must usually be established based on cognitive and physical characteristics. Students meeting eligibility criteria in a low incidence category will require, and receive, more costly supports (low incidence = higher costs; high incidence = lower costs).

The multidisciplinary team

A child with identified special needs will usually have the support of
a multidisciplinary team. The prefix "multi" simply means involvement of personnel from several disciplines. The most common team
is the IEP team, the educational team that meets to set and review
individualized education program goals. The team usually consists of
core members (e.g., classroom teacher, special education or learning
assistance teacher, parent, administrator) and others as necessary (e.g.,
psychologist, counsellor, speech and language therapist, occupational
therapist, physiotherapist). Each team member brings expertise from a
different discipline. The essence of teaming is collaboration for more
effective decision-making. The team meeting is the venue for sharing
concerns and seeking solutions. The collective wisdom is meant to
ensure a best practice approach.

Individual education plan (IEP)

It is the multidisciplinary team that is responsible for the development
of the IEP. The IEP is a requirement in order for the school or system
to receive special education funding for a child. The IEP is considered
to be a work in progress. Formats may vary by school or district. Most
importantly, it contains demographic and assessment data, and short
and long-term goal planning. Responsibilities are identified and review
dates established. Parents are required to be involved in the IEP planning. The process is formalized by the signatures of the participants.
While decision making is by consensus, parents have more power than
they often realize. Their lack of consent can veto others' ideas. To be
an effective team member parents need to become familiar with the
process and not be intimidated by the educators. To be effective as an
advocate on the team, parents need to maintain positive relationships
with the team members.

 The existence of an IEP means that the education plan is individualized. Goals will be modified, that is to say different from those of the
regular students. The student with special needs is evaluated against personal learning goals and not against the provincially authorized learning
outcomes which apply to the other students. One mother says:

> Ask early for an IEP. From our experience it can often be
> the end of October before it can be planned so we always
> try to do it in the second or third week of school.
>
> The other thing we always concentrate on, that we have
> learned from experience, is to make sure to include strong

academic goals in the IEP. It is easy to focus on behaviour
and not concentrate on academics.

The IEP allows for the identification of academic and non-academic
goals. It is the opportunity to introduce goals for behaviour, social integration, interpersonal relationships, crisis management, personal safety,
or whatever a parent would like to see as part of the school program.

Integration and inclusion

The majority of students with special needs are now integrated into
regular classes in neighbourhood schools. Generally, this works well
at the elementary level, but becomes more problematic as a child grows
older. The gap between the child with special needs and his or her
peers widens as curriculum becomes more complex and the physical
and intellectual demands increase at the secondary level.

Educators now talk about "inclusive" education. This implies
that all students have equitable access to educational opportunities
and interpersonal experiences in regular school environments. It
suggests that students are more than just physically integrated and
socially tolerated.

How has the evolution toward inclusiveness affected students with
PWS? Given that there is a considerable range in cognitive and behavioural performance within PWS it is dangerous to generalize. There
are two issues, however, which are frequently raised by parents.

First, many students with PWS require the support of an EA in
the regular classroom. In addition to learning needs (e.g., instructional
methods, modified materials, alternative curriculum) there may be
concerns for food access control, health and safety, and peer relations.
Educating staff about PWS needs and advocating for EA support is a
perennial exercise that is frustrating to parents. Decisions about EA
time may be made at a school or district level, depending on the
assessment of the child and whether there is a school or district-based
administrative model. Parents are advised to deal directly with special
education administrators in order to understand the process for the
allocation of EA support time.

Second, despite attending classes with peers of the same age, integration has seldom translated into meaningful long-term friendships.
This is most evident during the transition to adolescence. Students
with PWS, as with many students with special needs, do not receive
regular telephone calls or get invited to sleep-overs and birthday parties
to the same degree as their siblings. While it is not a popular thought
among integrationists, experience suggests that the opportunity to be

with peers who share common interests, based on cognitive ability or developmental level, has more potential for translating into meaningful long-term friendships.

Integration does not have to be an all-or-nothing process. There is scope for individual and small group work, resource room or learning assistance pull-out, work experience, or other community-based activities. Parents should ask three key questions:

- Is there sufficient support in the regular classroom to meet the individual learning needs of my child?
- Is there enough flexibility in the regular class environment to address the behavioural training that is desirable?
- Does my child have the opportunity at some point to be with peers with similar levels of intellectual development?

Integration is simply a strategy to achieve an inclusive philosophy. In any child-centred approach, a guiding principle should always be "the most enabling environment."

Union versus non-union environment

Parents do not always understand the implications of a unionized work environment. There are two important points to consider: first, unions exist to protect the workers and their jobs; second, seniority is usually the determining factor in job assignments. Parents have told "horror" stories about their children having had multiple EAs, as many as 4 or 5 during the course of a school year. Indeed, Susan recounts how her son had this many in the first month of school:

Last year in Kindergarten Evan had 4 different assistants during the first 4 weeks of school until that magical deadline of October 1 and his permanent person was actually put in place. I find this very frustrating and seemingly unnecessary.

This degree of change is not healthy for a child with PWS. Indeed, proactive parents argue that continuity is needed from year to year and they fight to retain a good EA long-term. So why are there problems?

The union is there to protect jobs and job rights for its members. Thus an EA job supporting a child with PWS is tied in with all other jobs in the bargaining unit. Rights to jobs are determined by seniority. In some bargaining units union and management have agreed that employees should not be able to bid or bump for a job across classifications. Where such an agreement is in place parents should be thankful as this prevents a janitor or bus driver or other bargaining unit member from taking a job as an EA. Yes, such situations have occurred.

Collective agreements emphasize seniority, provided that the applicant or a candidate has the "appropriate qualifications." When classroom aides initially became a reality in the public school systems there were only generic job descriptions. Progressive districts today have multiple job descriptions for differentiated EA job roles. This progress helps to ensure that students with special needs get the best qualified persons for support positions, not just the ones with the most seniority.

Twenty years ago one district used a staffing process described as resembling a meat market, where students with special needs had their names written on a blackboard. EAs were then brought in, according to seniority, and given their choice of assignment. This was an annual exercise with no protection for the a EA-student relationships. Today, the same district invites parents to have in-put in the process

Unionized work forces receive higher wages and usually enjoy a deeper pool of qualified applicants. In unionized districts today, most of the EAs are college trained in the human services field, some with specific programs for the preparation of special education assistants for the classroom. Conversely, EAs working in non-unionized environments may have less job security and fewer qualifications. There is greater turn-over as non-union employers compete with the general labour market for lower-skilled workers.

Parents are encouraged to be proactive in seeking to influence union-management agreements which will work for their situation. Progressive districts have:
- eliminated bumping during the year
- emphasized the importance of qualifications
- allowed multi-year assignments
- given parents a voice in the selection process.

Having a reliable and effective long-term EA is a dream of most parents. This alone would add to their quality of life by eliminating the anxiety of the annual staffing procedures, the annoyance of an ineffective or uncooperative EA, the trauma of a poor EA-child relationship, and the chronic need to educate the EA.

So how did Susan's initial concerns about her son's EA support turn out? By grade 4 her anxieties had abated:

This year he is in grade 4 and I am pleased to say he has been having his best year at school. He has a male teacher and male assistant who is wonderful. I can't say enough good things about him and I am advocating for Evan to have him again next year (his last year at his school), which the Principal has told me will be possible.

Key to Susan's successful advocacy was maintaining a positive working relationship with the school.

Special education administrator

All school jurisdictions have an administrator with the designated responsibility for special education services. This is the key individual responsible for the design of services and the allocation of staffing and resources. While in smaller districts special education might just be one part of someone's portfolio, in larger districts it has its own department and hierarchy of staff. In centralized models it is the district special education administrator, and not the school-based principal, who has the final say on most questions of great importance to parents, for example: placement and allocation of EA time, staff training, and special needs transportation. This administrator is often called upon to draft policy, or changes to policy, for the School Board, and is required to be current with legal considerations. It is important for parents to cultivate a relationship with the special education or student services administrator, either as individuals or as part of an association. In most cases, families will have a much longer-term relationship with this person than with any teacher, EA, or principal.

At the school level the principal is responsible for overseeing the day-to-day operations, including district special education programs housed within the building. One savvy mother said, "I make a very strong effort to get to know the principal, vice-principal and resource teachers very well so they understand our expectations." It is better to establish a relationship, and discuss expectations, other than in a crisis situation. Several parents indicated that they participated fully in school parents' activities because it gave them an opportunity to get to know the administrators.

Educational assistant (EA)

The position of the EA is a paraprofessional position, that is to say it is a position in support of the professional teacher. Trained or certified EAs are graduates of a one or two-year community college program. They have met the academic entry requirements, and in some cases, adequate community service hours. They have passed the academic courses and practicums. They have applied for, been screened, interviewed and selected by the employer for a position. They have usually taken courses related to: communications, behaviour management, health care principles, disabilities, technology, and classroom interventions. They are philosophically committed to the process of educational integration and conversant with student rights and responsibilities. Their training has included guidelines on how to work with parents.

EAs are assigned to a classroom or teacher in support of a student or students with disabilities. They are under the direct supervision of a professional teacher or administrator. They are prohibited from reporting student progress, as this is the realm of the professional teacher. While parents seek daily feedback on the performance of their child in class, they should appreciate that request for feedback should be directed to the teacher and not the EA. This is a confusing area for some parents who feel that the EA has a job because of their child and owes allegiance to the parent. EAs must be courteous to parents, and will engage in daily conversation as required. They will defer to the teacher, however, when there are questions that are evaluative.

In describing the good and bad experiences with EAs, one Manitoba mother looked back fondly on her first experience with the school system, saying that the person that her daughter had in Kindergarten "was dropped from Heaven. She was so wonderful. She had 20 plus years of experience but was very young at heart. She was so with it."

As discussed earlier, the assignment of EAs vary by jurisdiction. If unionized, seniority plays a critical role. In a centralized model, the district special education administrator, or human resources manager, is a key person in determining processes for staff allocation. In a school-based model, the principal must make the decision on staffing. In most situations, parents have little control or even in-put. Their concerns and requests, however, should always be respectfully heard.

Shared time. At times it is necessary to share EAs. The funding received in support of special needs students from the provincial governments is not enough to provide one-to-one coverage (unless the student is dependent handicapped, in a wheelchair, requiring toileting, feeding, and communication assistance). To the degree that class composition language (identifying the number of children with special needs that can be in a classroom) in teacher contracts will allow, administrators will try to allocate resources on a shared basis. For example, EAs may support two or more children simultaneously in a classroom, support students in more than one classroom by splitting their time between classes, or support multiple students who visit their resource centre on rotating timetables during the course of a day or week.

Sometimes a child may receive support from more than one EA. While some parents argue the need for familiarity and continuity, others recognize it might be healthier for the adults to share the load. In describing her son's move to junior secondary school, Cindy said:

> There were a couple of changes with aides but by late fall we had settled into a routine with two aides, each sharing half the morning with him, which worked very well.

Another mother described her son's introduction to middle school as quite disastrous. Initially he received support from four EAs, a different one for each block of the school day. It took months before support was changed to one male EA, which proved to be a much better solution.

Multi-year assignments. When there is a good relationship between the student and EA parents often advocate for an assignment continuing from year to year. Cindy was thankful that her son's elementary experience included a multi-year assignment:

> His aide in elementary school for 7 years (yes, unheard of, we were soooo lucky!) .... understood what makes him tick, why he did things the way he did. It helped us so much to have her completely on our side.

Others, too, have had the benefit of the same aide for multiple years. In a world of unionized staff and collective agreements, however, such arrangements would not be possible without the support of the special education administrator.

Anne, an EA, worked with Lindsay for six years through secondary school. For an EA to have to support a student in new courses every year adds difficulty to her job; but Anne chose to stay in the same role because she really liked Lindsay and enjoyed the challenges of the assignment. During this time her relationship with Lindsay's mother was very important. Today they are still friends. Although experienced as an EA, she knew nothing about PWS when she first took the assignment.

Job risk. EAs work closely with their students and are usually trained to manage difficult behaviours. They are expected to follow behavioural plans established in the IEP and have the guidance and support of teachers, psychologists and behavioural consultants. Being front-line, they can be exposed to risk on the job. For example, one female EA had her glasses ripped from her face and destroyed, another had buttons popped and her blouse ripped when pulled by the student. Another had bruises on her legs and arms from pokes and kicks. In one province, such assaults create a dilemma for the EA. On the one hand they are hired to manage behaviours and to admit that they are not being successful is a blow to their ego; on the other hand the union wants all incidents recorded and reported to the Workers' Compensation Board (WCB) as a job safety concern. However, the union and WCB are concerned solely with worker protection and not what is best for the student.

Teacher variables

Teachers are professionals who function with relative autonomy within their classrooms. Yes, they are expected to follow prescribed curricula or individualized education plans, but they do so with little supervision. Unless they hold a temporary assignment or are a probationary teacher, they have a great deal of professional autonomy and job security. Formal complaint or appeal processes will always consider whether a parent complaint has first been made to the teacher. Before a supervisor will intervene the teacher must be given the opportunity to address the complaint. Parents are therefore encouraged to document the purpose and outcomes of meetings with teachers.

In the words of one mother, "working with teachers has been about the most challenging thing - getting them to understand the syndrome and not overwhelming them either" (Kinash, 2007b). Working with teachers is a major complaint that hasn't changed over the years. There is the annual need to re-educate the teacher. Students change teachers yearly while teachers tend to teach the same grade year after year. The bad news is that this really does have to be done annually; the good news is that there are improved materials and resources available to assist today's parents.

Parents complain that they are often intimidated by a teacher or the system at large. This may be particularly so for parents who had bad experiences in the school system themselves. Parents must always be treated with respect and have a right to be involved in their child's education and have their concerns heard. They should not be confused with jargon; they have a right to have things explained in simplified language so that they can understand.

While teachers may have a say in "class composition," it is the principal who ultimately has responsibility for drawing up class lists. If there are peer or teacher placement concerns these should be addressed promptly with the principal. Even though inclusion is now mandated, there are still teachers resistant to the philosophy. Sometimes a classroom teacher is encountered who is not in tune with what should be happening. Some argue that they have not been trained to work with children with special needs, that they need in-service and assistance in the classroom. Some of their arguments may seem like political posturing on issues of working and learning conditions. Nevertheless, children with PWS have been integrated into regular, as well as special education classes with success for a number of years. Some parents have indicated that the teacher was "hand-picked" by the principal based on understanding of, and rapport with, the child.

Parent advocacy

Many PWS parents of school-aged children complain about their advocacy role with educators, that is to say the need to teach the teachers about PWS. Given that most schools and teachers have had no experience with PWS, advocacy is a perennial need. In the words of one mother, "my biggest effort is educating the educators." In an American study comparing parent perceptions of educational issues for children with Down syndrome, Prader-Willi syndrome, and Williams syndrome, the authors found that significantly more individuals (e.g., parents, school psychologists, teachers, speech-language pathologists) brought Down syndrome-related information to the classroom than for the other two groups (Fidler, Hodapp, & Dykens, 2002). They suggested that this difference might be explained by the greater understanding of the syndrome by the general public (e.g., television shows, books, and organizations) and by the amount of research (140 years worth). Earlier, James and Brown (1992) had suggested that PWS parents as a group are about 30 years behind parents of children with Down syndrome in their advocacy for awareness and services. Fortunately, over the last quarter century things have improved. While perennial advocacy is part of the PWS parent role, there are far more resources available for the younger parents today.

Regardless of the experience of the previous year, parents need to start each year afresh. Usually there are a number of staff changes. While change can be viewed as negative, particularly if one is happy with the previous personnel, it can also be seen as positive if hoping for a better experience in the coming year. It is important for parents to have a healthy working relationship with the school system. The following exemplifies a very positive approach:

> We approached the school year with the attitude that we would have a very open and friendly relationship with everyone involved and would trust their judgement and decisions, only interfering if we saw a problem or were concerned.

Parent rights

All too frequently parents are unaware of their rights relative to the education of their child with special needs. These can be found in the School Act, Minister's Orders, Inter-Ministerial Protocols, and special education policies at the provincial and local level. As education is a provincial responsibility there might be slight variations across provinces, but the spirit and intent are similar. In addition to rights, there are corresponding responsibilities. Parents are encouraged to do their homework on this topic when their child enters the public system.

Individual characteristics

Research is shedding increasing light on differences within PWS and in comparison to other disability groups. While some generalizations and trends may hold true, it is important to remember that children and adults with PWS have unique strengths and abilities, challenges and struggles. They must be understood in the context of their individual and family differences.

Cognitive ability and PWS

In a British study, Whittington et al. (2004a) found the distribution of the PWS IQ scores to be "approximately normal," but with "a mean IQ 40 points below that of the general population" (p. 172). In other words, while the mean IQ for the general population is 100, the mean for the PWS population would be about 60. According to the classification structure of the American Psychiatric Association (2000) a mean of 60 would fall within the "mild" range of mental retardation (IQ 55-70). The approximately normal distribution also suggests that some individuals would fall within the "normal" range, and others on the far end of the scale could be in the "moderate," "severe" and "profound" categories of mental retardation. In general, this means that there is usually subaverage general intellectual functioning along with significant limitations in adaptive functioning.

The term "mental retardation" has been used here because it is the language of the Diagnostic and Statistical Manual of Mental Disorders (4th ed.) (APA, 2000). Commonly the term has been replaced with less offensive synonyms such as mental handicap, cognitive impairment, or intellectual disability.

Learning disability or mental retardation? While the original descriptors for PWS included mental retardation (Prader et al., 1956), formal assessment data, as cited above, indicate that some individuals fall within the normal range of cognitive functioning. Whittington et al. (2004a) suggest that there is a global effect of having PWS, as well as the possibility of specific learning disabilities. Simplistically, a typical profile for someone with mental retardation will see subaverage scores across intellectual and adaptive behaviour subtests; a typical profile for someone with a learning disability will show characteristic strengths and weaknesses in specific subtests. For example, there are recognized learning disabilities (or learning disorders) in reading, mathematics, and written expression.

In some cases testing can reveal surprising results. There can be exceptional strengths which are not suggestive of mental retardation or learning disability. For example, a six-year-old girl with PWS scored at the 98th percentile on the Peabody Picture Vocabulary Test (a non-verbal test of receptive language). This translated into an age equivalent of 14.1 years. In looking for an explanation, it was learned that the family is highly verbal and read a lot. The daughter was described as having "an amazing memory" and "mimics well and uses the right vocabulary." Also, she had participated in a speech program that had "amazing strategies" that the parents took to heart. The home environment and school program reinforced a strength in the verbal area.

Assessment issues. The mother of the six-year-old said that she was "quite upset," however, by her daughter's IQ score last year, feeling that she had been "unfairly assessed." Herself a teacher, she did not think that the test results reflected a true picture of her daughter. Given that a psycho-educational test battery takes close to three hours to administer, a school psychologist should be aware of when the child last ate, the proximity to recess and lunch time, the arrangements for the recess snack or lunch, and the emotional state of the child that day. There should not be any food stimuli, particularly pictures or aromas, at the test site. Most psychologists will take time to develop rapport before begining the testing and may split the testing session. They should also note any conditions which might have influenced the score results. For example, one assessor noted that a 15-year-old female "chatted almost non-stop throughout the test situation....consequently the results, particularly those which required concentration, may be a little bit on the low side." It is important to note such observations as short attention span, refusal to complete tasks, distractions, and expressive language difficulties as these can impact the test outcomes.

Special class placement and academic achievement. In the U.K., Whittington et al. (2004b) investigated the extent to which children and adults with PWS reached levels predicted by their IQ and factors that might be associated with any under-achievement. The percentage of time spent in a special needs school was a significant predictor of under-achievement. The authors explain that some children with PWS are placed in special needs schools, not because of low IQ, but for behavioural reasons. They suggest that intellectual abilities may therefore be "masked" by immature social behaviour. In Canada, placement in neighbourhood schools is more the norm, however there may still be placement in special classes within these schools. If the observation of Whittington et al. is valid for special needs schools, it may well hold true for special needs classes as well.

As Whittington et al. (2004b) point out, under-achievement is not universal with PWS, although average attainment levels are generally below predicted levels.

Intellectual characteristics and PWS sub-type

In the U.S., Roof et al. (2000) studied 38 individuals with PWS (ages 10 – 49) to explore differences in intellectual functioning between those with a paternal chromosome 15 deletion and those with maternal uniparental disomy (UPD). This was the first report to document the difference between verbal (general knowledge) and performance (non-verbal) IQ score patterns when compared by subtypes. On average, the UPD group attained higher verbal IQ scores. They did better on tests of: numeric calculation, attention, word meanings, factual knowledge, and social reasoning.

Whittington et al. (2004a) compared cognitive abilities of the PWS sub-types and a non-differentiated learning disability group and reported that the UPD group had a relative strength in vocabulary and weakness in coding (making pairs from a series of shapes or numbers), In another report (Whittington et al., 2004b), they indicated that the differences in mean under-achievement between the deletion and disomy groups was greatest in reading, slightly smaller in spelling and quite similar in arithmetic. There was no under-achievement for the UPD group in reading. Interestingly, their deletion group demonstrated a significant strength with the Object Assembly subtest. This test measures visual-perceptual skills. The authors noted that this may explain the anecdotal accounts of uncanny jigsaw puzzle ability. Studies by other investigators have also found that individuals with the deletion sub-type have relative ability at visuo-spatial tasks (Dykens, 2002; Walley & Donaldson, 2005).

Of critical interest in the Roof et al. study is the fact that the average verbal IQ fell at the classification point for mild mental retardation as defined by the American Psychiatric Association. Fifty percent of those with UPD had an IQ equal to, or greater than, 70. This same classification point is used in most jurisdictions to determine eligibility for services. If a child does not qualify for a low incidence designation due to an IQ score over 70 there are usually other services which can provide supports (e.g., learning assistance), although not at the same service level. It is particularly problematic, however, in adult services where those with a Full Scale IQ score over 70 could be denied service.

Speech and language

"Speech articulation defects" is listed as one of the minor diagnostic criteria for PWS (Holm et al., 1993), however there may be more speech and language problems than just articulation defects. Lewis (2006) discusses speech and language disorders in PWS, explaining that there are several factors which may affect speech-sound development, including: "oral structure abnormalities, abnormal saliva, hypotonia, poor phonological skills, and cognitive deficits" (p. 273). Few parents in the present study identified speech and language as an issue. A few school children received service, with varying levels of intensity. There were no reports of adults receiving speech and language therapy.

Learning strengths

Learning strengths will be identified through psycho-educational assessment and teacher testing and observation. Understanding learning strengths is important from the teacher's perspective. It allows for the selection of appropriate learning materials and instructional approaches. Once identified, parents may better understand the learning style of their child, recognizing the manner in which the child learns best around the home.

Levine and Wharton (1993) identified the following learning strengths for school-aged children with PWS: "long term memory for information; receptive language; ability to learn from photos, illustrations, videos; ability to learn through actual hands-on experiences; reading ability" (p. 10). They noted, however, that these are "strengths relative to their own abilities, not necessarily relative to their peers." A decade later, Dorn and Goff (2003) summarized a similar list of learning strengths: "good long term memory skills, receptive language, good at puzzles, visual learners, basic math skills, reading skills, social and friendly" (p. 26).

As indicated earlier, recent research is finding differences in strengths and weaknesses according to PWS subtype. For example, Joseph et al. (2001) reported superior visual recognition memory for those with maternal disomy. It is now understood that being "good at puzzles" is not a universal characteristic of those with PWS, but rather a strength associated with a deletion and not UPD (Dykens, 2002).

Learning weaknesses

An awareness of learning weaknesses similarly assists the teacher in choosing material and designing instructional activities that will remediate. In the same way that they will require more focus from the teacher, they may become a focus for remedial strategies in the home.

Levine and Wharton (1993) identified the following weaknesses: expressive language, especially in preschoolers; short term auditory memory; fine motor skills, related to strength, tone, and motor planning; developing friendships; and gross motor development (pp. 11-12). Dorn and Goff (2003) list: poor short-term memory skills; expressive language, poor fine and gross motor skills; sequential processing deficit – difficulty understanding abstract concepts (p. 27).

It should be noted that while Dorn and Goff (2003) identify basic math skills as a learning strength, Bertella et al. (2005) concluded that "failure of mathematical skills is the most distinctive feature in the cognitive profile of PWS" (p. 159). Again, the variability within the syndrome must be emphasized.

Executive functioning

Executive functioning refers to the ability to deal successfully with novel situations which require the use of interrelated abilities. In a small study of teens and adults with PWS and a similar group with intellectual disability of unknown causation, Walley and Donaldson (2005) found the PWS group to have "a relatively intact central executive function" (p. 615). There are many stories of individuals with PWS in western Canada obtaining food in "creative" or "clandestine" ways. Parents have described them "casing" the place (e.g., determining the best access to the food), determining a schedule (e.g., to coincide when supervision is not present), "pre-planning" (e.g., wearing baggy clothes to conceal the loot), following multi-step procedures (e.g., finding the key, using the key, replacing the key), concocting a plausible story (e.g., why he has been sent to the store), having an alibi (i.e., why he couldn't possibly have done it), executing action with speed (i.e., with more than a normal speed of action), negotiating with others (e.g., in order to set the scenario to obtain what is wanted), using money to purchase (e.g., food from others or stores), stashing food for later consumption (i.e., determining a safe place to hide the food), and destroying evidence (e.g., hiding food wrappers or empty containers). Such descriptions suggest that some teens and adults with PWS are capable of executive functioning, that is to say dealing successfully with novel situations, particularly, where food is concerned.

Behavioural characteristics

How does a teacher deal with an obese student who defiantly sits on the floor and refuses to move, or one who has a full-blown tantrum in front of other students? Management of classroom behaviours is the biggest concern of teachers and administrators. Often they claim not to have training to deal with problematic behaviours associated with PWS and argue that the behaviours require a disproportionate amount of teacher time, thus depriving other students of their share of time. When classroom behaviours are difficult to manage, parent-teacher relations may become strained.

Having to deal with calls from the school regarding classroom misbehaviours is one of the most frustrating issues with parents. They dislike being called to come and get the child from school for misconduct. They feel that the school has a responsibility to provide a regular daily education program and should be able to cope with the behaviours. Parents advocate for EA support, believing that one-to-one support will help to maintain stability at school.

Levine and Wharton (1993) identified the following behaviours as problematic: difficulty modulating emotions; difficulty with unexpected changes or transitions; perseveration; sleepiness, low level of arousal, and sometimes difficulty sustaining attention; intense hunger with difficult behaviours around trying to get food. Dorn and Goff (2003) identified: food preoccupation, food seeking, uncontrollable food drive; compulsive tendencies; perseveration or obsessive thinking; tenuous emotional control; rigid thought processes; elopement (running away); lying and stealing. All of these characteristics, and more, can manifest in the school environment.

A review of teacher-identified behavioural concerns from the author's files follows in Table 9. These concerns were of sufficient severity to warrant the involvement of a behaviour consultant. In all cases there were multiple behaviours identified with each referral. This does not mean to suggest, however, that all individuals will display all of these behaviours. The list is representative of the type of problems concerning educators, and should not be considered exhaustive.

Table 9
Teacher identified behaviour concerns

aggression (hitting, pushing, biting, kicking, yelling)	non-compliance
	non-stop talking
anger	not following directions
argumentativeness	obsessive-compulsiveness
assault (on EA)	passive resistance
attention seeking	perseveration
avoidance of new tasks	personal hygiene needs
consumption of inedibles	politeness and manners
daydreaming	property damage
dishonesty	rejection of EA
disrupting the class	running away
distractibility	self-talk
emotional lability	skin picking
explosive temper	sleepiness
food foraging	social isolation
gorging	stubborness
high anxiety	tantrums
hoarding	theft (food and non-food items)
lying	difficulty with transitions
moodiness	

Educational interventions

Most schools are experienced in working with children with special needs. Few, however, have staff experienced in working with PWS. Common problems reported by schools relate to programming considerations, environmental controls, and behaviour management.

Programming considerations

At the primary level students with PWS can generally participate with their peers without many changes to their program. By the upper intermediate and junior secondary years they often lag behind peers and are recommended for special education supports.

Academics. Not all students can cope with the rigours of academic classes (homework, assignments, quizzes, mid-terms, final exams) and the competition for letter grades. Personal stress and low achievement may result. On the other hand, some may have the ability and interest to study academic subjects successfully. Sometimes students carry only one or two academic classes in areas of strength, while taking the rest as special education or lifeskills classes. Most students, however, receive special education supports by the high school years.

Lifeskills. When on an individualized education program the content may be modified to suit the individuals needs. Lifeskills focusses on the practical things that special education students will require to be successful as adults. The approach can be applied across all subject areas. Lifeskills includes such things as: personal safety, community awareness, social skills training, functional academics, leisure and recreation activities, and work experiences. A lifeskills approach considers the next environment (e.g., residential, vocational, social) and looks at the skills that will be needed. Lifeskills classes have less pressure as student progress is an individual matter and does not involve comparison with other students.

Food classes. Should students with PWS be programmed into foods classes? Some parents are adamantly opposed; others are supportive, with precautions. First, a distinction should be made between the types of food classes. "Regular" food classes teach such things as kitchen management, food safety, diet and nutrition, and recipe preparation. There is an academic and practical component to the class. Students must work cooperatively, integrated in a group of three or four to cook and bake. They are then given the opportunity to consume their products. The exposure to edibles, the academic focus, the need to work closely in a group with a time restriction, and the expectation of consuming the finished product can all be problematic for a student with PWS. Instructional kitchen areas have been identified as a source for food theft for some teens with PWS who are not enrolled in cooking classes. On the other hand, one young man took Foods 10 and a Commercial Kitchen course. He loved the kitchen and worked at all stations under the supervision of an EA. He now assists with vegetable prep at home. He collects items related to cooking and got a set of bowls for his birthday.

A special education life skills approach differs. Often it is done in an environment resembling a home kitchen rather than in a foods lab. The food topics can be relevant to the individual's needs, as outlined in the IEP. Given that many adults with PWS are now experiencing supported independent living it can be argued that a lifeskills approach should prepare them for this next environment. There is much that can be taught about reading labels, counting calories, food exchange systems, nutrition, healthy living, and low-calorie food preparation. Even where people are not involved in their own kitchen management and food preparation they often have their own small fridge for snacks and liquid refreshments. Something as simple as learning to prepare and enjoy a range of teas might add immediate enjoyment to a school program and add to lifelong quality of life.

Physical education. As described in Chapter 6, exercise is an essential element in the management of PWS. While there are some regular physical education activities which a student with PWS can accomplish, many will require adaptation, particularly as the gap in physical capacities widens with increasing age. It is possible to achieve the same learning outcomes with some changes to the ways in which competency is demonstrated, making allowance for short stature and extra weight. IEP physical activity goals, for example, have included participation in: the special needs swim program, therapeutic riding (hippotherapy), jazzercize, aquasize, bowling, and other life-time leisure opportunities. Some schools have created new P.E. options which may be more attractive to students, for example: dance options, rhythmic gymnastics, or community leisure activities.

Physical activity is essential. Once a child presented an excuse from her doctor to get out of physical education - "Please excuse this child from P.E. as she has Prader-Willi syndrome." Hopefully this would not happen today. Educators are more experienced at adaptation and modification to include all students; medical doctors should be more aware of the successes of integrated and individualized programs. In an American study comparing parent education-related wants, significantly more PWS parents wanted improvements and increases in adaptive physical education services, in comparison to parents of children with Down syndrome or Williams syndrome (Fidler, Lawson, & Hodapp, 2003). The successes of teens and adults with PWS who train and compete with Special Olympics give testimony to the enjoyment of, and commitment to, physical activity for some with PWS.

Work experience. Work experience can be part of regular or special education programs. Essentially, students are required to complete a certain number of hours on a job, usually unpaid, as an exploration of possible career directions. The placements are customized for each participant and require parental consent. Usually the classroom EA accompanies the student to the job to ensure success. There have been some very successful work experience placements which have raised expectations about future work possibilities. Jill enjoyed her placement in a hotel laundry, was delighted when she was able to stay on after graduation on a funded training program, but was saddened when there was no job for her in the end. Richard similarly enjoyed a placement in a hotel laundry and was disappointed when the union would not permit him to stay on after graduation. On the other hand, Sara's work experience in a hotel laundry did lead to employment after graduation, a position which she held for five years. Ben also got his initial exposure to library work through work experience, and had it work into a full-time job for him after graduation.

Field trips. Field trips can be highly problematic, both from the standpoint of destination and logistics. The parent of a primary student complained about the lack of appropriateness when a field trip was arranged to a bakery, where all children would receive a doughnut at the end of the tour. Why was it necessary to go to a bakery? If the curriculum focus was to learn about the community, then couldn't some other destination have been chosen? In another situation, just being able to physically get on and off the bus was problematic with short legs, excessive weight and the height of the first step. No one thought to bring a portable step.

Overnight field trips are particularly difficult given that EAs are hourly paid employees and may not be eligible for over-time pay. Parents have gone as a chaperone to ensure adequate supervision when an EA would only cover working hours. Other EAs have volunteered their time to provide all day and night coverage, and have been given time off in lieu at a convenient time when the student has been absent from school. Students have enjoyed overnight field trips involving: camp weeks, choir trips, and special cultural events. One teen even got to travel from BC to Ontario for a week as part of a national class exchange program.

Class bike rides and hikes can also be a challenge for someone with short legs and less endurance. To maintain good parent-teacher relations, a PWS parent may need to accept adaptations or alternatives for their child. For example, rather than thwart the class outing, the parent might agree to the child only biking part of the way and riding the rest of the way in an escort vehicle. The goal is to facilitate maximum participation. While a parent may volunteer to keep the child home from any event, it is not appropriate for the school to suggest that the parent keep the child home as a solution to difficulties in field trip planning.

Transitions. How periods of transition are handled definitely affects individual and family quality of life. Most children and adults with PWS have difficulty with change. Parents are polarized on whether to announce change early in order to prepare the individual, or whether to announce the change at the last minute in order to avoid the anxiety. From a system perspective, best practice provides supports through periods of transition.

Parent stories emphasize two important points. First, change increases the likelihood of stress, and second, that stress leads to behaviour issues. PWS literature also acknowledges that people with PWS have difficulty with transitions. Educational best practice involves transition planning as a means of avoiding or reducing student stress. Most importantly, transition planning also reduces parental stress as both parent and child have the same information and common expectations.

Consistent with current best practices, transition planning requires a team approach. It brings parents and professionals together to establish goals and processes to address changes to come. Key transitions include preschool to public school and from public school to the community. However, there are also important transition points within the education system. In most jurisdictions there is a change of facilities in going from elementary to middle or junior secondary school and then to senior secondary. Along with the change of facilities there may be changes of teachers, EAs, principals, vice-principals, janitors, secretaries, and classmates. New schools may be in new neighbourhoods and involve new bus routes and bus drivers. Lots of things may change at key transition times.

Parents can take some proactive steps to assist transitions. For example, with respect to the EA, they can:

- request an EA change in the year before or a year after a transition between levels with the same system (i.e., change the EA at the beginning of the grade 6 year if the student must move to a junior school for grade 7); this will ensure some continuity of familiar support.
- request that the EA agree to take this position as a minimum two-year assignment in order to bridge the transition.

Table 10 presents additional transition strategies that parents can discuss with school personnel to assist with transitions.

Table 10
Some transition strategies

- observe at the new location
- meet with key staff at the new location
- meet with the new administrators
- provide a PWS information package for the new staff
- provide a written profile and picture of your child
- invite new staff to an IEP meeting with current team
- have key new staff observe student in current location
- have the child visit the new location and meet new staff
- have the child observe the arrival or departure of the school bus that he/she will be riding at the new location
- have the child attend at new location on a part-time basis before the end of the school year
- have the child attend at the new location for year-end social events
- invite the new teacher to meet the student at home before the school year begins
- identify a buddy in the new class and arrange for the child to get to know the buddy for next year
- volunteer to assist with staff training
- provide PWS videos and professional reading material for staff to use at their leisure over the summer
- provide, or recommend, a PWS resource person for staff training
- ensure that team members have met with their counterparts at the next level and have passed on information
- invite key new staff to attend regional or provincial PWS conferences
- offer to take the old and the new EA for coffee, where you can guide the sharing of information

At about the time of graduation there will also be a change from child to adult social services. This will bring a difference in funding levels, available services, and a different social worker. There are major decisions to be made at about this time, involving:

- day programs or employment options
- post-secondary education or other training
- residential options
- recreational opportunities.

For many services there is no urgency for the child to move from the family home at this time. This is a decision that can be deferred for some time. Most important is the question of major daily activity.

Transition planning helps to make for a seamless move to an adult role in the community. It is important for parents to be proactive in planning for adult services. This involves educating oneself to what programs and services are available. Without this planning individuals in need of social services may be placed on waiting lists.

Environmental interventions

By manipulating the educational environment, potential triggers and stressors can be removed. Environments include: the bus line-up, the bus, hallways, coat room, locker room, gym, classroom, lunch room, playground, and any other area frequented by students. The following guidelines are derived from the school experiences of many families:

- *implement food access controls.* There are two aspects to food access controls. First it is necessary to ensure the security of food (e.g., lock the teacher's desk and filing cabinet, lock food storage areas), and second, it is necessary to limit access by the student (out-of-bounds areas, EA supervision, total staff awareness).
- *remove food stimulation.* Remove visual and olfactory stimulation caused by food which can trigger or reinforce the food seeking behaviours. For example, locate classroom and locker away from a kitchen, cafeteria, foods lab, or vending machine. Pictures of food and pleasant cooking odours are torture according to some teens and adults.
- *enlist team allies.* It is essential to enlist the help of, and give direction to, the janitor and secretary as part of the support network for a student with PWS. The janitor should keep the garbage containers emptied immediately after recess and lunch breaks in order to prevent food foraging. The secretary, who usually has the vantage point of being able to see those who enter and leave the school, often has a view of the hallways as well. She is able to visually monitor if a student is lingering or "hovering" in the hallway or escaping from the school.

Classroom management

Parents generally have high expectations of a school system to be able to manage the behaviours of a child with PWS, After all, they have all those professional people! What seems like a straight forward management issue in the home, however, may be more complex in the education setting.

Management policies

Teachers and administrators are required to follow student conduct policies adopted by boards of education, and school behaviour codes, often jointly developed by school parents and staff. Teachers and administrators exercise professional judgement in the way in which they invoke rules and policies. Worst case scenarios have seen students with special needs subjected to rigourous policies such as "zero tolerance" and "three strikes and you are out," without due consideration for their individual needs. Parents are reminded that they always have a right to appeal any decision of an employee of a board of education. There are always policies that ensure due process and protection for the rights of children and parents. The reality is, however, that children with PWS do receive school suspensions. Sometimes this is with the consent of the parents, at other times it causes them great consternation.

Individual versus group rights

While all children have a right to an educaiton, there is always a point at which an educational system will not tolerate one student's behaviour if it is interfering significantly with the rights of the other students to get an education. Rather than have their child formally suspended and removed from school for behavioural reasons, some parents have agreed to their child being sent home when having a bad day, or their child attending part-time when the pattern of behaviour suggests that the regular school day is too long. One grade 10 student, for example, was programmed for only 3 out of 4 blocks daily, going home at 2:00. While the school suggested only half-time attendance, the mid afternoon dismissal was a compromise. The parent did not want to "give in" to the school, feeling that "more should be done at the school." But the parent also recognized the value of working with the school in a problem solving mode rather than having to face the administrative consequences of behavioural incidents.

Individualized behaviour plans

While behaviour is almost always a consideration in an individual IEP, some students warrant a more detailed behavioural intervention plan. The plan is proactive in anticipating behaviours, rather than just being reactive to them. A behaviour plan allows for the identification and defining of problematic behaviours and the establishment of conditions necessary to change the behaviour. A behaviour plan is particularly important if the child is likely to be: removed from the classroom, excluded from activities, limited in privileges, sent home from school, suspended for a period of time, or referred to outside agencies. The behaviour plan involves parents, assuring them of appropriate process.

Parents and educators should expect compliance to school rules and teacher requests. PWS should not be used as an excuse for poor behaviours. Parents should be reassured, however, that most individuals with PWS perform quite adequately in the school and classroom environments for most of the time.

When there is no plan...

Without a plan, staff will react to behaviours according to their own knowledge, skill, and background experiences. Consistency and consultation will be lost. Administrators will be more likely to respond without consideration of the individual needs. With a plan, behaviours will be seen in a more objective manner. Parents should pay particular attention to:

- *threats and bribes:* threats of removed privileges, suspensions, and other punishments have been used by teachers to increase compliant behaviours, with little success. Threats without carry-through are quite meaningless and encourage the behaviour. Bribes teach that non-compliant behaviours will be rewarded with something wanted. Both are very poor strategies and should be avoided.
- *recordkeeping:* insist on recording data about specific behaviours, for example: frequency and duration of the event, time of day, class subject or period, personnel involved, antecedents to the event, and consequences to the behaviour. Such data aids in identifying patterns and potential causes of the behaviour. It also gets away from vague descriptions of behaviours which "always" or "frequently" are said to occur.
- *incident reporting:* unions want events to be reported for the protection of the workers. The frequency and severity of incidents reported can work against the child's reputation and be limiting to future staffing and opportunities for the child. Some teachers and assistants may be too quick to want to report events which should be routinely handled. Parents should insist on a clear understanding of what is a reportable incident, and to whom it would be reported.

Behaviour as communication

It is important for everyone working with PWS to recognize behaviour as a form of communication and to try to understand what is being expressed. For example:

- A highly verbal grade 4 student constantly sidetracked adults at school with excessive conversation. He relished adult attention but overwhelmed the staff. He engaged adults less after a daily "walk and talk" time with an EA was used as a reward.

- A grade 5 student didn't like to go into the boy's changing room and hid behind the curtains on the stage or in an out-of-bounds area during PE time. Participation improved when he went to the swimming pool on an individualized PE program.
- A grade 7 student fell asleep daily at school. He was tuning out to academic classroom instruction. When his program was modified by decreasing academics and adding work experience and community-based activities his somnolence disappeared.

In each instance, there was a message: the grade 4 student needed some one-on-one attention, the grade 5 student tried to avoid the discomfort of the PE experience, and the grade 7 student tuned out because he found the load of academic work too difficult. In each case there was already EA support, but it required agreement between parents and educators to make programming changes in order to change the behaviour.

Restraint procedures

Some school districts are sponsoring non-violent crisis intervention training for staff. The Crisis Prevention Institute (CPI) is "an international training organization committed to best practices and safe behaviour management methods that focus on prevention." (CPI, 2010). CPI emphasizes verbal and physical intervention techniques to prevent escalation of behaviours. The Institute maintains that, "other than to provide medical or nursing care, individuals should be restrained only when all of the following guidelines are met:

- the person is an immediate danger to self or others
- other ways to manage the person's dangerous behavior have failed
- staff members are trained in the proper use of restraints" CPI, 2006, p. 2)

CPI has produced an ebook (available free of charge) on *Risks of Restraints: Understanding Restraint Related Positional Asphyxia.* The PWSA-USA (2007) has produced an *Advisory for Care Providers Exploring the Dangers of Positional Asphyxia* (2007). The use of face-down restraint procedures increases the risk of positional asphyxia, where the restrainer's body position interferes with the restrained person's ability to breathe. Individuals with PWS, because of their poor muscle tone and excess weight, are at increased risk if prone restraint is employed. Parents should query school district policy on the use of physical restraint procedures.

Toward the end

Most of the seniors with PWS did not have the opportunity to attend high school, graduate, or go on to college. Today, however, students with special needs get more supports to stay in school through twelfth grade, and continue with post-secondary education if they desire.

When public schooling does not work

Education is a provincial responsibility in Canada and each province protects the rights of parents to choose how their child will receive an education. Some parents have chosen to remove their child from the public system, usually in response to issues around behavioural management and educational programming. After many years of frustrations in dealing with the local school system in a small community, one mother withdrew her son from school at the end of grade nine. "The teachers just don't get it," she said. She was drained from the chronic problems that they both had to face.

Private schools may, or may not, offer the types of supports necessary for a child with PWS. One teen was admitted to an academy specializing in learning disabilities, where she attended from grades 7 through 12. The classes were smaller. but there was no EA support. There she experienced "peer issues every day." The academy was able to cope with the food issues better than the public school had been doing. At the end of her grade 12 year she weighed 115 pounds.

The options of home-schooling or on-line courses afford a good degree of control for parents. Educating a child with special needs at home, however, requires extreme patience. Parents must be prepared to provide: daily instruction, supervision, and alternative activities for socialization. Such parent and child proximity on a daily basis can create heavy stress for both parties.

Graduation

Graduation is usually the culmination of thirteen years of education. It is a rite of passage that students look forward to; it is an event that is emotionally charged for parents.

There are usually two types of graduation certificates. The names given to the certificates may vary by province and jurisdiction. Some students may receive the "regular" graduation certificate, meaning that they have met the provincially authorized course requirements for graduation. The majority of students with PWS, however, receive an alternative certificate indicating that they have been enrolled in special education and have been on individualized programs. The latter certificate will limit opportunities for academic post-secondary course work.

The pioneer parents never had the opportunity to see their sons and daughters with PWS walk across the stage and receive any certificate. Many parents themselves never had the opportunity to stay in school until grade 12. Today, however, parents can anticipate a range of graduation activities for their child. Most schools start early in the grade 12 year with grad fund-raising events such as carnivals, music concerts, and fashion shows. At some point in the year there are traditional cap and gown photos taken.

Graduation may include a banquet, ceremony, dance, and after-parties. It is a time of family celebration. Kevin did an "awesome job" at his graduation, according to his mother, "The whole family was there and everyone was proud." It is often expected that parent and child will have a dance together. Of course grad is a fashion affair. David modelled in the grad fashion show and went to the prom in a rented tuxedo, just like his peers. Parents are advised to anticipate clothing requirements well in advance.

Graduation is also a time for special recognitions and awards. For Krystin, graduation was extra-special as she received a scholarship from the Lieutenant-Governor. Shelagh, received a special piece of original art from her art teacher which has been a lasting memory. Of course, families usually recognize this milestone with a special memento or activity.

Post-secondary education

After graduation from secondary school, some young adults with PWS choose to continue with post-secondary education at the community college level. They have registered in the following options:

- regular course (for credit or audit)
- academic upgrading
- adult special education
- leisure learning.

When a student has high interest, but lacks the prerequisite skills to be successful in a regular academic or vocational course, it may be possible to audit the course. This permits the student to participate fully in the class but provides exemption from the exams. Adult special education is similar to secondary special education, usually with a focus on functional academics and lifeskills topics. Leisure learning is also known as continuing education. These courses have more of a recreation and leisure focus.

Students will encounter a more liberal atmosphere at the post-secondary level. One Alberta mother related visiting a potential college where there were some courses of interest to her son. However, she said that she had "never seen so many vending machines," and that the cafeteria staff "wouldn't do half portions." They decided against sending their son to that college.

All students are considered to be adults at the college level. In contrast to secondary education, parents may have no rights to progress reports. Unless the young adult is in a special program, it may be difficult to gain access to the instructor. Post-secondary education is an adjustment for the parents as well as the students.

∽

This book has emphasized that there is a range within PWS, Students do not all exhibit the same characteristics, nor do they perform at similar levels. They are individuals with differing interests, abilities, and challenges to their learning. They come from unique home environments and family circumstances. They all come to school with their personal "baggage" of past experiences. What they do share, however, is untapped human potential. Those working with these students, while encouraged to learn about the syndrome, must realize that PWS is something that they have, but it does not define who they are or who they will become.

In the DVDs produced by Kinash (2007a & b) parents reiterate that they want communication with educators. They feel that they know their child best and are willing to share the information with teachers. Their hope is that the educators will take the time to listen.

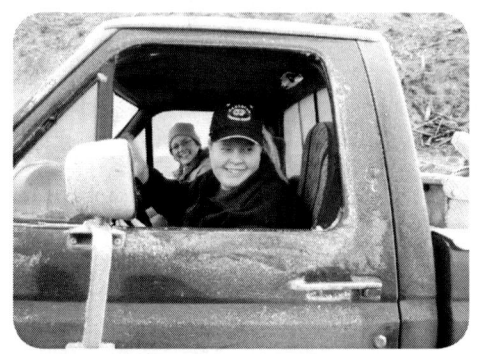

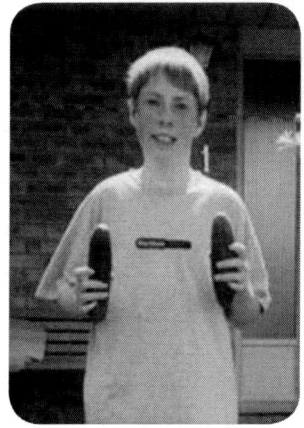
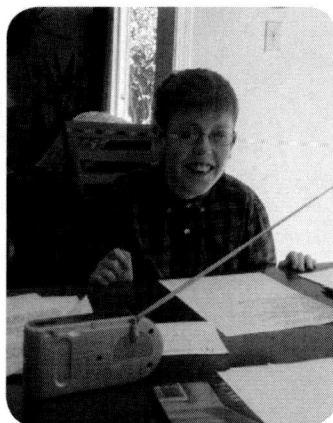

Teens

8

Leisure

L eisure is an important aspect of quality of life. Everyone seems
to crave discretionary time, which can be used in leisure pursuits.
Fine (1996) suggests that the overall goal of leisure is to improve quality of life by enabling the freedom to make choices that will improve
lifestyles in healthy ways. Appropriate leisure activity

> seems to be very relevant to the development of positive
> self-image, gross and fine motor skill development, physical
> stamina and health, and adequate motivation. Balanced leisure
> activity can also lead to the development of appropriate social
> behaviours and planning skills. It is [with] the development
> of these areas, and what may be called the 'self starting' of
> such behaviours, that PWS children and adults have great
> difficulty (James and Brown, 1992, p. 175).

Thus any restriction to the development of leisure skills may contribute
to the development of secondary handicaps later in life.

Leisure considerations

The low levels of employment amongst adults with PWS suggests that
leisure time should be more available, hence the importance of leisure
skills to quality of life. Unfortunately, there are often limitations placed
on leisure pursuits which diminish quality of life.

Lack of opportunity
The lack of opportunity to participate in leisure activities for children
with PWS is usually related to:

- presence of food
- difficulty with behaviour management
- energy level of the parent, and
- cost.

Food is central to so many childhood recreational experiences, and is a constant issue for PWS parents. Some parents have admitted restricting their child's participation in special events such as birthday parties or extended family celebrations because of the presence of food. Similarly, participation in well-established children's activities such as Brownies, Cubs, and church youth groups have been denied because of the presence of food.

Food often triggers behavioural issues. Parents of preschool and elementary age students, in particular, have acknowledged the difficulties in controlling behaviour when food, with or without restrictions, is present. The lack of awareness by a hostess, other parents, or activity leaders creates tension, with little time and opportunity to explain about PWS and the child's needs. Once embarrassed by the food behaviours or tantrums, drained from the constancy of supervision requirements, or fed up with the complaints from group leaders, parents are less likely to want to repeat the experience. Declining an invitation and staying at home, or not registering a child for an activity, may become the preferred option for the parent, however it contributes to a lack of opportunity for the child.

Oftentimes parents coping with severe behaviour management issues simply don't have any energy left for social invitations, whether for the child or themselves. This is particularly so in single parent situations where one individual must carry the full brunt of the day-to-day management of the child with PWS. Other demands, such as employment, family, church, and community responsibilities, also require energy. Sometimes there is simply not enough to go around.

For some families cost can be a deterrent to child participation in leisure activities. Single parents and large families are often at an economic disadvantage. Costs associated with integrated activities are usually more expensive than those sponsored by groups specifically supporting children with special needs.

Integrated versus segregated programs

Parents are split on whether they want their child to participate in integrated leisure experiences or whether they prefer the more protective environment of a special needs program. Summer camps are a good illustration. Some parents prefer to send their child to a regular camp program for their age group such as those sponsored by a church, Scouts, or a local recreation association. Others, however, prefer special needs programs which are often sponsored by service clubs such as the Lions Club, Kiwanis, or even a provincial PWS association. In the former, children must associate with non-handicapped peers and participate to the best of their ability in a range of activities, some of which will be novel and some of which will challenge the limits of physical endurance. While there may be sympathetic support for the special needs, it will be incidental to the main focus of the camp experience for the others. In the latter, they will have the benefit of appropriate activities, staff trained to support children or adults with special needs, and supervision levels appropriate to the individual needs.

Osteoporosis caution

Exercise is important to health, particularly for maintaining sturdy bones. Weight-bearing exercise is very important. Thune (1998), however, points out that individuals with PWS are prone to the development of osteoporosis (condition in which bones become brittle) due to a "lack of hormones, lack of weight bearing exercise, and lack of diets high in bone building nutrients" (p. 6). Therefore, participation in physical activities should be "appropriate activities." Contact sports (e.g., football), high-risk sports (e.g., skiing) and physically demanding sports (e.g., some track and field events) would not be suitable for someone with weak bones. There are other forms of exercise, however, which are suitable because they do not stress the joints and bones. Developing an interest in lifetime leisure activities such as walking, swimming, and dancing, for example, can safely contribute to physical health and quality of life.

Types of leisure activities

Brown and Brown (2003) assert that leisure activity is a major learning dimension and that a range of activities is necessary for adequate learning and performance in later life. Thus it is important that leisure activities be included throughout the developmental stages, particularly for the generalization of skills to subsequent activities.

Sellinger, Hodapp, and Dykens (2006), in a survey of leisure activities with Prader-Willi, Down, and Williams syndromes found that "individuals with PWS chose activities related to their etiology-related strengths in visual activities" (p. 68). More specifically, they participated in visual-spatial activities (colouring and drawing, arts and crafts, jigsaw puzzles, board and card games) and visual strategy activities (electronic games, computer games, word searches). It is important to note that the authors used a leisure activities questionnaire that had been designed for persons with mental retardation, to which they added several items that were hypothesized as areas of interest for those with PWS. In contrast, the following section identifies actual activities identified by children and adults with PWS and their parents/caregivers.

Table 11 lists leisure activities experienced by children with PWS known to the author. All with PWS enjoy some sedentary activities; not all enjoy physical activities. Physical exercise, however, is a necessary component of comprehensive weight management. Parents endeavour to provide community experiences that will involve either physical activity or socialization. They provide lessons in physical activities such as dance, gymnastics, and swimming. They engage in physical activities with the family such as walking, hiking, swimming, bike riding in order to model and encourage physical activity. They encourage their child to participate in activities that are provided at school. These are more likely to be in the area of the arts (drama, choir, other music) and special events (theme days, fundraisers) than in sports.

Table 12 is a similar composite list for adults with PWS. Walking and swimming are the two most popular physical activities. All adults with well-managed weight seem to have an on-going interest in some form of physical activity. Some of these activities are unique to females, for example: jazzercize, aquasize, and most dancing. Consistent with the observation of Brown and Brown (2003), females also tend to do more of the creative pursuits, such as: knitting, crochetting, rug hooking, painting, and crafts.

One young lady described herself as "an active couch potato," indicating her preference for sedentary activities at home such as: television, Game Boy, word puzzles, and jigsaw puzzles. Yet another, who once had a BMI in excess of 70, was very disciplined about walking to work daily, walking the dog, and and participating in weekly Special Olympics activities. Most adults, however, enjoyed a combination of sedentary and active leisure pursuits.

Even the oldest group, that is to say those over the age of 40, maintained an active lifestyle. Physical recreation activities were built into everyone's program. For example, a woman who had two knee operations rode a stationary bike daily, and a woman with leg braces and scoliosis attended a gym regularly.

Table 11
Leisure activities experienced by children with PWS

activity books	fishing	singing
ballet class	Girl Guides	soccer
ballroom dance	gymnastics	softball
beading	horseback riding	Sunday School
bike riding	ice skating	summer camp
board games	jazz dance	swimming
bowling	jigsaw puzzles	T-ball
card games	mini-golf	tap dance
choir	movies	television
collections	music lessons	therapeutic riding
colouring books	oragami	trampoline
crafts	Pathfinders	video games
Cubs	playing with toys	weight training
day camp	playing with a friend	youth group
dog walking	reading	
drawing	Scouts	

Table 12
Leisure activities enjoyed by adults with PWS

animal care	fishing	reading
armchair sports	floor hockey	rhythmic gymnastics
aquasize	fly-ball	rug-hooking
ATV riding	gardening	sewing
bingo	going for a beer	shopping
board games	going for coffee	skiing
bowling	going to the cinema	soap making
boys' night out	golf	social dancing
camps	guitar	Spanish dancing
card games	home movies	Special Olympics
ceramics	horseback riding	spectator sports events
church activities	horse shows	swimming
clogging	jazzercize	table games
collections	jigsaw puzzles	television
computer games	knitting	therapeutic riding
concerts	line dancing	TOPS
cooking	listening to music	video games
crafts	mini-golf	visiting with friends
crochetting	movies	walking
curling	music therapy	watching hockey
dog walking	painting	weaving
drawing	People First	woodworking
Facebook	piano lessons	word searches

Children and adults with PWS have participated with some frequency in two well recognized national special needs programs: Special Olympics and Therapeutic Riding. The Special Olympics organization offers a range of competitive sports opportunities which have enhanced physical well-being. Therapeutic Riding offers the physical benefits of hippotherapy along with a chance to learn about and provide care for a horse. Both organizations provide an opportunity to socialize with peers with similar interests in a supportive, structured environment.

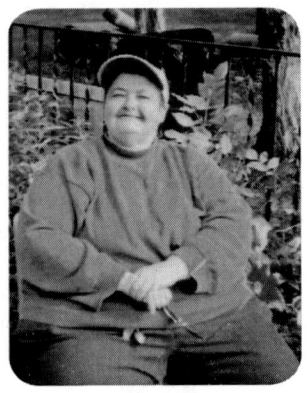

LeeAnne enjoying time in the park

Special Olympics

The Special Olympics organization provides opportunities for individuals with intellectual disabilities to participate in a variety of sports in many communities across Canada. At the community level the organization is run by a local volunteer executive and volunteer coaches. Coaches must be certified by the National Coaching Certification Program (NCCP). Sports offered in any area vary according to the availability of facilities and coaches. Participants enjoy training and competitive opportunities at the community level and travel to compete at their level of ability at organized competitions up to an international level.

Special Olympics Canada recognizes the sports listed in Table 13. Any sports which potentially place athletes at risk, because they do not meet the minimum health and safety standard set by Special Olympics Canada and/or Special Olympics International, are prohibited.

Special Olympics bowling is a sport which appeals to a wide range of ages and ability levels. In some communities it has become the main activity for training and competitive opportunities, and social-recreational enjoyment.

Competitive sports

For the more able athlete, there is the opportunity to compete at regional, provincial, national and international competitions. Special Olympics Incorporated hosts the World Games competitions every two years, alternating between summer and winter sports, and amongst countries. Special Olympic World Games are held in the years following National Games. More than 175 countries participate in the Special Olympics World Summer and Winter Games. For athletes representing their region, province or country at competitions, the majority of expenses are covered,

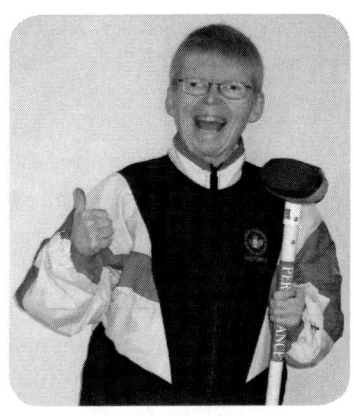

Bill as a Team BC curler

There are some athletes who enjoy competitive sports and rise to a high level of challenge. At 47, Bill, pictured on this page, competed in his second National Games competition in 2008 as a member of Team BC in the sport of curling. A profile of Corrie Carlile follows, describing her success at the international level.

In order to compete beyond provincial level events it is essential that an athlete be able to travel and live with the team, without one-on-one support. In some cases PWS parents have been annoyed when they learn that their son or daughter cannot stay with them but must sleep and eat with the team. In some cases this has discouraged or limited participation. In other cases athletes with PWS have been able to fully participate, and with success.

Table 13
Special Olympics sports

Summer	Winter
athletics	alpine skiing
aquatics	Nordic (cross country) skiing
power lifting	figure skating
bowling (5 and 10 pin)	speed skating
rhythmic gymnastics	snowshoeing
soccer	floor hockey
softball	curling

Source: Special Olympics Canada (2009)

International success

Special Olympian Corrie Carlile was diagnosed with PWS in 1980, at 15 months of age. She began participating in Special Olympics at age 12, competing in several sports, including: swimming, rhythmic gymnastics, track and field, snowshoeing, and bowling. Her parents supported her activities and her mother became involved with coaching.

Corrie had a goal to some day represent her country at the Special Olympics World Games. In 2000 her hopes seemed dashed when she fell and dislocated her left elbow. She got her brace off just before the Provincial Games qualifier in Prince George, allowing her to compete in swimming. She qualified for the National Games in Prince Albert, but then suffered through a bout of mononucleosis, limiting her training prior to the games. She persevered and competed, and was named to Team Canada for the Special Olympics World Summer Games in Dublin, Ireland, in 2003. There she won two gold medals, in the 25m backstroke and as a member of the 4 x 25m relay team. She also had a fourth place finish in the 25m freestyle.

In 2004 she competed in snowshoeing at the 100, 200, 400, and 800 metre distances at the National Games in Charlottetown and was selected to Team Canada to compete at the Special Olympics World Winter Games in Nagano, Japan, in 2005. In November of 2004, however, she tore the ACL in her left knee while taking part in a Special Olympics training camp in Winnipeg. Fitted with a leg brace she was able to continue training and to compete in March. She won silver medals in the 200m and 4 x 100m relay snowshoe events. She also had a fourth place finish at the 400m distance.

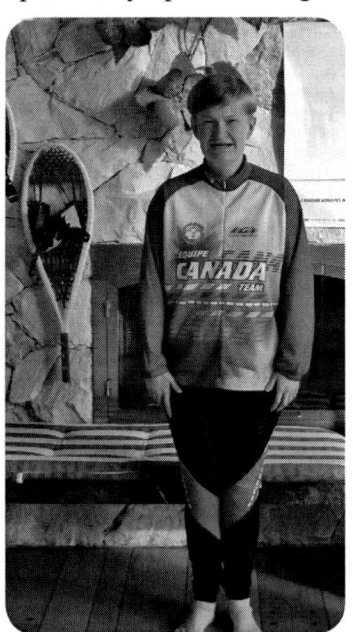

Corrie as a member of
Team Canada 2004

After returning from Japan Corrie kept up her training regime as she was preparing to go to Comox for the B.C. Special Olympics Summer Games. There she competed in 100, 200, and 400m track events, winning two silver and a bronze medal. Later that summer she underwent ACL reconstuctive surgery to repair the torn ACL. After working extremely hard at her rehab she is now back to swimming in top form. Her next goal is to qualify to go to another international competition.

Earning a spot on Team Canada is not an easy task. Corrie has to progress through a series of regional, provincial and national competitions. Today she trains almost every day of the week, year round. At 4 feet 11 inches and 103 pounds she is very fit. She has a hectic schedule as she also works 20 hours per week as an administration clerk with the RBC Cash Operations Centre in Vancouver.

When asked if she had any advice for young athletes, she gave a threefold response: "Keep active, watch your foods, and never give up." Competing in Special Olympics has allowed Corrie to meet lots of people, make new friends, learn new skills, and travel widely. This young lady is a role model and inspiration to other athletes, not only those with PWS.

Individual PWS leisure activities

The following section illustrates some of the more common activities enjoyed by children, teens, and adults with PWS.

Animals

Families often have animals for companionship and responsibility training. At 14, Robbie enjoys his dog, Dublin, and is responsible for walking him daily. Dogs are perhaps the most common family pets. David taught his pug, Oscar, to play fly-ball and enjoys taking him to tournaments. Christa shares her apartment with her dog, Barkley. Several people with PWS enjoy dog walking as a recreational or paid activity for friends and neighbours.

Erin works in a pet store and has two cats of her own to care for in her apartment. Another Erinn also has two cats. LeeAnne has a pair of finches in her apartment. And although she doesn't own one, Jill loves horses. Her room is decorated with pictures and memorabilia on an equestrian theme and she delights in attending horse shows. Anne Marie doesn't have any pets, but loves animals, so other tenants bring their cats to visit, and a staff person brings her dog once a week and they go dog walking.

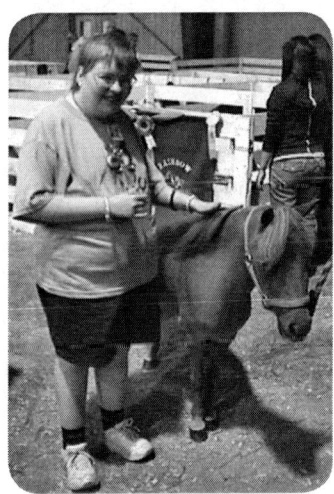

Jill likes to attend horse events

Collections

Reference is made in PWS literature to the propensity to collect things. According to Ziccardi (2006), this inclination "for both collecting and hoarding" is accompanied by "an extraordinary sense of protectiveness for these collections" and secure space requirements (p.

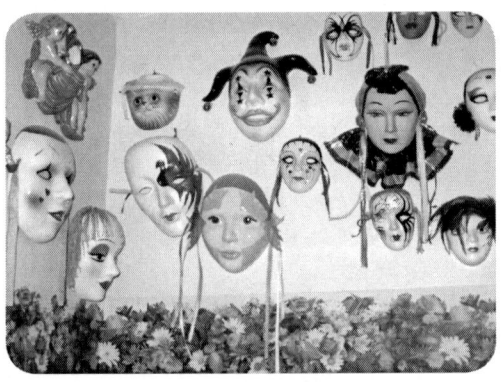

Lindsay's ceramic mask collection

386). Not everyone is a collector, but those who do collect as children seem to continue as collectors in adulthood. Some children begin to collect things when they get to school, taking pencils, erasers, and other collectibles from classmates' desks. With the support of parents, however, collecting can become a positive experience, teaching: orderliness, pride in having possessions, and self-confidence in sharing their knowledge.

Collecting brings joy at any age. At 6, Janine has a large collection of stuffed animals, all with names. Dicdre, a 20-year-old from Newfoundland, is known in her community for her collections and has been featured in the local newspaper. She has a collection of 569 bottles of nail polish as well as CDs. At 45, Margaret has a collection of 451 videos, all neatly arranged on shelves in her living room, and international dolls displayed in her bedroom. Lindsay collects ceramic masks. Collecting isn't just a female activity. Ben collects baseball caps and models of cars and motorcycles. Darcy collects dog figurines, and another man collects mugs. Another young man reportedly collects "everything."

Crafts

Despite generally low muscle tone, some individuals with PWS enjoy fine motor activities. One mother described how her son, as a child, spent hours in the basement doing crafts and using up all of her "buttons, macaroni, or whatever else caught his eye." (In later years she learned that he exchanged his art work around the neighbourhood for cookies!) Now as an adult he enjoys making cards for special occasions. Some adults have become proficient at crafts and even make some pocket money from their creations.

In Calgary, Erinn sews stuffed dolls to sell. When Lindsay from Courtenay first met Anita from Australia they exchanged crafts which they had made. Lindsay sews and her mother proudly displayed the table cloth and napkins that Lindsay had made for her at Christmas. Margaret won a prize for her rug-hooking at the Calgary Stampede and sold an oil painting and ceramic bowl that she had made.

Community leisure programs

Some children and adults with PWS participate in fully integrated community leisure programs. Informing the instructor, and in some cases other participants, about PWS seems to be an important element for success. One parent related that her daughter Joined TOPS for weight control:

> She volunteered to give a talk - so I suggested that she share PWS information with the group. Her topic was 'PWS, dieting and me!' She outlined PWS, expressed her personal thoughts about herself and ended with 'It seems I have been dieting all my life!' I had several people tell me that they had a change of heart once they were aware of the syndrome and the challenges she has encountered. One lady told me that the talks opened the eyes and the hearts of those present.

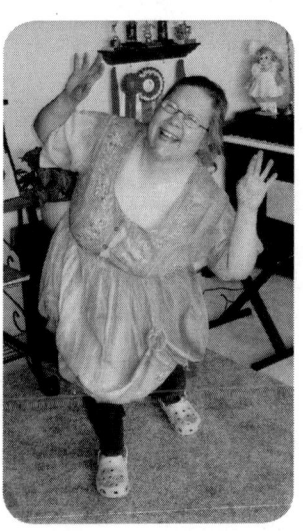

Blossom the clown
(without her hat)

In Red Deer, Angela took a clown course and adopted the name "Blossom" at the end of the course. She has used her new skills to entertain in hospitals. "She is reliable, flexible, goes out of her way to help others and is a genuine asset to our health care team" (Huston, 2006). Angela also took a course in self-defense for women, enjoys clogging with a community group, and is developing her public speaking skills with Toastmasters.

Computer

For school-aged children the computer can be a tool to assist with written output. Teens and adults with proficiency at keyboarding enjoy recreational use of computers. Brenda uses e-mail and Facebook daily. She also enjoys playing games on her PC. Another young woman "loves the Internet," and is very good with e-mail, but her parents expressed a concern for safety. For a young couple, who cannot see each other regularly, e-mail has become important to maintain their relationship.

Lindsay e-mails her friend with PWS in Australia. Her friend, Anita, uses the Internet as a a tool for encouraging others. She sends birthday and anniversary greetings and forwards humourous and inspirational stories to a list of contacts she has made in North America as well as Australia.

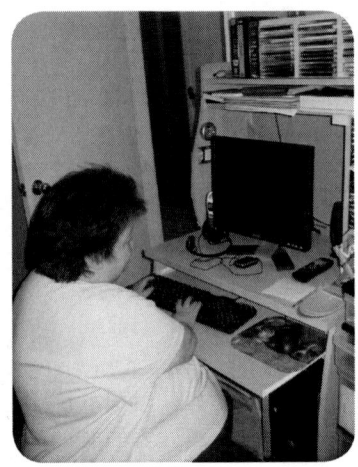

Brenda uses her computer daily

Fishing

In an essay in *The Globe and Mail* (January 8, 2008) a father described fishing with his PWS son:

> He is a good fisherman. He has patience, tenacity, a formidable capacity to concentrate and an uncanny ability to imagine where the fish may be lurking under the dark waters of the lake.

The pair do a lot of fishing around Toronto with meager results - hence the title of the essay, "Fishing, not catching."

Fishing on the west coast is likely more productive. In Sooke, David does both fresh and salt water fishing with his dad. His largest salmon was 26 pounds. His mother described a recent trout fishing trip with his worker - "He was so proud that he brought home supper that night!" According to his mother he has preferences and doesn't eat all fish.

Fishing isn't just a male activity. Trout fishing is Lee-Anne's favourite activity and one that she would do every day of the week if she could. She cleans her own fish and has her favourite recipes for cooking.

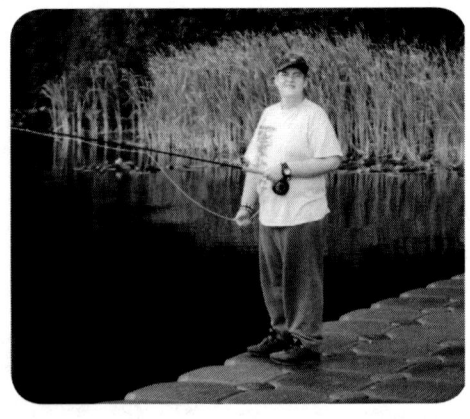

David enjoys fresh and salt water fishing

Jigsaw puzzles

Jigsaw puzzles are a table activity which deserve special mention. "Unusual skill with jigsaw puzzles" is one of the supportive criteria in the clinical diagnosis of PWS (Holm et al., 1993). Dykens (2002) reported that children with PWS far outperformed normal peers on jigsaw puzzles, "placing more than twice as many pieces as the typically developing group." This puzzle proficiency "was not predicted by age, IQ, gender, degree of obesity, or obsessive-compulsive symptoms, but by genetic subtypes." Dykens concluded that deletion PWS is associated with exceptional jigsaw puzzle skill. Whittington et al. (2004a), however, reasoned that the initial interest in puzzles may arise from a natural relative ability in visuo-spatial skills which is stronger in those with deletions.

Some of the individuals with PWS in this book enjoy the challenge of jigsaw puzzles and can handle complex puzzles up to 3,000 pieces. There are also those who dislike puzzles and won't tackle more than a 20 piece puzzle. For those who like doing jigsaw puzzles, the final product is often mounted and displayed or put away to be tackled again at a later date.

Music

Some children show an interest in music at an early age. At 4, Cody "loves to sing and dance." When the author first met Trevor at this same age, an "exceptionally strong interest in music" was noted. Although he could not read, Trevor identified the singers on seven tapes that his parent showed him. At 25, Trevor still loves to listen to music, particularly heavy metal. David is very musical and enjoys his tapes, "everything from the Irish Rovers to bagpipes and hymns."

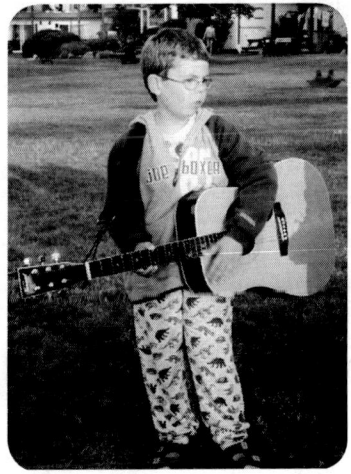

Evan sings in his elementary school choir ("the first thing he can do by himself") and performed in the school production of the Wizard of Oz. He takes cello lessons and hopes to take the strings program when he goes to junior high school. He is also learning to play the guitar.

Evan is learning to play the guitar

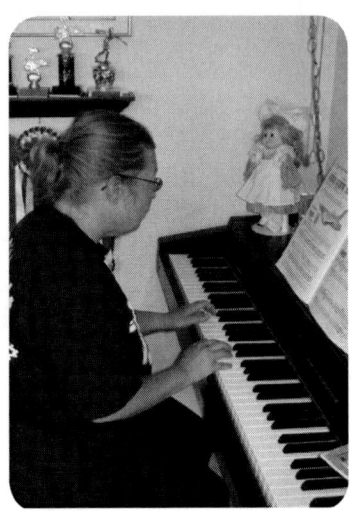

Angela plays the piano at home

Angela has taken piano lessons for many years and enjoys playing the piano for recreational enjoyment. Lee-Anne learned to play the accordion but now likes to strum the guitar. At 46, Ann has recently begun taking piano lessons, her "new passion," and can play some simple songs.

Not everyone who enjoys music plays an instrument. Some like to sing. Margaret will "break into song spontaneously at times." The late John Symons is remembered by the writer for his a cappella rendition of El Shaddai while on a picnic at a park in Langley. And Ray, also deceased, enjoyed singing along with a gospel song when riding in a friend's car (Jamin, 1990). A story from Saskatoon described a 16-year-old with PWS who sings "in near-perfect harmony as his dad plays the guitar." They were helping the annual telethon by busking for donations and performing at the event (Mario, 2008).

Physical exercise

Physical exercise is an essential part of a weight management program at all ages. Exercise helps to increase coordination, balance, strength and agility. Physical activities may also provide opportunities for socialization and peer acceptance.

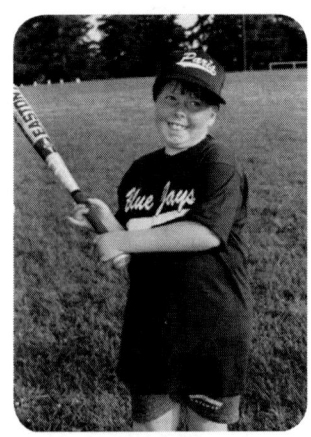

Stephen played community softball

In Kelowna, Isabelle, age 4, jumps on her back yard trampoline, an activity that she can enjoy with her brother. At 10, Lauren swims laps, walks 2 kilometres each day, and plays soccer in a non-competitive league. Robbie, in addition to walking his dog, lifts weights at school and goes horseback riding. When he was younger, Stephen played organized softball.

Dance lessons are often encouraged in childhood to develop coordination, poise, rhythm and social skills. Kate, age 9, takes ballet. "She is no better or worse than anyone else in the class and she enjoys it." Most adults with PWS enjoy attending dances sponsored by the local Associations for Community Living.

Spectator events

Joel, seen on this page in BC Place Stadium, when interviewed claimed to be the biggest PWS Vancouver Canucks fan. At just over 6 feet in height and 300 pounds, he was likely correct (He has since lost 120 pounds!). He is a sports fan and also enjoys watching football games.

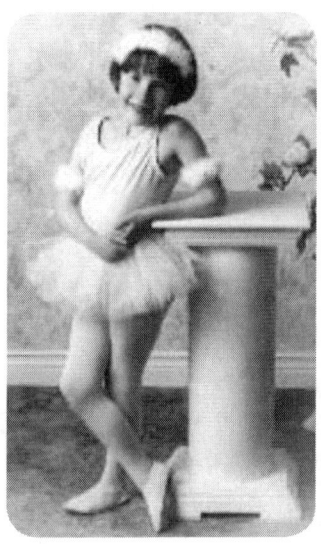

Kate takes ballet classes

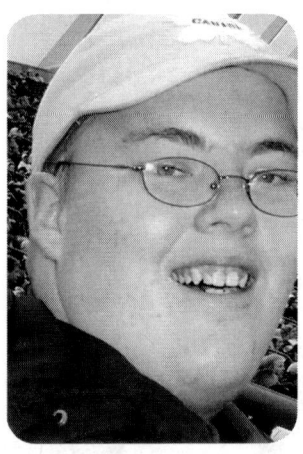

Joel at BC Place Stadium

Anne Marie likes to attend special community events as part of her individualized day program. Jill likes to attend horse events at the fair grounds. Others cite attendance at concerts or church events as meaningful spectator activities. One young man has been to concerts by Britney Spears and the Backstreet Boys, as well as to the theatre to see South Pacific and Phantom of the Opera. Spectator events can provide cultural enrichment.

Swimming

Swimming is a lifetime recreational activity that is enjoyed by many with PWS. Some have had particular successes in the water. Corrie won medals at the Special Olympics World Games swimming the backstroke. Ben successfully completed a swim across Okanagan Lake with 300 swimmers. Erinn competed in a cumulative 40 km swim challenge in Calgary.

Others swim as part of their individual exercise program. At 10, Lauren is an avid swimmer and swims daily in the family pool. Kevin enjoys recreational swimming in the lake when the family is at their float house. He also takes part in recreational swimming with Special Olympics.

Table games

Table games include favourite board games and card games. There is a range of favourite games that reflects the range of abilities within the syndrome. Some are very basic, some are complex. Games identified as favourites include: Crib, Monopoly, Snakes & Ladders, Yahtzee, Crazy 8's, Fish, Scrabble, and Bingo.

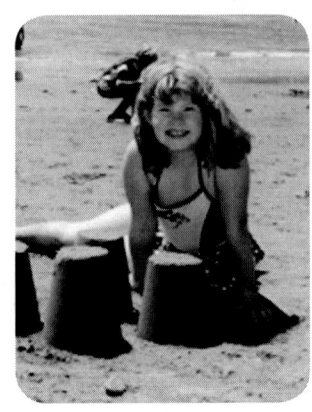

Lauren enjoys swimming and the beach

Some families promote a "culture" of games which begins in early childhood with educational toys and games. Games become a family activity which continues when the adult returns home for a visit. One mother shared that when her 27-year-old daughter came home to visit on weekends she could give her sister and parents a run for their money playing scrabble. She is an excellent speller and "We've been beaten at the game more times that we can count," she said. Table games can be an excellent vehicle for spending quality time together. Games can be found to challenge developmental concerns such as reading, spelling, arithmetic, and problem-solving skills.

Television/DVDs/videos

Almost everyone enjoys watching television and can name their favourite programs. Favourites represent a wide range of interest: soaps, game shows, cartoons, sitcoms, reality TV shows, and dramas. Some have amassed large collections of DVDs or videos which they enjoy.

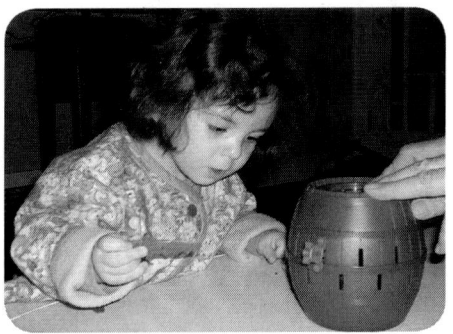

Amaia playing and learning

For some, these media are a form of relaxation at the end of a work day. They may also be a tool for social interactions. One young lady and her worker engaged in an on-going dialogue about the Survivor show as they cheered for the success of their favourite personalities. Some looked forward to an evening of sharing a home movie with friends or family.

Word puzzles

Word searches and crossword puzzles were described almost as often as jigsaw puzzles. Small word search books are convenient to carry in a purse or bag and are a favourite to fill idle time. Adults have been observed to do word searches while watching television or engaging in a social visit. Ann has a special clipboard with a compartment to carry her word search materials.

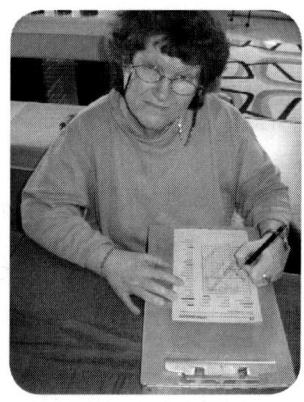

Many adults with PWS enjoy reading and certainly have functional reading levels. Word-based activities help to develop vocabulary and general knowledge.

Ann enjoys word searches

Dykens (2002) reported that children with PWS scored on a par with normal peers on word searches.

PWS family leisure

Family modelling is an important factor in developing lifelong leisure interest. Corrie, the Special Olympian profiled earlier, came from a family where leisure experiences were enjoyed together. As Corrie became interested in Special Olympics her mother became interested in coaching. Her parents still support her sports interests and attend all of her competitions. In North Vancouver, Paul became proficient as a skier because skiing was a family leisure activity.

Active living

A number of younger families embrace an active living lifestyle where physical activity is valued and integrated into daily routines. There is an expectation that *all* members of the family will be involved in daily physical activity.

While parents and children do not necessarily share all of the same activities, the parents model the importance of, and encourage participation in, physical activity. At least some activities are shared. Most commonly they include simple activities like: walking, hiking, biking, or swimming. With increasing age of their sons, fathers often pass on their recreation interests such as fishing and golf.

Families that embrace the active living concept enjoy holidays together as well. The most frequently mentioned family holiday activity is camping.

Family time

Family time refers to that time set aside for family members to do things together, without interruptions from the outside world. It is time that parents may use to create positive learning experiences for their children, or simply time to spend enjoying each other's company. Indoor activities have included: video/DVD nights, favourite TV programs, card games, board games, and popcorn nights. Outdoor activities have varied by climate and geography, for example: beach walking, hiking, bike riding, fishing, camping, swimming, and sledding.

The Wiens family has a seasonal tradition involving jigsaw puzzles. Each December they set out a Christmas theme jigsaw puzzle on a special table in the living room to facilitate family leisure interactions. This is an enjoyable family activity which incorporates one of their daughter's strengths. When one member chooses to work on the puzzle others are attracted to help.

PWS conferences

For many families attendance at a PWS conference becomes an annual affair. The Willotts from Calgary attended almost every PWSA-USA conference and were the driving force in hosting this annual American conference in Calgary in 1989. Their daughter, Madeline, attended every conference with her parents.

Most parents who have attended a regional conference in Canada, the American national conference or a world congress have enjoyed the experience. The parent networking is often as important as the latest research presentations. Several parents gave testimony to the importance of the conference experience to them. For example, the MacDonalds credit attendance at the PWSA-USA conference in Minneapolis in 1979 as a turning point in their son's weight management; the Willms family attended the PWSA-USA conference in Calgary in 1989, which resulted in the diagnosis of PWS for their son by Dr. Suzanne Cassidy; and

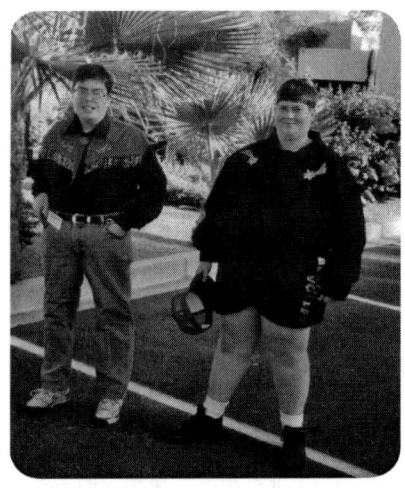

Old friends meet - Richard and Trevor at the PWSA(USA) conference in Scottsdale, Arizona

Kim felt empowered to educate police and transit workers in her community after attending the same conference in Columbus in 1998 (Nicholas, 1999).

Attendance at PWS conferences is not just for parents and professionals. Children and adults with PWS attend annually with their parents as well. Richard and Trevor, coming from different regions of British Columbia, are pictured renewing their friendship at a PWSA-USA conference. After Trevor's death, his mother described the importance of the affiliation with the American PWSA and attendance at the conferences:

> For the past 13 years, The Gathered View has been among the most popular mail received, and attendance at conferences was eagerly anticipated. Because we live in northern Canada, Trevor was only able to attend two conferences, but those were highlights in his life. He was eagerly awaiting his trip to Seattle. In Trevor's words, 'it is always neat going to conference, because I know that I am not alone.'
>
> Without the association, Trevor's life would have had less quality; his family would not have had the understanding or support which was so crucial. The information, guidance and friendship resulting from an affiliation with the PWSA was and always will be appreciated (Thom, 1995).

Summer camps

While camping is a great Canadian tradition, it is understandable that parents will have concerns about sending their child away from home for a week, particularly the first time. They will have questions about diet, food access, supervision levels, and behaviour management strategies. By visiting the camp to meet the Director and getting a sense of the lay-out, some of the fears can be alleviated. Talking to other parents about their child's experience can also be helpful.

Summer camping is a great way to enhance social and recreational experiences in a safe environment. It also addresses the need for independence, the need for the child to function without immediate parental supervision. For children with PWS, summer camp can be a major event, a rite of passage. For adults, it may be the only break that they get from their highly structured life.

PWS-specific camps

In Ontario, there is the opportunity for some young people to attend an annual PWS-specific camp at Shadow Lake, sponsored by the OPWSA. This camp offers a chance to meet new friends and experience independence from parents while parents are assured of strict diet management and physical activity. The camp follows a strict 1200 calorie Red Yellow Green diet. Chris, a 28-year-old with PWS, says that "the activities are awesome." He cites swimming, paddle-boarding, riding water bikes, and biking the trails as favourite activities. Campers reportedly

> cry when they go home knowing how much they'll miss the camaraderie, the high fives and group hugs. They fit in at camp. They don't always fit in at home (Ferenc, 2007).

Unfortunately, Ontario is the only province at present which offers a PWS-specific camp.

Under the former leadership of Geoff and Margaret Willott, the PWS Alberta Association in 1986 began an annual family camp at the William Watson Lodge in Kananaskis Country of the Rockies. The annual family event became a meaningful tradition, on hold only in 1989, the year the the Alberta Association hosted the PWS-USA national conference in Calgary. In 2006 the annual summer camp experience was temporarily moved, and then suspended pending a new location.

The camp weekend was truly a family affair. Extended family members (grandparents, aunts, and uncles) attended with parents and siblings. Families were responsible for meals within their cabins ensuring diets and routines were continued. Common time included singsongs, games (cards, board games), and informal group activities. There was lots of time for visiting, walking the trails, and the favourite treasure hunt. It was a chance to renew old acquaintances and to meet new friends.

Special needs camps

Summer camps for children and adults with special needs are offered by various organizations across the provinces. Chris, the young man mentioned in the previous section, has attended camps at Shadow Lake, for nine years. This camp is owned and operated by Community Living Toronto for those with intellectual disabilities (Ferenc, 2007).

For the last two years Evan, age 9, has attended an Easter Seals Camp at Shawnigan Lake on Vancouver Island. Susan recalls her anxiety at the thought of him being away from her for five nights and then admits that he had an "awesome" time. "He had no home-sickness gene," she quipped. With a ratio of one staff person for every three children there was good supervision. Being a special needs camp they were willing to accommodate Evan's dietary needs. Evan loved the arts, crafts, music, campfires, and camp rituals. And, of course, one of his greatest memories was of the camp food. Evan is very social, according to his mother, and "camp brought out the best in him."

Lindsay, now an adult, attended the same camp as a teen, and commented that "it is not fair that we can't go anymore." As an adult Carrie enjoyed going to a similar camp in another part of the province, sponsored by the Community Living Skills Association.

Of course not everyone enjoys the camp experience. One Alberta teen went to a special needs camp and "hated it." She didn't like to be associated with others with special needs. This reaction was consistent with her exposure to others with special needs elsewhere. According to her mother, "she would prefer to walk at 40 degrees below zero rather than get on a special needs bus."

Special needs camps are focused on the unique needs associated with people with disabilities. As such, they are staffed enabling a higher supervision level than would be experienced in regular summer camps.

Integrated summer camps

Regular summer camp programs may or may not take children with special needs. It is important that camp organizers understand the nature of the individual's needs before they make a decision. Where a child is already a member of an integrated group (e.g., Brownies, Scouts, Guides, youth group), and leaders already have awareness of the individual support needs, it will be easier for the child to be included in the summer camp experience. Given a philosophical commitment to integration, leaders will work with parents to create the greatest opportunity for success. Where the child is unknown to the camp organizers, the ways in which the query and application are made, and PWS information conveyed, will be critical.

Many communities offer day camp opportunities for children during the summer. These generally run for four or five hours each day. Usually the children take their own bag lunch. Often children will be attending day camp activities with classmates from school or other peers from their neighbourhood. One parent of a preschooler valued the day camp socialization experience and chose to use her community support hours to be able to send her child with a worker.

Church camps

Churches often include camp programs as part of their ministries to families. Camps commonly target, boys, girls, teens or families.

One camp leader described how a lad with PWS was accommodated in a week long Boy's Camp. Prior to his arrival, all personnel were made aware of his needs, "especially the cook and her assistants." With their help, "he very quickly realized that he was not going to get any extra food and so it did not become a problem." Trevor took part in all of the activities and was accepted by the other campers. "He volunteered as group leader of his cabin," without issues. "He was over-zealous in some activities, such as 'elbows on the table,'" where he enjoyed deliberately plac-ing his elbows on the table, in order to be get the attention of the others while he experienced the penalty of running around the perimeter of the dining hall. Staff had to put an end to this activity. He was active in the chapel activities and the eve-ning campfires. He reportedly "glowed with happiness" dur-ing the singing and skits.

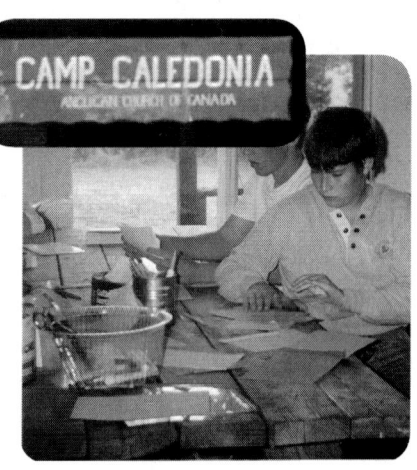

Trevor loved his involve-ment with the church and camp as just a continuation of church life. Familiarity with the lead-

Trevor at church camp doing a craft

ers lessened stress associated with the new experience for him and gave reassurance to his mother that appropriate care and supervision would be provided.

Vacations

Regardless of age, individuals with PWS enjoy their vacations. For children, vacations are part of family life. Some families find safety in camping experiences. They prefer being away from crowds and in a setting close to home in case they have to suddenly change plans. Others venture to child-centred destination spots like Disneyland or Disneyworld. These family vacations often continue into adulthood, even when the adult with PWS no longer lives at home.

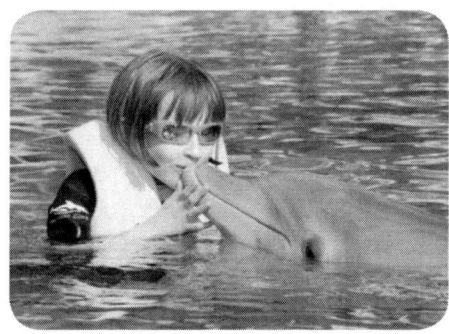

Kate and dolphin while on family
vacation at Discovery Cove

For adults living in the community, there may or may not be the possibility for a vacation. In some cases agencies include vacation planning in their services. Christa, from Olds, went on a Caribbean cruise and a trip to Disneyland with the local Association for Community Living. She also toured Sweden as a member of a Special Olympics rhythmic gymnastics team. From Edmonton, Anne Marie went to Disneyland with another client and two Skills Now staff. Years earlier she had been to Japan and South Korea with L'Arche.

From Calgary, Tyler took her sister Margaret to Mexico to an all-inclusive resort for a week. While they shared a great experience, she recommends caution when considering an all-inclusive vacation or a cruise. The availability of food requires constant supervision.

Vacations do not always require international travel. At 38, Angela took her first holiday without her mother. She travelled from Alberta to Vancouver Island with her hired staff.

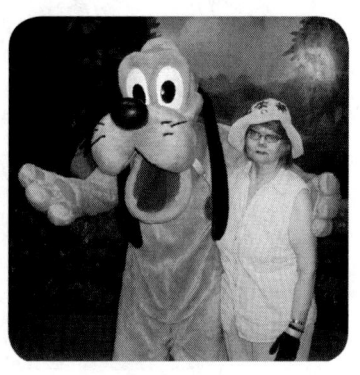

Margaret at Disneyland

They rented a car and visited the Butchart Gardens and the sites of Victoria, and even drove up to Nanaimo.

Vacations should be a time of relaxation, a time to enhance quality of life. For some parents, however, increased stress leads to avoidance. Some concerns and cautions mentioned by parents include:
- staying close to home in case there is a need to suddenly curtail the holiday
- checking policies of public carriers (e.g., air lines and bus companies) as there can be seating issues with someone who is obese
- learning to enjoy activities and events which are not too public if behaviour is problematic (e.g., camping)

- choosing an "all-inclusive" holiday will create extra food related and supervision stress
- going to a hot climate is not wise for someone with excessive weight.

Vacations live on in memory but are enhanced with photos and souvenirs. Adults with PWS enjoy sharing their vacation experiences with others. As with most adults, their homes usually display momentos from their travels. The enthusiasm of their vacation stories suggest that travel and vacation opportunities add richness to their quality of life.

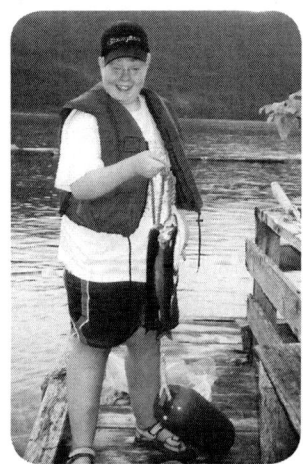
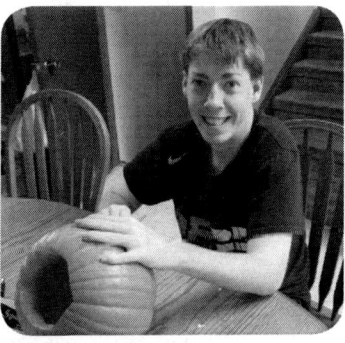
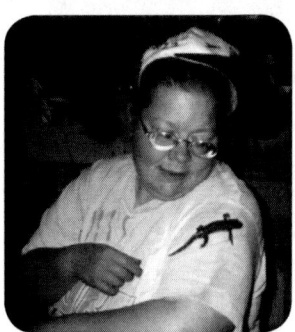
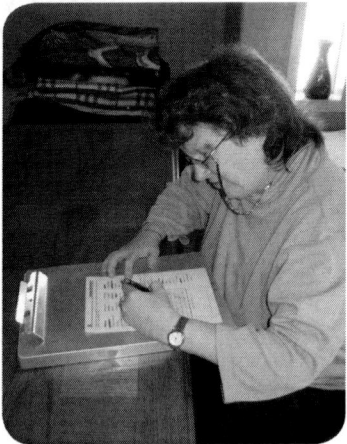

Enjoying leisure time

9

Residential options

Generally, where a person chooses to live is an indicator of the qual-ity of life desired. For people with developmental disabilities, however, there may be little choice. In some cases, parents do not know all the options available. Or, being over-protective, they may choose to ignore the options, hence, limiting the choices available to the young person with PWS. Over-protective parents tend not to listen to the child on the matter of residential options. They may see their offspring as an eternal child in need of their protection.

Some considerations

The residential options available, and the attitude toward out-of-home placements, have changed in the last 25 years. Today it is accepted that a young adult should be able to leave the parents' home and live more independently in the community. While moving out of the family home is often a difficult process, laden with emotion, it is a milestone which affects the quality of life of all concerned.

In general, research with developmental disabilities has found that residential options that resemble family homes, that are located in communities where individuals have a social network and have well-organized and directed levels of supports, promote quality of life (Community Living Research Project, 2008).

Desire for independence

Like their siblings and peers, most teens and young adults with PWS express a desire to move out of the family home. While parents may initially be aghast at the thought, there are many success stories about individuals with PWS who have moved out. Most noticeably, the relationship between parent and child improves when the child moves. No longer faced with the daily food access controls and behavioural strains, parents can enjoy visits. The child, independent of parent controls, can come home to visit like other adult siblings. As one parent expressed after her daughter left the family home, "I no longer have to be the food Nazi!"

While few with PWS go into full independent living situations, any move away from the family home represents greater independence from the viewpoint of the young adult with PWS. Semi-independence may contribute to self-worth, more than total independence. Under the supervision of caregivers or support staff the young adult with PWS can grow into new relationships with parents, family, and the community. If left completely unsupervised, there are usually tragic consequences.

Paternalism versus autonomy

Paternalism has to do with control through the perpetuation of a parent-child type of relationship. Young people with PWS want to be treated as adults, like older siblings and peers. In general, there is more chance of this happening while living elsewhere in the community. At 38, Angela emphasized her adulthood when she said

> I am not a child; I am an adult. I am short. Some people
> also call me *cute* - as an adult, I consider this word insult-
> ing and degrading. Sometimes it takes me longer to get my
> words out, even though my ideas are there. Add these things
> together and people think of me as a child. I am not a child.
> Do not treat me as a child (Kinash, 2007c, p. 63).

After fighting paternalistic attitudes most of her life, Angela has become an advocate for others with special needs. She states that she must fight for the little children with PWS who need a friend, because they "need someone who believes in them, so that they too can have a voice." Autonomy means that one has a voice. She concludes her section on Prader-Willi misconceptions by saying, "there is one thing I want you to remember. I threw my crutch away years ago. Please do not give it back to me."

Social policy has closed institutions, embraced normalization, and protected individual rights. Today, children with special needs attend neighbourhood schools and participate in their community. They have similar aspirations as peers and siblings to work and live in the same communities. Social policies promote their right to self-determination and independence. And then there is PWS!

> The promotion of autonomy for people with ID [intellectual disabilities] is not easy, and gives rise to ethical dilemmas. Caregivers are regularly confronted with situations in which there is a conflict between providing good care and respecting the client's autonomy. This becomes evident in the case of prevention of obesity in people with Prader-Willi syndrome (Van Hooren et al., 2002, p. 560).

In a study in the Netherlands, Van Hooren et al. (2002) found that the dichotomy between autonomy (respecting freedom of choice) and paternalism (guardian determination of what is best) is too simplistic to do justice to the care process. They interviewed parents, professional caregivers, and adults with PWS and "did not find parents or professional caregivers who were prepared to leave choices completely up to the child with PWS" (p. 566). This does not mean that caregivers necessarily take a paternalistic stance, but it does acknowledge the resistance to autonomy for people with PWS.

Some teens and adults with PWS resent, or rebel, against the constancy of parental supervision and control. They want to be independent, to be treated as adults. Evidence of conflict in alternative residential situations suggests that they also resent and/or reject paternalism by other caregivers as well. Success in the supported independent living model, to be described shortly, is largely due to the empowerment of individuals to have control over their lives and support for individual choice making.

In-home versus out-of-home placement

When first considering the question of adult placement, the protective urge of some parents dictates the choice of options. They consider existing space and even contemplate home renovations to accommodate continued living in the family home. While there is an acknowledgment of the need for more independence, it is viewed more as the provision of increased space or of more private space. When contemplating keeping an adult with PWS at home, parents should consider the following points which have been made by many parents:

- *financial support:* A common complaint from PWS parents in the past was that in-home care was not financially supported to the same degree as out-of home care. They argued that they knew their child best, so why should the government pay strangers to provide out-of-home care and not provide help to parents for in-home care? Now individualized funding may permit more equity.

- *future care:* A long-term problem associated with in-home care is the question of future care when the parents are no longer able to continue their caregiving role. Aging parents must consider who will take care of their child when they cannot, and where this care will occur.
- *relationships:* There is considerable testimonial evidence from parents and adults with PWS that parent-child relationships improve with out-of-home placement. Put simply, the quality of life of both the PWS adult and the parents often improves when a move is made to another residential setting.
- *respite:* Parents considering keeping their adult child at home must also consider the matter of respite. Usually the level of respite available decreases significantly when the change is made from child to adult services.
- *supervision:* If the individual with PWS is not working, attending a day program, or otherwise occupied in a supervised program during the day, the burden of care can become onerous and around the clock.

All of this is not to suggest that out-of-home placements do not have issues for parents. Parents who have remained vitally involved in the life of their child during an out-of-home placement have also had issues, for example:

- *caregiver use of respite:* While the parent would like to see respite used as an additional opportunity for structured learning, or participating in new experiences, they have been critical where it appears more as a "babysitting" service.
- *social experiences:* While parents formerly structured participation in social-recreational activities, new caregivers argue that respecting the client's right of choice permits them to choose more sedentary activities like sitting at home watching television.
- *sexual experiences:* Where parents would not permit intimate experiences in the home, other caregivers may respect the PWS adult's choice to experience such relationships.
- *weight management:* While parents previously valued longevity of life and restricted access to food, in some settings the matter of individual rights has superseded the need for protection.

- *smoking and drinking:* Residential workers who smoke and drink are more likely to support these activities as normalized behaviour. One parent was very upset that residential support workers accompanied her son to a bar where he was allowed to smoke, drink, and experience a lap dance.

Whether an adult with PWS should continue to live with parents or move out is sometimes just a matter of timing. Assertion of independence and deterioration of relationships, for example, may suggest that the time is approaching. Despite the level of in-home stress, however, some single-parenting mothers have resisted a move, more out of fear of abandonment or the need to maintain their co-dependence, rather than on the needs of their child.

While social service policies support independence and autonomy there is much to be said for the teaching of inter-dependence as well. Learning to live in a relationship that relies on others is realistic, particularly for people with special needs. Some adults with PWS have continued to live with their parents, or have returned to live with their parents after a period of living in an alternative residential model. When interviewed in 1986 one mother said her daughter "will never leave home." In 2007, at age 31, she is still living at home. In 1986 another mother thought that a basement suite would be an optimal environment for her son. Today he lives at home in a basement suite at age 32. In both of these examples, there is very protective family support. For these families this is what works best, for the present.

The support of the family can provide security and a nurturing environment which allows the person to continue to accept new challenges and grow without stresses associated with more independent living. Again, every personal and family situation is unique and should be considered in its present and future contexts.

Rural versus urban

People with disabilities have restricted options when it comes to where to live. Once they leave home, they generally live close to their parents or family, or they live where the appropriate services can be provided. Rural families tend to be more tied to their land and less mobile.

After years of living in Calgary, Doris moved to the outskirts of Innisfail with her daughter. The nearest neighbour is a mile away. Angela has several animals and enjoys flower and vegetable gardens. Growing up in a coastal logging community one teen has enjoyed many rural activities - the family summer float house, driving his ATV in the woods, operating his dad's crew boat on the lake, and helping his grandfather at his logging yard. In the small community of Sooke on Vancouver Island, David attends a day program with only three other young people. He enjoys the benefits of a large organic garden and the opportunities to go fishing, but must travel for an hour to be able to see his girlfriend.

Often rural communities offer a closeness and neighbourly spirit not enjoyed in a city. Living on a small island with only one commercial establishment was attractive for one family. Neighbours visited and welcomed the daughter into their homes. Neighbours trusted each other and didn't lock their doors. Unfortunately this lifestyle also offered temptations to obtain food.

Small communities, however, do not always have the range of services and amenities that are desirable. Out of town trips are required for specialist medical appointments. There are fewer community-based options for adult day programs. And there are fewer peers available for social activities.

Factors influencing alternative residential options

Many young people leave home when they go off to college, university, or work. Young people with PWS, like others with special needs, however, usually stay at home longer than their siblings and seldom leave their home communities.

Residential options will vary across provinces and amongst communities depending on social services funding policies and the desires and resources of the community. Ideally, there should be a range of residential options, representing varying degrees of independence and support in any community or region. Each family situation must be considered uniquely – there is no universal "best option" for persons with PWS.

The age at which a young person leaves the family home can be dependent on many factors. Some families plan for a move from the home soon after graduation, others do not plan for such a move. For some families it is a crisis which brings about a move. For example, uncontrollable behaviours, assault on a parent, chronic running away, sibling conflicts, and deteriorating parental health have been cited as contributing to the decision. Despite the trauma associated with a move from the family home, relationships are maintained and, in most cases, there are improved long-term relations as a result. A move out of the family home is seen by most adults with PWS as a significant step toward independence and adult status.

One mother related the background to the decision for an out-of-home placement for their son. At age 33 he had become too difficult to handle. The mother was so exhausted all of the time that all she could do was cry and sleep. If she was left alone with him she could not control him. He had become aggressive toward her and would try to push her. He would get very angry, have temper outbursts, and throw things. The son is now stabilized on Prozac and happy in his supported independent living situation. The parents are still intimately involved in his life, and their quality of life has greatly improved with his placement outside of their home.

American influence

American PWS literature strongly supports PWS-specific group homes. In discussing current residential options in the U.S., Ziccardi (2006) identifies PWS-specific group homes ranging from small (3 to 5 bed) to large (up to 16 beds), but goes on to state that due to budget constraints "many states now encourage families to keep the adults with developmental disabilities in the family home with supportive services provided as needed" (p. 393). While commenting on the transition to adulthood, Kazemi and Hodapp (2006) state that "many parents and professionals feel that specialized Prader-Willi group homes are particularly beneficial for most adults with this disorder" (p. 262). It is interesting to note that these same authors admit that "few studies directly compare Prader-Willi syndrome group homes to generic group homes or to home living for adults with the syndrome," yet they say "the consensus is that Prader-Willi groups are most beneficial" (p. 363). The only evidence cited for the possible beneficial effects of PWS group homes was lower BMIs.

Certainly lower BMIs can be obtained under other residential models, as illustrated in the individual weight loss examples presented earlier in this document. Research is needed to compare the continuum of options that exist in Canada. The majority of adults with PWS in the current research neither live at home with parents nor in PWS-specific group homes The satisfaction expressed by individuals with PWS, and their parents, suggests that several other models may produce reduced BMIs, afford greater independence, and substantial satisfaction with quality of life. This may be particularly so with supported independent living.

When considering residential options, the safety and security that parents seek for their child will contribute to their own quality of life. More structure and security for the young adult equates to greater freedom and relaxation for the parents. While PWS-specific group homes meet the requirements that many parents are looking for, do they present the optimal environment for continued growth and development for the young adult? And do they meet the young adult's desire for independence? They are a valued option in the residential continuum that will be most beneficial for some family situations, but until there is research comparing other models, they cannot be considered to be the "best" model.

Family care

Family care may be provided in the home of parents, relatives or complete strangers. Family care is seen as the most normalized residential model for children and teens. To have their young adult with PWS continue in the family home is the preferred option for many parents. There is often a struggle, however, with issues of independence, diet management, and behaviour. Whatever the burden associated with providing care, however, it is easier for some parents to accept than the uncertainty of care that would be provided elsewhere. Others parents, recognizing the preferability, or the inevitability, of an out-of-home placement for their young adults, favour the family care model in another's home because of the more personal relationships and lifestyle. Living in the home of paid caregivers is closest to the model of the natural family.

Parent care

In the U. K., Waters et al. (2007) reported that 48% of adults with PWS live at home with one or two parents/guardians. In the author's files, only 33 % of adults over the age of 18 live with their parents. In both cases this category included the household of close family, including parents, step-parents, or siblings. In other words, family are distinguished from professional caregivers who are paid to provide care.

Childhood bedroom. Simply keeping the childhood bedroom in the parents' home seems easy. Privacy and the need for independence, however, can be a problem, as can space for adult possessions. In some cases it works, in others it creates strained relations.

At age 30 Brenda returned to live in her parents' home. She has a bedroom large enough to have her desk and computer, which she uses daily. Brenda was previously married for four years, lived in a community two hours distant, and was used to complete independence from her parents. Her return to her parents home required some adjustments. She borrows the family car at times to go to her meetings at the Legion. She has an easy relationship with her parents and they keep an eye on her medications. Food is not considered to be an issue.

Not all situations are as comfortable as just described. Having lived independently, Brenda had adult status. Where children are living at home in their twenties there is often a struggle to establish adult status, involving issues of: space, privacy, lifestyle choices, and independence of activities.

Basement suite. For some families a basement suite in the family residence is seen as ideal. Of course, the physical structure of the house dictates the possibility of this option. Here the physical separation provides a degree of independence, while the proximity still allows for daily supervision. This in-home option affords the greatest degree of privacy for all parties.

David, age 22, has his own suite in the basement of his parents' home. "I love it," he says, and describes it as "cozy." He has a bedroom, kitchen-living room, and bathroom. He has his meals upstairs with his parents but has some refreshments in his own fridge. David says that he likes the privacy while still being close to his parents. His pug, Oscar, shares the suite with him.

Ben lived for 3.5 years in a basement suite in his parents' home. A worker came in to teach him healthy living concepts. For example, he had to make three dinners from scratch each week, clean his suite, and do his laundry. Then he began cooking one or two nights each week for his sister as well. This was in anticipation of him moving out of the family home. Today he and his sister live independent of their parents, sharing a condominium in the same section of town. Thus the basement suite was a stepping stone to a more independent lifestyle.

Sharing the house. At age 40, Angela shares the house with her mother. She contributes her share to the finances and is involved in all decision making. The kitchen has been divided, with the food storage and preparation area, including the stove and fridge, behind a locked door. While Angela is involved in all aspects of menu planning, shopping, and food preparation, she does so with supervision. She vetoed her mother's desire for a glass door to the pantry, preferring a solid door so that she would not be tempted by what she could see. She has equal use of all areas of the house and shares responsibilities for housekeeping and care of the animals.

Private care homes

There are differing terms used across provinces for private homes taking in adults with developmental disabilities, for example: private care, proprietary care, and host families.

At 44, Ann has lived in several different types of residential situations (parents' home, residential school, PWS-specific group home, integrated group homes, rural and urban, and in two countries). Currently she lives in a private care home and spoke positively about this model. Her bedroom is on a different level, away from the traffic flow to the kitchen. Food is not under lock and Ann knows that she is not to be in the kitchen unless supervised.

Carrie, age 34, also lives in a private care setting. After an unsuccessful group home experience and a period of hospitalization, she went to live with a worker who knew her well. Carrie credits her dramatic weight loss to the dedication of her caregiver. She says "they treat me like part of the family. They have two kids, who have become my brother and sister." She has her own suite in the basement and goes upstairs for meals with the family. She adds, "I am happier than I've ever been."

Private family care homes provide daily supervision, meals, housekeeping, and assistance with activities of daily living. In most cases the house parents are considered to be professional caregivers. As such, they usually belong to a local or provincial group of care providers and take advantage of training opportunities. The homes are inspected and required to meet health and safety standards.

Group living

Group homes provide accommodation for a small group, usually less than six residents. They may be disability specific or cross disabilities. Group homes were the preferred model after the closure of institutions. Many of the older individuals with PWS have experienced living in a group home at some point. For example, 12 of the 13 people over the age of 40 had at least one experience of living in a group home (James, 2010). The only one without this experience had lived most of his adult life in a large institution.

Integrated group homes

Prior to supported independent living, the integrated group home was the most popular out-of-home placement. Weight loss and improved

relations with parents were commonly cited as benefits with these placements. One mother reported that her son left home at age 21 when he
left school, and moved into a group home with three other males and
two females. She went on to explain:

> he lost 135 pounds in two years with this move. Has a
> girlfriend. Spends weekends at home every second week.
> Goes to the Legion for games and a light beer once a month
> with a worker. He is very involved with his church where
> his Pastor has been very supportive of him. He is also in-
> volved in People First. He enjoys his guitar, table games,
> rug hooking, dancing and music.

A young lady with PWS left home at age 25 to live in a group home.
She is proud of her bedroom and enjoys the residence. With a severe
language impairment, she never used the telephone when she lived at
home. Now she initiates telephone calls home and can receive calls
from her parents.

On the other hand, there are also negative stories associated with
this model. Maureen stresses the ongoing need for parent vigilance
once a placement is made. She describes a group home placement
where her son, a diabetic requiring insulin, was not given his injection
because the relief worker didn't know how to administer it. Because
of the shortage of workers in Alberta the agency was using untrained
immigrant workers. Also, despite getting funding for one-on-one there
was no day program schedule and he spent most of his time sitting in
his room with his Playstation. After another resident came into his
room and pulled some feathers out of his pet cockatiel, he put a lock
on his door. This became a safety issue and the supervisor said that
it had to be removed. Her son reportedly uttered threats and hit the
supervisor, at which point the police were called. Charges were laid
and he was then given a 90-day eviction notice. Other parent issues
included a lack of dietary consideration, poor behaviour management,
lack of parent involvement in goal planning, and loss of his personal
possessions.

Several parents criticized the lack of physical exercise in group
homes. One parent complained that there was no follow through after
a physiotherapy assessment. Another complained that her daughter
was putting on weight, but the staff nutritionist refused to cut the
calories further.

PWS group homes

PWS-specific group homes are championed by many parents and professionals in the U.S. and the international PWS communities. At the time of writing, however, Ontario is the only province with PWS-specific group homes. There are six homes with 34 residents (N. Goldband, personal communication, March 19, 2008). PWS-specific group homes can offer highly specialized care. It is not just a matter of diet control:

> Food access is limited to staff only and diets are regulated by healthy eating. Food is structured and set; all menu items have the distinction of being low fat and low calorie...weight loss does not come from diet alone. Daily exercise is also a regular part of the Prader-Willi home routine. For at least an hour a day, clients are exposed to a variety of activities, from aerobic videos or stair climbing in the house, to walking outdoors... they make use of the gym, take part in aqua fit programs and other activities like bocce... all staff follow the same diet as the clients, nutritional needs are met with large portions of low calorie food.

The home described here opened in 2004 under Vita Community Living Services (Villa Charities, 2005) and is managed in partnership with North York General Hospital and the Ontario Prader-Willi Syndrome Association. Of the six residents, three were quite obese upon entry and had lost over 60 pounds each within the first year.

David has been a resident of Headon House, a PWS-specific home in Burlington, for 12 years and works at ARC Industries. According to his mother:

> I feel our son has the best of all possible worlds - work that he likes, the safety net of a home (and workplace) with 24 hour security and programs built around Prader-Willi syndrome, and a community of caring people who understand his syndrome but appreciate David for the person he really is.

Headon House and ARC Industries are both under the same parent organization. The Community Living Board hired a psychologist to set up behaviour programs for both the workshop and the home, which have been very successful. The Board also engaged a nutritionist familiar with PWS to set up the food program and give cooking lessons to staff. David is responsible for making his bed and keeping his bedroom neat, personal cleanliness and grooming, and maintaining his weight at an appropriate level by exercising. Staff conduct a weekly weigh-in with charted records and provide a Friday night games night.

Is a syndrome-specific group home the best residential option? From the standpoint of resource allocation, expertise, and economics it might look very attractive. From a parent's perspective, it provides the food access control and diet regulation that are essential, with a knowledgeable staff. While regional parent groups have entertained the idea of a PWS-specific group home only one attempt has been made in western Canada. A home in Vancouver, in the mid 1980s, failed after 18 months due to a lack of economic viability, with only three residents. John, one of the residents from this home later wrote:

> I used to live in a Prader-Willi Syndrome group home where I almost died. I was told out in British Columbia I did not qualify to receive assistance from workers so while I was living there I was cast out on the streets to fend for myself, which of course I could not manage by myself! The other two clients I was told were able to be accompanied by our caregiver to their work placements. I was told in B.C. I could not because I was not labelled developmentally delayed like I am considered here to be in Ontario. While I was in B.C. I ended going to shopping malls – you guessed it – eating Laura Secord Chocolates and Ice Cream. Boy did it taste good. It was so yummy! When I was in a care home before this time for acutely brain damaged grown-ups where I weighed over 333 pounds I lost weight to 177 pounds. When I was forced to fend for myself out on the streets I gained back to 318 pounds (Symons, 1997).

In this passage, John raises the issue of eligibility for service. While eligible for placement in the group home, he was not eligible for additional funding, which would have provided assistance for a work placement or day program. In pragmatic terms, there weren't enough workers to support everyone - and John was the one who did not receive needed support.

One woman in her forties lived in a PWS-specific group home in California for four years, which she described as a "terrible" experience. She disliked: the locks on cupboards and fridge, another girl who fought and pulled hair, and abusive staff. The home relied on immigrant workers who were under-qualified to provide the care required, resulting in on-going behavioural issues. While the model is important, the economic stability of the agency and the qualifications of workers are very important as well.

There are pros and cons to a disability-specific group home. On the plus side are: an appropriately designed facility, specialist staff, and required support services. Negative opinions have to do with congregating people on the basis of a medical diagnosis, the incompatibility between people with PWS, and limitations placed on their personal development.

Supported independent living

The supported independent living model enables an individual with PWS to live a more self-directed life in the community. There is greater freedom than in the family home or group home models. It offers live-in attendant, itinerant, or on-site support. In the first case someone lives in the unit and usually has responsibility for the kitchen, including: grocery shopping, food preparation, food storage, and garbage disposal. This live-in helper may, or may not, be involved with other important areas such as: finances, transportation, recreation, and work supervision. Itinerant support involves less time. Here the worker is primarily responsible for the provision of meals, which are brought in daily. Under this model, the person with PWS must have a high level of self-care and personal management skills. The third variation has staff on site for all residents of the building, but not specifically assigned in support of one individual.

Supported living offers a high degree of independence. It can occur in an agency operated facility (i.e., a small block of apartments), in a regular apartment, or in a condominium. The supports are recognized as necessary, and offer peace of mind to the resident with PWS and the parents. Where this type of support is provided by an agency, however, there may be issues with continuity and staff changes.

Apartment with live-in support

In the following examples there is a similar level of support provided. The difference has to do with the identity of the employer. In the first example, with the availability of individualized service dollars, the parents became the employer. They were responsible for the rental agreement and the supervision of the worker. For some parents this is feasible, for others it would be too onerous. In the second example an agency is responsible for the hiring and supervision of the live-in worker.

In the first situation, the Calgary parents found, rented, and furnished a townhouse. The worker was hired by the parents, through a service broker who drew up contracts for each party. The worker was responsible to the parents and was to contact them with any problems she might have in dealing with their daughter or her restricted 900 calorie diet. The situation was comfortable, except for escalating weight. However, they went through three workers in less than two years. Each new worker had to learn about PWS, the specialized way of cooking, and enforcement of a low-calorie diet. As the employer, the parents had to be very involved.

In the following two examples an agency is the employer and provides the accommodation. In Manitoba a man is grateful to have his own place after living in shared accommodation and a group home. His agency purchased a mobile home in a trailer park for him to live in. He has the master bedroom. The wall between the two small bedrooms was knocked out so that an office and sleeping area could be made for staff. The trailer was an economic solution for accommodation. The only downside is concern about the increased tornado activity in the area.

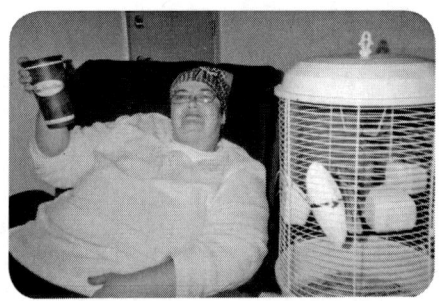

LeeAnne in her apartment with two favourite things - her birds and a drink from Tim Hortons

In Stony Plain, Leanne enjoys her current apartment which is shared with a support worker. "This," she says, "was worth fighting for." She previously lived in a group home and shared accommodation, and is adamant that she would never live in a PWS-specific group home. As hers is a one-bedroom apartment the worker must set up her own bed each night in the living room.

Apartment with part-time support

Not everyone requires, or is deemed eligible for, full-time support. In the first example, the young lady began with full-time support but then moved to more independence. According to her parents, at

age 17 she moved into her own supported apartment with 24-hour care at first. At age 18 she was weaned off night time care. She has been able to handle the responsibility of getting up and getting to work on time very well.

In the next example, a 34-year-old woman who had years of shared living arrangements, finally moved into a more independent situation.

She shared a basement suite with her dog, under agency care, an arrangement that she preferred over previously shared accommodation. She had found staff and roommates to be obnoxious and disrespectful when they would eat in front of her. Now menus are set weekly and staff come in to unlock food at meal times.

In Edmonton, Erin shares an apartment with another woman with special needs. The two of them have less than full-time support. Erin has more freedom than previously in a group home, although food is still under lock. She says that she feels safer when food is locked up. It improves her quality of life and independence. She has to clean the apartment and care for her two cats. The worker walks with her to the bus. She rides to work independently and works part-time in a pet store with only employer supervision. She maintains a very active lifestyle, which she says is necessary in order to help to keep the weight off.

The part-time support model does have its difficulties at times. From the parent perspective it may not provide enough supervision; from the young adult's perspective it may still represent too much intrusiveness. Pat wrote:

> Would I recommend this type of living arrangement to younger families? I am not sure. If there was any way to get them used to more supervision yet minimize the hassles, I would say 'do that.' But this is an option if your person is so unhappy all the time under more supervision that their life becomes intolerable and unmanageable for themselves and others around them. Now that Sara has been independent for so long, there is no way we could ever take that away from her.
>
> I have to be honest and tell you that there have been lots of problems and heartaches with this arrangement. Its not all roses and cream, believe me. But she was SO miserable in the group home that we just had to explore another way for her.

Attached suite

In Cumberland, Lindsay has her own suite, a former garage that was remodelled, which is attached to her caregiver's home. She has a kitchenette, living room, bedroom, and private bathroom. She has a fireplace and ample space to have a computer, television, her birds and cats. She has her mask collection on her bedroom wall and various wall-hangings elsewhere. Her meals are brought in for her, although she eats with her caregivers and other residents on special occasions. She is allowed to have tea in her own suite. Lindsay is one of several individuals being supported in independent living by the same caregiver. Her suite is private and secure. Supervision is always present, but not intrusive. In Lindsay's words, "I like being independent."

For 12 years, Madeline had a similar arrangement with a bed/ sitting room in the basement of her caregiver's home. She shared the downstairs bathroom with another member of the family. She could take all of her meals upstairs with her caregiver's family, but she chose to eat some meals in her own living room area where she could relax and enjoy her favorite television programs while eating.

Again, supervision was always available on-site, but it was not intrusive. Madeline appreciated her private area and the fact that she could make her own decisions about when to participate with the family and when to enjoy her privacy.

Staffed residence building

In the staffed residence building model each individual has a private apartment in an affordable housing building sponsored by an association. The building has comprehensive staffing for the benefit of all residents and is very secure. Christa has her own suite, but takes her meals with the other residents. There is no temptation of food in her apartment. Anne Marie, on the other hand, is involved in food shopping and preparation and is responsible for her own breakfast and lunch. Each apartment in her building has an alarm to monitor night activity and the building has a night supervisor on duty.

In both examples just cited there is a high degree of independence. Both individuals value the privacy of their accommodation, but benefit from the meal support and security of the environment provided.

Personal residence with attendant support

In Alberta, close friends and relatives incorporated Joel's Friendship Society (JFS) under the Societies Act. With individualized funding from the Ministry of Seniors and Community Supports, JFS provides 24/7 support for Joel. JFS also undertook fund raising in order to purchase a personal residence for him. The Rehoboth Christian Ministries Foundation technically owns the home, but Joel has the right to live in it for as long as he has need. All donations receive a tax receipt through the Foundation.

Joel moved from his parents' home into his new residence three years ago at the age of 23. "He has lost 130 pounds and is now at his goal weight. He no longer has to take insulin for diabetes, only a few pills." His behaviour is more manageable and he feels good about himself. This arrangement provides supported independence and long-term residential security for Joel, and peace of mind for his parents.

Shared PWS accommodation

It cannot be assumed that because two or more people share the same condition that they will be compatible for living together. In Calgary two young woman with PWS shared accommodation for a period of two years. While the arrangement provided an economic base for providing live-in support for the two women, it was not viable long term. Both sets of parents finally agreed that the two were not suited to sharing with each other. One father wrote:

> After two years together I was trying to see acceptance between the girls and I'm sure there has been some, but mostly it has been only a tolerating situation with each one respecting the other's territory – with a pathetic lack of territory being available in the shared living area. This has resulted in more friction, not only between the girls but also with staff.

In Manitoba, two young men with PWS shared a home under Hearthstone Community Services. The former Executive Director of the Association explained that two is an awkward number because there is no sense of community. Also, the size of house that can be acquired to support only two people is small, not allowing much private space given that live-in attendants are required. And, if the two individuals have personalities that clash, there can be daily difficulties. When alternate accommodation was found for one of the two young men both experienced reductions in their stress levels.

Independent living

Independent living refers to living in the community without formal agency supports. It means living as most others do, with support coming only from family and friends. Few with PWS have experienced this model successfully.

Living alone

There are few stories of individuals with PWS living in a completely independent fashion. In Vancouver, a 35-year-old woman was living on her own. With support from a dietitian she was able to reduce her weight from 197 to 167 pounds. She worked one day per week in a video store, to supplement her social assistance. She got to and from work on public transit. She handled her own finances. Her mother visited weekly. She expressed concern that her daughter was always "close to the line" with finances and that she "paid through the nose" for clothes and shoes as there were few bargains because of her size. Her mother felt that there should be more supervision from the social worker, and that there should be a homemaker. She felt her daughter was vulnerable when in public and that she spent too much time alone at home. She admitted, however, that her daughter was very happy in her apartment and that "you couldn't get her to move if you wanted to."

One young man was placed into an apartment in a major city, without agency supports. Unfortunately, there were many fast food outlets within walking distance of his residence. In four months his weight went from 170 to 240 pounds. Tragically, he died within a short period of time.

After episodes of living on the street, a 23-year-old woman with PWS was moved into an apartment by her parents. Thereafter she would not let a social worker go in, although she would let her mother in weekly. She tried to clean up as much as her daughter would permit. The mother admitted that it was not the best arrangement and that she was frustrated by the lack of support. Unfortunately, her daughter died three years later.

Shared accommodation

In Kelowna, a young man shares a two bedroom condominium with his sister. The two have a good relationship and his sister helps to keep him accountable. They do not have agency involvement but do have the strong support of parents. Assistance is provided for weekly meal planning and shopping. Lots of salad and raw vegetables are a must. As he does not want to be on a diet he understands that he must stay physically active. He shares all of the costs of his accommodation and has a disposable income of twenty dollars per week. This situation allows him to retain control of his life, but with some structure.

Marriage or co-habitation

Many young people with PWS aspire to be married, however marriage is rare. Only one woman in this study was married. There were four examples (3 female, one male) of individuals with PWS co-habiting in a common-law relationship. While this arrangement may not have been the preferred one in the minds of parents, it was respectful of the individual's expressed desires. Two mothers said that they were thankful that their daughters had found love, intimacy, and commitment, even though it did not work out in the end.

In two cases there was some parental hope that the partner would be able to understand the food issues and help to provide supervision. In both cases, however, the male partners had their own special needs and limitations, and were unable to manage supervision.

Institutional care

Institutional care can be either short or long-term. Placement in provincial institutions for mentally handicapped persons occurred for a number of adults with PWS in the past. Today institutional placements are more likely to be for a shorter duration for assessment or intervention. Institutional care is not generally an alternative long-term residential option.

One of the major issues in any institution has to do with food. As illustrated in the following examples, teens and adults entering institutions may not have limitations placed on their food intake. This is an important issue. Social services policies usually uphold the right of adult clients to make their own decisions. Despite having access to full client records, including the medical diagnosis of PWS, decisions have been made to allow full diet privileges. Presumably the institutions in the following examples would have had a qualified dietitian in charge of the kitchen, nursing care available to residents, and medical personnel available on-call. Even in the absence of a medical diagnosis, the eating habits and excessive weight gain should have been a clue to investigate the file more thoroughly and consider dietary interventions.

Institution for the mentally handicapped

A 1991 issue of British Columbia Report (Carter, 1991) carried the story of a young man who had lived for ten years in Alberta's Michener Centre, an institution for 1,000 residents with mental handicaps. The young man wanted to leave the institution - he wanted to be able to go to the movies and to a football game. He became his own advocate, "writing to the local newspaper, lobbying government officials, and contacting Legal Aid for advice." It was reported that a doctor had said that his patient was "depressed and possibly suicidal because his desire to leave the institution has been frustrated by the lack of funding."

Institutional life is highly regulated. Wake-up, meals, activities, and bedtime are all governed by schedules. Personal space and privacy are limited. Possessions are minimized. Behavioural compliance is expected and aberrant behaviour is dealt with. Meals do not resemble home cooking. Social interactions are limited, sometimes restricted and often not "normal."

So what happened to this young man? With the advocacy of a young woman with PWS and her mother, he eventually left Michener Centre in 2006, 15 years after the article appeared. Today he shares a house with another young man with special needs in a nearby community, with live-in support, enjoying a quality of life that he had dreamed of for years. When he left the institution he weighed 255 pounds; one year later he was down to 183 pounds and no longer required constant oxygen. His story is unusual in that he became his own advocate to get out of the institution.

A woman in her senior years similarly spent a decade in the same institution. While she did not receive her PWS diagnosis until several years after leaving the institution, her weight was permitted to climb to 280 pounds by the time she left at age 20. Today her weight is maintained at around 137 pounds, a weight much more agreeable to her 4 feet 6 inch frame.

In both of these examples there was excessive weight gain while in the institution. They were both discharged with a level of morbid obesity.

Youth custody centre

In the 1980s, a 13-year-old teen entered a provincial custody centre in British Columbia. She was high functioning, very verbal, and socially quite competent. She entered the institution weighing 116 pounds. Four years later she was morbidly obese and discharged at 226 pounds. During her stay she had been allowed to double her weight.

Forensic assessment centre

Trevor, at age 19, volunteered to undergo a 30-day forensic assessment (i.e., an assessment for the purpose of the courts) after having been picked up for attempted arson. Initially he was upset when, as a result of a clerical error, he was told that his stay would be for six weeks and not the 30 days that he had agreed to. When he went into the institution he was obese, but when he returned home he had put on a significant amount of weight and had serious breathing and incontinence problems.

He was admitted to the hospital with a seizure within a few hours of returning to his home town, and died less than two days later.

Excerpts from the medical inquiry indicated that he had experienced a considerable amount of stress from inmate teasing while in the institution. A week before he was released, he recognized that he was "losing it" because he was being teased so much and he telephoned his friend to get help coping. His friend immediately went to visit, only to be denied access because he was in solitary confinement. Trevor had indicated that he was sometimes afraid to tell the staff about the teasing, because he was intimidated by them:

> During this time, Trevor was upset because he had requested being returned to his medication Paxil, and had not been given it. He knew that this was a great help to him in coping with the teasing, etc. He had been taken off it temporarily, to see if it was contributing to periods of passing out that he was experiencing. This would have reduced the stress that he was under.

The staff at the institution took him off his diet, as they felt they had no choice - "Because he was an adult, and he had requested that he be taken off!!" Despite a diagnosis of PWS, a well-documented file history and obvious excessive weight gain, there was no focus on appropriate PWS interventions. The involvement of health and medical personnel did not help to address his condition.

Self-managed programs

Traditional home care has been based on a medical model, with agencies or health care professionals determining care needs and how support should be delivered. In many areas this model is still predominant. However, in the last decade or so, an alternative model, based on self-managed care, has evolved in each of the provinces. Self-managed care may be known as "direct funding," "individualized funding," or "family managed care." Program names vary across provinces.

Instead of a government funding professionals and agencies to deliver services to clients, it directly funds the clients, who then decide which services they wish to purchase. The funding can also be received by families or support groups to manage on behalf of an individual. The self-managed care model gives the individual requiring care an active role in determining care needs and choice of services.

Alberta: Family Managed Supports

Alberta's Individualized Funding program became Family Managed Supports in April of 2009. Under this program families may hire their own staff or contract with an approved service provider. Administrative responsibilities remain with the family, the guardian, or the individual with PWS. They involve: accounting for funds expended, maintaining the necessary bank accounts, paying the staff and/or service providers, and submitting invoices accordingly (AACL, 2009). This funding is provided by the Ministry of Seniors and Community Supports and administered by the Persons with Developmental Disabilities Alberta Provincial Board (PDD).

Angela, age 40, is her own administrator. With the support of her mother she hires her own staff and has put together a one page hand-out titled "How to support me," which is given to all staff. She states her expectations very clearly and provides a rationale. The hand-out talks about eating, setting her up to fail, degrading and condescending attitudes, boredom, shopping, and walking together. Finding suitable staff is one of her greatest challenges.

Previous experiences with the adult care system were not positive for Angela. According to Doris, Angela's mother, the adult system deluded them. It convinced them that Angela would be better off living away from home in a more independent fashion. The service levels, however, vacillated between total freedom, which demanded impossible self-control, or structured external controls, which stripped her of her dignity and inner discipline. The resulting obesity placed her health at severe risk.

Angela now shares a house in a rural setting with her mother. Staff provide support for her responsibilities in the home and activities in the community. Angela says, "I finally feel that I have freedom and less controls and more choices now."

Manitoba: In the Company of Friends (ICOF)

This program is funded by the Department of Family Services, through the Living in Friendship Everyday (LIFE) organization, which provides assistance with applications and on-going support. Funding is not available to family members, rather the consumer receives the cheque in their own name. Thus the consumer becomes the employer of their personal support workers, and must abide by all employer regulations.

Michael, age 24, lives in a home of his choosing with a support network of his choice. He directs his own program, hires his own staff, and is involved in all decisions. His staff support him 24/7. Michael participates in staff interviews and has the ultimate say in their selection. According to his mother, "there were difficulties retaining staff in the beginning but we have all experienced that learning curve and are having very good success now....It is more difficult to acquire staff because we live outside of Winnipeg."

Michael has a support network to assist him with paperwork. His team leader does the scheduling, his accountant does the payroll, and his resource person from LIFE, or his mother, addresses staffing concerns if Michael or his team Leader are uncomfortable. In his mother's words:

> it comes down to this. Michael's staff are told that his home is his haven. It is his safe spot. If he curses and swears in it (not at them) and that is going to make them uncomfortable, then they aren't a good fit. They are silent support and teachers by example. Michael is 24 - not an age to be handheld and directed. Michael is a business man (he must have a business number in this program) and he is to be represented as one in the community....We tell staff that Michael will do as much as he possibly can and they are the support in the areas that he is unsure of. When Michael says, 'he's the boss,' it's true.

"I can't say enough about this program," says his mother. People with special needs are supported in this program with time ranging from 4 hours per week to 24/7 care.

British Columbia: Vela Microboards

A Vela Microboard is "a small group of committed family and friends that join together with a person to create a small non-profit society that will address the person's needs in an empowering and customized fashion" (Vela, 1997). Capacity for self-determination is an underlying assumption. Board members have a personal relationship with the individual and pursue supports "based on the person's needs, not availability of services." Vela Microboard Association of B.C. is a non-profit society which provides "direct, ongoing, hands on assistance" to Vela Microboards throughout the province. It also hosts an annual conference and provides a regular newsletter.

A Vela Microboard provides structure for the use of individualized funding in support of a person with disabilities. There are several individuals with PWS in B.C. who receive support through microboards.

For one family member providing care, the recognition of her own advancing years was the impetus to form a microboard. For another it was the need to spread some of the workload associated with support. In both cases, there was an over-arching commitment to empowering individual choices over the long term.

Child services

While this chapter describes residential options for adults, a few comments regarding child residential services seem warranted. A few decades ago, parents were often encouraged to place children with special needs into institutions. Today, this is not an option. When a family can no longer cope, however, there may be the possibility of an out-of-home placement. Provinces make provision for the care of children under extra-ordinary circumstances.

One family agreed to the placement of their eight-year-old daughter with a foster family. Her autistic-like behaviours were too difficult to manage within the home. In another example, a single parent allowed her daughter to move into a group home at age sixteen. Her behaviour wasn't conducive to home living; she needed a higher level of care than could be provided by her working mother.

To make the decision to place a child in someone else's care is a big step. It is a wrenching decision which can leave parents doubting their values, parenting skills, and motivation. On the other hand, it can stabilize a family home, a particular benefit for siblings. It can also provide a fresh start and new opportunities with skilled workers. One family placed their 15-year-old daughter in care. She lived in a home with three other children, all with different diagnoses, and live-in house parents. In the mother's words:

> We have been on a roller coaster set of emotions lately but overall we're sure it was the right decision. The calm at home the past two weeks is almost disorienting!!!

Every family situation is unique. Parents should always be encouraged to seek assistance when the load is too heavy. In each of the cases just cited, there is an on-going relationship with the parents. In each situation the child immediately benefited from a consistent structured approach to management and the family experienced a much needed reprieve.

Children with PWS are sometimes born into circumstances which are less than acceptable. At such times, child services will step in to provide protection if necessary. One young man, subjected to alcoholism and abuse in the home, was placed into foster care by court order. Despite his fears and aggression, experienced foster parents provided a loving and supportive home environment that encouraged his successes through Special Olympics. He proudly shared his medals and ribbons from competing in multiple sports and his special award for perseverance. Living outside of the family home provided him with new life opportunities which he would not have otherwise received . . . . and a better quality of life.

Pets

The presence of pets can be very therapeutic. Brown, Bayer, and McFarlane (1988), in a major study of quality of life of developmentally handicapped adolescents and adults in the three western provinces, noted that clients identified the availability of pets as one of the reasons for enjoying where they were living. Many PWS parents recognize the value of pets for their children, particularly for companionship, exercise, and responsibility training. Children growing up with pets are more likely to want pets as adults.

Family pets

Children and adults living with their parents, and adults living in family care homes, may enjoy the family pet. One parent described her daughter as having a love for animals, and added that "they like her." The family had cats, dogs, and rabbits. A young adult with PWS was auditing an animal health technology course at an institute of technology as a result of her long interest in animals. And one young man identified the two family dogs first when asked about his "best friends."

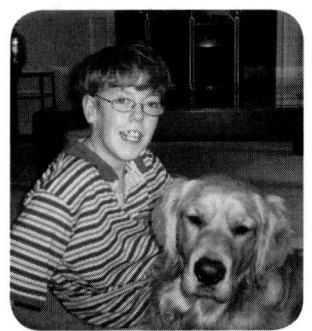

Robbie and Dublin

"Getting Dublin was one of the best things that we have ever done," wrote Cindy.

> He came from PADS (Pacific Assistance Dog Society) and is a well trained, beautiful animal that is a huge part of our family now. Robbie loves him so much and as part of his

exercise routine, walks him daily, usually twice on the weekends. The love that Robbie has for Dublin is so amazing.

Approaching their senior years, some older individuals with PWS also enjoy animals. Madeline lives with a family and enjoys walking the family dog with her caregiver. Bill also enjoys walking the family dog and has responsibilities for cleaning the bird cages as well.

Pet ownership

The type of residence is a major factor in determining whether or not someone can own pets. Adults with PWS, living in their parents' home or in a supported independent living model, are more likely to have pets than those living in group living situations, although some group homes may have a house pet.

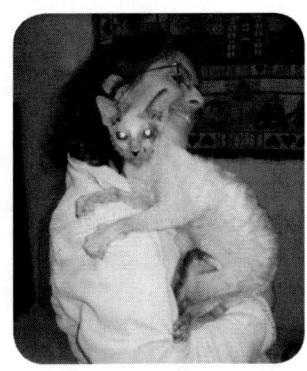

Cats, dogs, and birds are the most common pets. David shares his basement suite in his parents' home with his dog,

Lindsay with one of her cats

Oscar. This faithful companion sleeps on his bed at night. Leanne has her own apartment, with attendant support, and has two finches. Lindsay lives in a supported independent living situation and has a pair of lovebirds and three cats. Trevor had a cat when living at home and was allowed to have a cockatiel when he went into a group home. Living on acreage in a rural area, Angela has dogs, cats and a pair of llamas as pets.

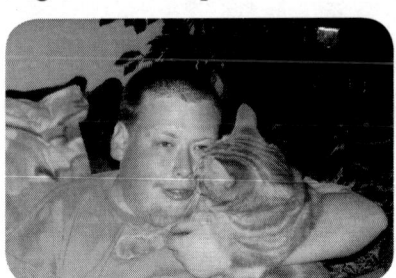

Trevor enjoying his cat

Pets fill the role of companions and give and receive love, with a disregard for disability. There were no reports of individuals with PWS abusing or disrespecting their pets. The presence of pets enhances the self-worth of those providing care and enriches the quality of their home life.

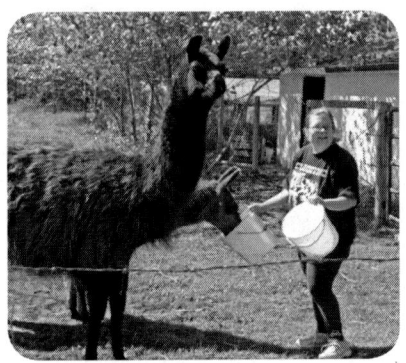

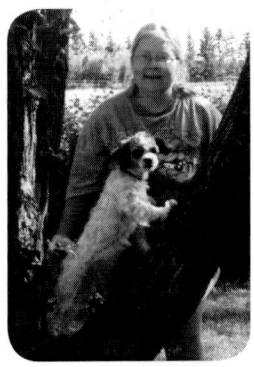

Angela lives on a small acreage
and enjoys animals

10

Vocational experiences

Parents of children with PWS, like all parents, hope that their child will some day be employed and contributing to their community like everyone else. By the high school years, when students begin to select vocational courses and/or participate in work experience placements, a potential worker profile begins to emerge. By the time of graduation, parents should have a clear understanding of the next environment to expect, whether that be competitive employment, sheltered employment, day program, or individualized activities. In some situations, due to local circumstances such as wait lists or a lack of other opportunities, volunteering may be a realistic option.

Most teens with PWS aspire to have a job, like their older siblings, and peers. Many, however, have unrealistic expectations. Vocational guidance for students with special needs is an area of specialty often overlooked by school districts. As a consequence, it is usually left to the special education teacher rather than the school counsellors, neither of whom have any particular training in the area. Often it is not until eligible for adult services that the young person with PWS finally receives service from an employment counsellor with rehabilitation training.

Apart from the need for supervision for food access control, adults with PWS are similar to many other workers with developmental disabilities. They may exhibit issues with: attention span, following instructions, quality of production, behavioural outbursts, comprehending complex tasks, changes in routines, perseveration, sleepiness, and stubbornness. However, with counselling, training, or on-the-job supervision these may be overcome or minimized.

For most of the population, having a job helps to define self-worth, social role, and status. Often adults with special needs understand, and aspire to, the social norms and expectations. Unfortunately, there may be a variety of situational factors hindering vocational success. For example, stereotyping, employer bias, economic conditions, employment regulations, collective agreements, and union protectionism have little to do with the ability of a worker with special needs being able to perform the required job tasks. However, they may have a lot to do with the individual with special needs getting the opportunity to try to perform the job tasks. Many times, individuals with special needs must struggle with a system which limits their participation, in addition to coping with their own disability.

Levels of employment

Opportunities for employment vary by community and are related to economic circumstances. Urban centres usually have the benefit of a wider range of options, rural possibilities are generally more limited. While this section outlines the range of job experiences, it must be noted that almost all of the individuals expressed satisfaction with their own level of employment. Only a few attending day programs, or staying at home doing nothing, expressed dissatisfaction. They wanted a real job.

Competitive employment

Competitive employment implies the ability to obtain, and hold, a job, whether full or part-time, seasonal or year-round, without special consideration or supports. It also requires remuneration, equal to or greater than the minimum wage. In other words, there is a legitimate job that would be done by someone else, if it was vacant.

In Vancouver, Corrie works at the RBC Cash and Operations Centre. After high school she went to Capilano College for a year in a career preparation program. It was at this time that she started riding public transportation. She received work experience placements at a dog kennel, day care centre, and nursing home laundry, but nothing lead to a job. Then she took a pre-employment program for two years with the North Shore Association for Community Living. During a field trip to Vancouver Community College she was attracted to, and subsequently registered in, a core skills course for office workers. She was recommended for employment and hired before graduation as a result of a work experience placement. She has since been employed for six years by RBC as an administration clerk, working 20 hours per week. To get to work, Corrie leaves home at 6:20 a.m., rides public transit and then transfers to the sea bus. After crossing the harbour she takes the sky train and then another bus in order to be at work at 7:15 a.m. She gets home from work at 4:20 p.m. after reversing this routine.

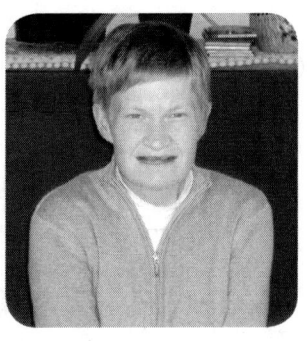

Corrie works as an administration clerk

In Winnipeg, Sara held a part-time job with a major hotel chain where she was assigned to the housekeeping department. She washed, dried, and folded laundry. She also bussed in the restaurant for five hours each week. Despite holding this job for five years, when the hotel came under new ownership Sara quite suddenly lost her minimum wage job. This was Sara's career, and it was arbitrarily terminated due to circumstances beyond her control.

In Calgary, a young woman prepared a resume with her mother's help and approached a women's fashion chain store in a large mall. At the time of writing she works part-time doing stock work for minimum wage. A young woman in B.C. held a paper route for two years, a job which helped to keep her weight under control.

While the hours worked may be less than full-time and the pay only minimum wage, these are nevertheless examples of real jobs done by individuals with PWS, without the need for extraordinary supervision or support.

Sheltered employment

Sheltered employment provides a sympathetic environment for individuals unable to procure competitive employment. While there is pay, it may be minimal, or based on piece work or an honourarium to supplement disability benefits. A sheltered work site understands and makes allowances for the disability but does not usually require the presence of an individual support worker. Accommodations may include such approaches as: working a small number of hours, scheduling work at low stress times, working under the supervision of a particular employee, or saving specific job tasks for the individual. It is still real work in a real work environment.

Ben, a graduate of a private Christian high school, now works five hours each day in the library of the same school from which he graduated. This is a job which was created for him through the advocacy of his special needs teacher. Ben receives an honourarium which supplements the disability benefits which he receives. At 26, Ben has been at his job for five years. He enjoys his job and feels competent at his tasks: repairing books, laminating covers, shelving returns, and checking out books. Ben gets to and from work on the school bus.

Erin works in a pet store in the West Edmonton Mall as the result of the advocacy of the Alumni Support Program. She also receives an honourarium to supplement her assured income. At 30, Erin has held her job for two years. She loves animals and enjoys washing and grooming dogs, cleaning cages, and occasionally helping with customer service. She previously worked for five years in a kindergarten. Erin rides public transportation to and from work.

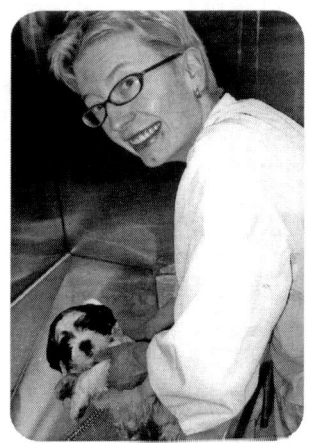

Erin at work in a pet store

Christa works as a cleaner for the Olds Association for Community Living. She has a schedule that she follows each day; at 4.15 p.m. daily her performance is checked. She receives a contract wage per month to supplement her disability benefits. Christa enjoys her job because she does it independently and without interference.

In Manitoba, a man worked for a popular restaurant chain for 12 years as a busboy, clearing tables two afternoons per week. The employer was understanding of his needs and provided an honourarium. In the same province, another young man worked for two years in a day care centre where he also received an incentive.

Supported employment

Supported employment involves work done in the community with the assistance of a personal support worker. Without the presence of the worker there would be no job opportunity. Some individualized day programs have the potential for supported employment. For example, some individuals who get paid for dog walking are accompanied by their support worker. Contract work in the community may also fall into this category. For example, one young man participated with a supervised crew cutting firewood and kindling which was sold in the community.

In Alberta, a woman has a weekly paper route in a small town. Her worker drops her off at the beginning of the route and then moves her vehicle down each block, maintaining visual contact. The route provides exercise, weekly pay, and forty dollars in tips at Christmas.

Entrepreneurship

In some locales the best work option has been an entrepreneurial model. Here the individual is able to make money through the provision of goods or services. This model works well where there is funding to support an individualized day program. For example, one young man provides a neighbourhood recycling service where he collects, sorts, and redeems waste products for cash, with the assistance of a day program worker. A young man, living with his mother, was proud of his well-equipped woodworking shop where he produced simple wood products, without any assistance. He was well-known in the small community and articles were placed in the driveway for sale. Another young man supplemented his disability allowance with a seasonal lawn mowing service in his neighbourhood, which he did without supervision; and another offered a power-washing service in his neighbourhood.

Day programs

Historically, training centres replaced institutions as places of care providing day programming. Originally, these centres had a vocational focus with the purpose of job training and work placement. With few opportunities to move into the labour force, however, the training centres often accumulated older trainees who had little likelihood of employment. Social policies and economic circumstances of the day kept adults with mental handicaps in sheltered environments. Today, some day programs still have a training focus, while others have significant recreation and leisure components. Most day programs also include other elements such as community-based volunteer work or contract work, cultural outings, life skills instruction, and physical exercise.

Sheltered workshops

Not long ago, sheltered workshops operated by local associations in support of people with developmental disabilities were the norm. They were typically engaged in entrepreneurial activities involving crafts or woodworking, contracting out small manufacturing or assembly operations, or providing food services. They provided a stable, safe work environment.   Workers were usually paid a piece-meal rate based on productivity, or an honourarium, rather than an hourly wage. Sheltered workshops were eventually closed in many jurisdictions and replaced by a range of contracted services providing training and support for community-based activities.   In some locales, however, they still remain as one of the options. Some parents favour sheltered workshops when they deem their son or daughter incapable of regular work productivity or unable to work in a regular work setting.   Others, however, find the workshop setting limiting. The highly repetitive tasks offer a lack of stimulation. In some cases individuals with PWS must participate with lower-functioning co-workers (Kazemi & Hodapp, 2006).

David goes to work at ARC Industries in Burlington, where contract work is done for local businesses. For example, they take on assembly line projects such as packaging knives, forks, spoons, and serviettes for fast food restaurants. When candies and seasonal Christmas foods are packaged he is given a different type of work to do in another area where he will not be tempted.   In Stony Plain, LeeAnne attends a workshop operated by Rehoboth Christian Ministries. She enjoys contract jobs and crafts. She works best alone and has been acknowledged by staff for her attention to detail.   Her program also involves a recreation/leisure component.

At 48, Bill attends a workshop where he has the opportunity to elect to participate in a range of community-based activities. He has enjoyed working at a radio station, at a soup kitchen, and displaying animals in shopping malls.   He laments, however, that he has never been trained to have a real job like some of his friends. He would like to bus tables in Starbucks or work in a pet store. At 28, a young woman also questions why she cannot have a real job.   She had good work experience reports when in high school, has developed good worker characteristics and some job related skills through her day program, but an individual community-based placement has never materialized for her.

Individualized day programs

Increasingly, adults are receiving individualized funding in order to have a unique day program suited to their interests and needs. Rather than being required to fit into existing workshop programs focussed on group activities, individualized funding allows for the creation of a program unique to the individual and community. For example, Paul gets physical exercise in his daily work schedule of cleaning tasks at several churches. On Fridays he gets to include a swim with his worker. Anne Marie's program involves some volunteer activities for non-profit groups, exercise, social/recreational activities, and life skills activities. Gardening is an important element in Tammy's program, along with leisure and recreational activities. Carrie, on the other hand, has a strong life skills component where she gets instruction in cooking, money management, hygiene and grooming, along with a day of farm work, where she is involved in fruit and vegetable harvesting and weeding. In each case, the family is involved with the individual to help determine the nature of their program. Individuals may receive incidental remuneration or other perks (e.g., small gifts, discounts) from an appreciative employer on occasion.

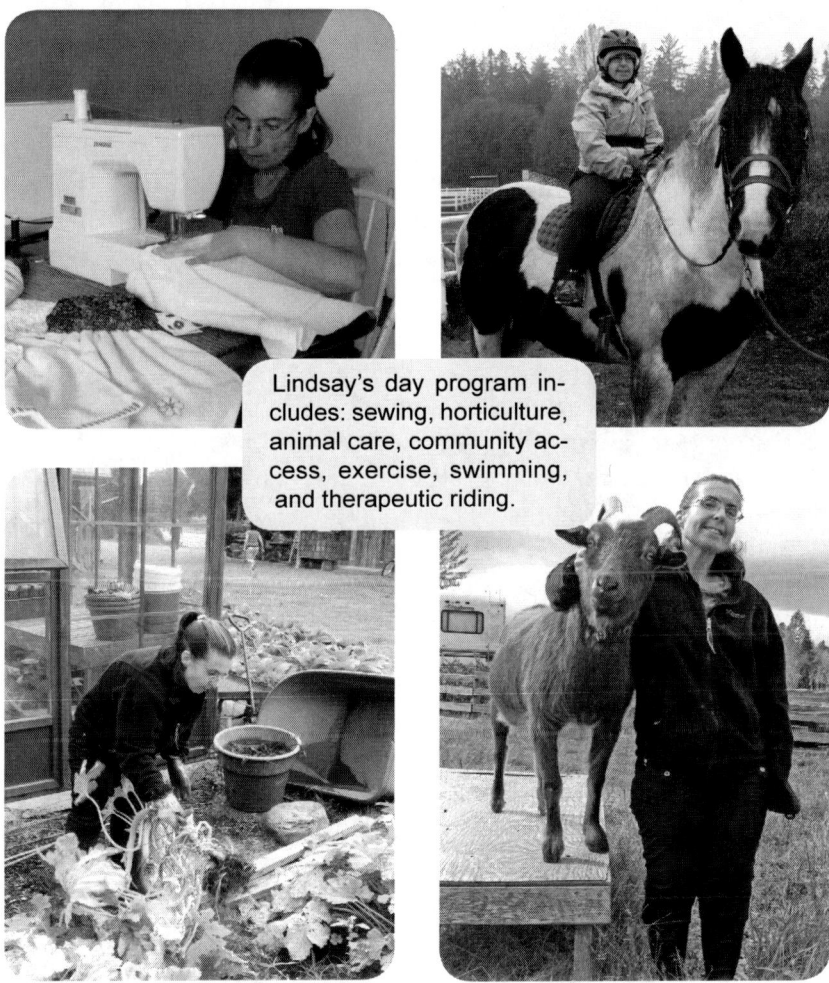

Lindsay's day program includes: sewing, horticulture, animal care, community access, exercise, swimming, and therapeutic riding.

Volunteering

For some, the only opportunity for real work is to volunteer in the community. The only differences with volunteer work are the lack of remuneration and the relative uncertainty of the workload. Schedules may be part-time, intermittent, or on-call. Employers still expect regularity according to their scheduled needs, satisfactory performance levels, positive relationships with co-workers, and allegiance to the organization. Volunteer positions can be successful, or not so successful, just like any regular employment opportunity.

Madeline arranges her own volunteer work schedule each week with several nonprofit agencies. She does clerical tasks, stuffs envelopes and prepares the mail. While she is competent in these tasks, her support worker provides social and emotional support. Volunteering is an important part of Madeline's lifestyle and she is disappointed if there is little work to do. Another woman in the Okanagan does similar office work three days per week, but with only one agency.

Some volunteer jobs may offer small perks. In Winnipeg, Jeff volunteers at the YMCA. He looks after the gym equipment from 8:30 a.m. to 2:30 p.m. daily and he and his support worker are given free use of the gym in return.

Vocational training

Most students get their first exposure to vocational training through high school work experience or special education programs. Beyond secondary school, they may get training through their day program or government funded employment training programs which are offered from time to time to target groups such as women, people with special needs, or ethnic minorities. Funded programs usually cover a period of on-the-job training, and then fade out, or terminate with the expectation that the employer will retain the new employee.

Work experience

Work experience is offered through most secondary schools to give students the opportunity to explore career interests. In B.C. it is a graduation requirement for all students. Richard's mother was enthusiastic about her son's work experience placement in the laundry of a seniors' care facility. She was hopeful that he would be able to continue there after graduation. However, she and her son were both disappointed when the union prevented this from happening.

One young lady received encouraging work experience reports from the school district program and also from a summer supported work program while in high school. She enjoyed placements in a museum, garden centre, and thrift shop. Her reports indicated that:

> she can work on projects independently, shows a good deal of initiative, is very motivated, has a strong work ethic, is very focussed, has excellent organizational skills, likes to complete tasks on time, is somewhat of a perfectionist, and knows when to ask for help.

The work experience program encouraged her expectations as a worker. Despite such strong good worker characteristics and successful work experiences, however, she has not been able to get a job in ten years since leaving high school.

For some students, work experiences do result in employment or training opportunities. Sara, the young lady from Manitoba who worked in the hotel laundry had received her initial placement there through her high school work experience program. Likewise, Jill also participated in work experience in a hotel laundry, which lead to the opportunity to participate in a funded job training program after graduation.

On-the-job training

On-the-job training addresses the need for skill development for a specific job. Participants get paid while training. Young people with PWS have benefitted from government subsidized training targeted for special needs populations.

Jill enjoyed her job in the laundry and was keen to take the training program that was offered. Eventually, however, the training had to end as there was no real job available. Her parents would have been happy for her to continue, even if not paid, but it was explained that liability issues precluded her from continuing to work as a volunteer.

Another young woman tried several jobs through a disability training program. She liked doing stock work and was given employment by a major chain store. Unfortunately she was not able to meet the employer's expectation and was let go after one month.

David works part-time on a subsidized training program. He gets $8.50 per hour while doing two three-hour shifts each week, stocking shelves in a grocery store. When he started he was assigned a job coach, however, "she was only with him once because he seemed to fit right in with his job description and could handle the responsibility so well." He had previously done well at this placement on the school district work experience program.

Worker training programs

Most community colleges with special needs programs offer worker training programs of a more generic nature which focus on exposure to work possibilities and the teaching of good worker characteristics. For example, in Vancouver, Carrie took a two year career awareness and work experience program at Kwantlen College, and Corrie did a similar one year career program at Capilano College.

Some colleges also allow students with special needs to audit courses in specific employment training programs. In Calgary, Erin enrolled in MacEwan College's College Connection Program which allowed her to audit early childhood education classes. She subsequently worked in a kindergarten class for five years in Edmonton. At the time of writing, another young lady in Alberta is auditing an animal health technology course.

Vocational success

It is essential that vocational success be viewed from the perspective of the person with PWS. In addition to directly asking about work enjoyment, parents might consider the following:
- Does the individual look forward to going to work?
- Does the person identify with other employees and/or with the employer?
- Does the person feel valued in the role assigned?
- Does he/she benefit from occasional perks from the job?
- Does the person participate in social or recreational activities with co-workers?

Frustrations with the job may manifest as: poor performance, expressed dislikes for the tasks of the job, behavioural disturbances, task avoidance, feigning illness, or refusal to go to work. Lack of success on the job may reflect situations which are remediable with knowledgeable guidance, for example: clarifying instructions, providing hand-over-hand training, changing rewards, lowering expectations, or changing work stations. These fall within the domain of the job coach or rehabilitation counsellor.

Vocational success does not just apply to competitive employment. In the present study, individuals enjoying supported or sheltered employment positions felt very successful and proud of their worker roles. Entrepreneurs and volunteers also expressed satisfaction with their roles. Higher functioning individuals who had to attend day programs expressed the least job-related satisfaction.

Entry level work

All of the positions held by those cited in this chapter would be considered entry level positions. Only one person, who was assigned to work as a quality control checker in a workshop, received what might be considered a promotion on the job. No one else related any opportunity for advancement and few had opportunities for variation in their duties. Nevertheless, almost all expressed satisfaction with their jobs. The fact that they had a job seemed more important than the duties performed.

Skill levels

There is a range of skill development amongst adults with PWS. While some may only be capable of simple tasks, others are capable of understanding and handling more complex instructions; while some require one-to-one accompaniment, others can work with minimal supervision.

Vocational skill levels are related to cognitive ability and physical capacity, both of which have a considerable range within this syndrome. Vocational skills develop best where there is high interest, and suitable personality characteristics. In the U.S., Goff (2006) observed that many individuals with PWS choose to work with animals or children, because they are very nurturing. There are examples cited in this chapter of adults doing such jobs. There are also a few examples where individuals have worked in the food services industry, another obvious high interest area and one which would give many parents concerns. They have worked long-term at such tasks as bussing tables, serving coffee, cleaning, or stocking shelves. Three individuals had school work experience success working in laundries and pursued the possibility of future work in this setting, suggesting that the job tasks of a laundry worker are a reasonable match for some adults with PWS. Whether working with animals or children, or working in a restaurant or laundry, job success seems to be based, at least in part, on manual activity, simple tasks, and clear routines.

Some individuals with PWS also possess artistic and creative skills and have been able to use them to make gifts or creations for sale. Lindsay sews with a sewing machine and has made gifts and simple clothing for herself with minimal guidance. LeeAnn makes wooden wind twirlers which she has sold at craft fairs. Margaret sold a painting and a piece of pottery through Indefinite Arts in Calgary. LeeAnn and Lindsay have both crocheted baby blankets as gifts.

Job success

There was no formal measure for job success in this study. Factors related to job success, however, were identified by a number of individuals with PWS and their parents or guardians.

Personal satisfaction. One measure of vocational success is personal satisfaction with the job. For example, a woman who began her work at a restaurant on a gradual entry basis, complained of boredom. When she was moved to full-time she became much happier. She liked to be busy. And even though David is only working part-time stocking shelves, he is happy to be given that chance, saying "I was designed for this job!"

The words that workers use to describe how they like their work are also indicators of personal satisfaction. For example, Erin says that she "loves" her work in the pet store; Ben "loves" his job in the school library. The pride with which they talk about their jobs affirms strong job satisfaction

Longevity in position. One correlate of job satisfaction may be the longevity enjoyed in the position. There were numerous examples of job situations being terminated after a short duration by the employers for a variety of causes, for example: lack of productivity, the need for greater supervision, theft, and food issues. On the other hand, there are examples of individuals who have remained with employers for a long term. For example, one man bussed tables in the same restaurant for 12 years; a woman worked for 8 years serving coffee, cleaning, and doing vegetable preparation; Corrie has been with RBC for 6 years; Ben has worked in the school library for 5 years. Such longevity on the job is surely an indicator of both worker and employer satisfaction and job success.

Remuneration. Relatively few adults with PWS have the opportunity for remunerative employment. Those that do, usually work for minimum wage or an honourarium to supplement their disability income. The fact that they are working, however, contributes importantly to their self-concept and social opportunities. Remuneration is not necessarily viewed as a correlate of job success by those with PWS. Some individuals, having experienced their only job tasks through day programs, also expressed satisfaction with their jobs, despite not receiving any pay. This seemed particularly so when doing contract work for other companies in the community. Performing real work tasks that were valued by established businesses gave them a high degree of satisfaction.

Self-worth. Marion reports that David has "such a positive attitude" toward his job and plenty of social interaction. He lives in a small community and many people know him. "He wears a uniform (shirt and vest) and always does his own laundry." She says:

> The spin-off benefits have been so positive. He has just purchased his own brand new couch set for his suite with his earnings. But his self-esteem is the most valuable...he is so proud of himself that he has a REAL job. This has made a huge difference in his life and he looks forward to going to work.

Most adults can understand such benefits from a job. Can they appreciate, however, what it would be like to never have the opportunity for a meaningful vocational activity? Having a job, something meaningful to do, regardless of the level, type, or hours worked, is important to self-worth and individual identity.

Transportation. Being able to get back and forth to a job without incidents along the way was viewed as an indicator of employment success by some parents. While some individuals can ride public transit unsupervised, others need support. One woman gets walked to the bus stop daily by a support worker who sees that she gets on the bus. She is on her own, however, when she gets off the bus and transfers at a busy mall. Another woman, who had to similarly transfer at a mall, got into difficulty when she was tempted by food in a grocery store. Some with PWS require a drop-off and pick-up service to eliminate such problems. Getting to and from the job in a timely manner is a requisite for all jobs. Transportation may require more support than the job itself.

Parent advocacy

Parents, used to advocacy while their son or daughter is in the school system, hope that it will no longer be necessary in the adult system. However, just as they advocated for better residential options, they may find themselves advocating for better vocational opportunities. One mother described an application process which "almost turned into a disaster" for her son:

> It was a very nasty experience for [our son] and us as parents to see how badly he was being treated and not given the respect of giving him a chance. I made a phone call to a friend well-known in our community and she immediately called a meeting with the head manager....I was at my wits

end, so it was very helpful to have this advocate. We certainly had to have a lot of patience because there was this
huge bump at the beginning that I was not expecting....but
everything is positive now!!

How to best advocate for an adult child is a question that all parents
face. In this case, third party advocacy was helpful and "the red carpet
was rolled out."

When a young lady lost her job, the father and employment
counsellor both became advocates. The mother wrote:

We have had several people who say we should let the
media know, but we are more inclined to try to sort it out,
or just say FORGET IT to the whole affair. Sometimes we
are aware of just how awfully burned out we have gotten
in our old age.

The last sentence reflects a reality of the advocacy process - it takes
time and energy. In this case there was already a responsible third
party to take up the fight. Deferring to a third party, while it may not
necessarily get the result wanted, does have the potential to relieve
some parental stress.

Retirement

A discussion of work should also consider the cessation of work, that
is to say "retirement." At what point does someone with PWS retire?
Who makes the decision to enter retirement? What happens during
retirement? What impact does retirement have on quality of life? At
this point in time there is little in the literature about senior status and
retirement. Given that most services for seniors are provided through
the disability system and not the seniors system, retirement activities
may not look much different from pre-retirement activities. For most,
individualized programming will continue to meet their needs in a
balanced manner.

In two interviews, with individuals over the age of 40, the word
"retired" was used as a descriptor. A male retired from a long-term
part-time position held in a restaurant. Physical difficulties with his
legs precluded working any longer as a bus boy. As with other adults,
physical limitations brought on by age or accident may precipitate a
change in status.

A female, with some health concerns, no longer had any expectations of seeking employment. She was not involved with any agency

and self-directed her own activities while living with her parents. Her self-declared retirement status included volunteer activities with the women's auxiliary at the local Legion. Like non-handicapped peers in retirement mode, she also enjoyed her computer, reading, hobbies, and family.

As the current population of people with PWS ages the questions about retirement will gain importance and challenge service providers to meet the needs of this stage of life.

The future?

Over the last few decades there have been many improvements in supports for people with PWS. This chapter, however, represents the one area where future focus is sorely needed. In the words of Drago (2006), "in the continuum of effective services for people with PWS, successful job placements have evolved to the status of 'the last hurdle' to be cleared. For this population, jobs remain the 'final frontier'" (p. 370).

During times of economic downturn, employment opportunities for workers with special needs are harder to find. Employers are concerned primarily with productivity; workers who cannot contribute to the business making a profit will not last. Nor will workers whose supervision requirements take a disproportionate amount of time. Minimum wage legislation and a very competitive labour market create a substantial employment hurdle for adults with PWS.

The integration of students with special needs, the participation in work experience programs, and the promotion of inclusionary practices while in high school raise expectations of students and parents about work in the future. While most individuals with PWS become resigned to what evolves as their lot in life, there are some who lament the lack of meaningful opportunity for employment.

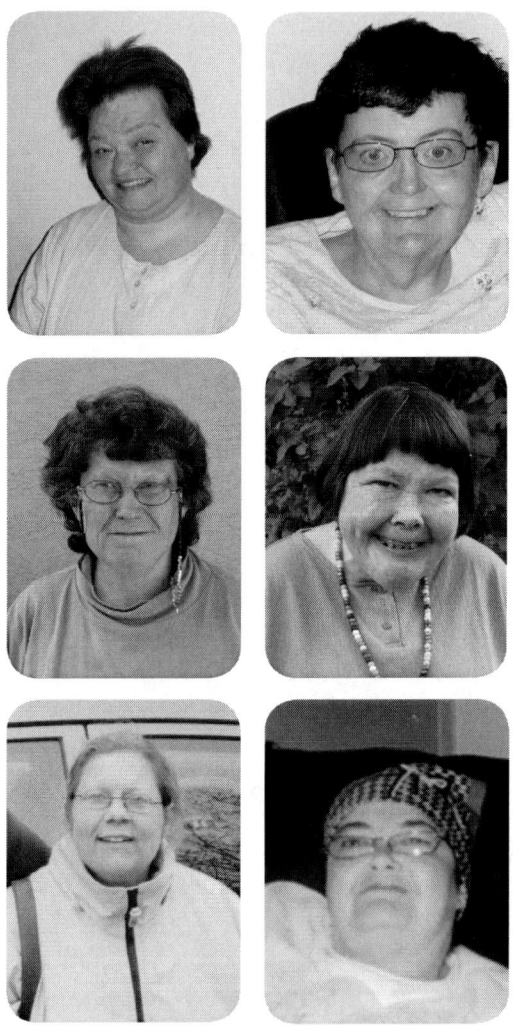

Women over 40 years of age

11

Religion and spirituality

Most models of quality of life include a spiritual dimension. In recent years there has been an increasing interest in the spirituality of people with developmental disabilities and how this contributes to their quality of life.

Children with PWS are born into families of all faiths, as well as to those who claim to be atheists or non-religious. The practice of religion is an important element in the quality of life for families of faith. These families seem to have an additional quality in their life which helps them to cope. Most often it is observed as a peace and confidence amidst the chaos associated with PWS. It begins with an easier acceptance of having a child with special needs and gives evidence as a strength of character that seldom despairs. While others may cry out, in desperation "Why me?", families of faith begin with a heart thankful for their newborn blessing. While others seek answers to assuage their fears, families with faith approach the future with confidence, believing that there is a divine purpose in everything.

"Religion" and "spirituality" are not synonymous terms. All humans are spiritual beings, but not necessarily religious. Spirituality encompasses man's search for meaning, whether it be in inter-relationships or exploration of that which is sacred. Religion, on the other hand, is the institutionalized approach for people to explore their spirituality. Most often, spirituality is expressed through the practice of religion in a group, however, it can also be a very personal and non-religious exploration as well. Each religion offers an organized belief system and social structure.

At some point most adults wrestle with spiritual questions of significance. Often the wrestling is prompted by personal or family crisis, such as the death of a loved one. Questions such as "What is the meaning of life?" or "Why are we here on earth?" are inherently spiritual. Most parents will also seek spiritual answers as to why they have been given the responsibility to parent a child with PWS.

Religion and disability

There are a number of religious and non-religious groups working in the field of disability in Canada. Historically, the great faiths have shown a concern for the dignity of persons with disabilities. While reference is made in this chapter to "church" it is done so because the majority of those with religious beliefs in this study attend a Christian church. Readers of other faiths are encouraged to substitute the words temple, synagogue, or mosque as is appropriate to their situation.

Calling out to God

When all hope seems gone, when in the depths of despair, or when otherwise reaching the end of one's tether, it is not uncommon to cry out to God for help. In times of desperation some will cry out to God, looking for answers or intervention, even when they do not profess belief in a God. One PWS mother, describing a positive turn in relationship with her husband, wrote in her diary, "Once again, thank God for that. (For someone who doesn't believe in God, I am thanking him/her a lot!!)" (Johnson, 2004, p. 41).

Others call out to God as a matter of course. With prayer as a cornerstone of their faith they turn to their Creator seeking personal peace and understanding. One mother described how her faith helped her immensely in the early months when she was struggling with her son's failure to thrive. While there were so many uncertainties her faith was constant.

Acceptance of disability

Religion offers an answer to the plaintive cry of "why me?" or "why us?" Most religions provide a framework which helps in the understanding and acceptance of disability. All children, regardless of abilities or disabilities, are seen as blessings from God. As one parent asserted, her son's life "has a purpose." She went on to explain that "he brings something important to our family" and "we have learned from him." One mother described the "unconditional love" that was given to her son. She was giving testimony to her biblical understanding of a love that expected nothing in return.

Personal strength

Belief in a God, who hears and responds to personal prayers, is a comfort to parents needing strength to cope with daily struggles. Harriet wrote:

> There were so many times when we were coping with Trevor related problems that seemed insurmountable. With prayer, solutions were found. The 'peace that passes understanding,' as the old hymn says, is very real to me, and it's been a significant factor in my life.

Parents of a young adult exhibiting some particularly difficult behaviours explained that their common faith was a basis for their marital cohesion, which was important for their parenting. Acknowledging the difficulties they were facing, the father went on to say "we take one day at a time, relying on our faith."

Future hope

Wanting a secure future for their child, parents of faith often turn to a faith-based agency for the provision of future services. Many denominations are involved in providing services for people with developmental disabilities. In most cases, the family does not have to be a member of a congregation, or even of the same faith, in order to receive services.

Knowing that their child will be cared for by others who share their faith offers hope for the future. Parents want the foundation that they provided to be continued to be available, and hope that those who give care will do so in the spirit of love and not just as a job.

For those believing in heaven, there is solace in knowing that they will be with departed relatives once again. As one parent explained to his son, "There will be a banquet in heaven." His son was encouraged, believing that he would not have PWS in heaven.

Family resilience

Resilience has to do with the ability of a family to successfully meet the challenges that they face. To what extent does the practice of a personal faith help an individual or family to cope with the challenges of raising a child with special needs? While there are no studies that address this issue with PWS families, there is an emerging literature across several disciplines which suggest that religious practices contribute to resilience. Certainly the testimonies of parents in the current study who profess a personal faith suggest that they receive a strength from their faith that helps them to cope in times of crisis. As one parent said, "as a family you feel vulnerable." Families must be resilient to withstand the daily vulnerabilities along with the periodic crises. Acknowledging the many difficulties over the years, one father stated, "It is by God's grace that we have been able to keep our son at home."

Church and disability

Identification as a member of a group within a community may be a factor in the quality of life for people with developmental disabilities. The local church can be a player in the community integration of people with disabilities (McNair and Smith, 2000). However, while the church may acknowledge the importance of including individuals with disabilities, it is often difficult to include them in a meaningful way. According to Poston and Turnbull (2004), families look for three things from their religious community:
- acceptance of their child
- spiritual and emotional support for themselves, and
- supports for their child during services so that both their child and themselves have meaningful participation in religious activities (p. 103).

As will be seen in this section, religious communities provide these, and more, in support of families with a PWS member.

Church as family

The practice of their religion is an important element in the quality of life for both parents and children. This is particularly so where an adult with PWS has maintained an active commitment to his or her faith and faith community since childhood.

Madeline was raised in a devout Catholic family. Now in her forties, she enjoys regular participation in the spiritual and social activities of her faith community. Paul, a Lutheran of about the same age, similarly participates in church activities with his parents, often volunteering to assist with setting up chairs and tables for special functions. In both of these examples going to church was a family experience which has continued into adulthood, even though the individuals no longer live in the homes of their parents.

Trevor's mother described how her son grew up with family church involvement:

> Trevor started going to church when he was a tiny baby, so he never knew a life without church affiliation. As he grew older, he participated in Sunday school and church functions of all kinds - and he particularly enjoyed those involving food, and many of the functions did involve food. As a young teen he became an altar server, which he continued the rest of his life.

She then described how the congregation was an extended family to her son:

> He was accepted as he was; he knew this and felt free to fully participate in all aspects. One good example was an annual hymn sing to which parishioners from other denominations had been invited. The cathedral was full. During the service, Trevor walked up to the priest at the front of the church wanting to help and was simply incorporated into the service. He was not robed in church garments, and not even particularly clean and tidy, but that didn't matter to him (his mother felt like crawling under the seat). He simply wanted to help, and did so. He had total confidence that he belonged, and that his assistance would be welcomed.

As with all families, many of the activities of a church centre around food. There are pot-lucks and community meals multiple times throughout the year. There are also weddings and funerals where food is common. As one father explained, in order to accommodate his son "the choir doesn't have cookies anymore."

Church as community

Adherence to a religion also provides a sense of community. The community can be a vehicle of support for the parents, providing solid values-based family-oriented activities, emotional encouragement, and at times respite. The benefits of a religious community are often in stark contrast to what some parents described as a "lack of understanding and support," or a "sense of isolation," and "loneliness." The personal peace exhibited by parents of faith is contrary to the anxiety and anger that some other parents confess.

The church is not just a place to attend on Sundays. It is a group of like-minded people who come together as an intentional community, committed to supporting one another. This is well illustrated by two parishioners, working at a church camp, who volunteered to supervise Trevor so that he would be able to have the church camp experience. Even in a supportive community, however, individuals with PWS will exhibit their uniqueness. As Trevor's mother related:

> Church affiliation also saw some of the same problems for Trevor as other areas of our community. At one point the collection plate presented too much temptation. Another time, the bread and wine disappeared inappropriately.

Churches usually have Sunday school, youth, and young adult programs. By the teen years there may be limitations to participation. One couple described how they hired a teen to accompany their daughter to youth group so that she might get the opportunity to participate. Another set of parents indicated that their son could not identify with the young adult group and chose not to attend. He was high functioning, enough to be aware of the differences. Another set of parents became leaders, choosing to work with young people with special needs in their church. They created a social environment for their daughter and others to enjoy table games, sing songs, and have Bible lessons.

The resources of the church community can also extend beyond existing programs; they can play a role in solving other difficulties, as illustrated in the following two examples. In an early parent article (King, 1988), a mother from Ontario described the experience of trying to find respite. It was not until the couple put a "help wanted" notice in their church bulletin that things turned around. She related:

> I will never forget how uncomfortable I felt the first Sunday it appeared in the bulletin. Typical of most parents of offspring with challenging needs, one rarely, if ever asks for help. Well, not only were we swallowing our pride and asking for help, we were asking in bold type in our bulletin. **HELP WANTED.**

To her surprise and delight they ended up with four new families and one single person involved in the support circle around their daughter. She concluded by saying: "church communities are a valuable resource. There are many people in our communities just waiting to be invited into your life, but the first and often biggest step is to swallow your pride and ask" (p. 32).

In Alberta, one church community has rallied to support a young man with PWS with a long-term commitment. As described in chapter 9, Joel's Friendship Society was incorporated under the Societies Act by family and friends from the church in order to raise funds to purchase a home for Joel. The home will be owned and administered by a Christian ministries foundation.

Church as service

Being a member of a church community presents opportunities for service. Two young men in different denominations serve as ushers. One of the parents reported that this role is a "source of pride," and that there are "no issues in this role."

Trevor loved to participate as an altar server, assisting the priest. He took pride in the fact that he had been there longer than any of the others. He pushed the point a bit when he started instructing the younger members, without necessarily being correct. His assistance was simply redirected. His mother remembers fondly the way in which the Minister reached out to include him in service:

> There was a particular gift that Trevor was exceptionally proud of. During the last year of his life, his weight gain made the normal servers' robes too tight on him. His mother was considering making him a robe of his own; instead, the Minister made him a gift of one of his own, which was cut differently and of an adequate size. He wore that robe with such pride.

Just like the community at large, churches may have difficulty finding ways in which people with PWS can serve. While they may not hold positions, some are given the opportunities to be helpers. For example, Paul helps by picking up hymnals, straightening pew items, and putting away library books. The church has also recognized his gift of singing. He has sung solo in church and at his brother's wedding. One mother reported that her son attends his girlfriend's church twice a month, but that "people at the church have not gone out of their way to make him feel involved." The easiest way to make someone feel involved is to give them something meaningful to do.

Faith of a person with PWS

The practice of a personal faith is an important element in the quality of life for some children and adults with PWS. Children describe their participation in church and the practice of their faith in the context of their family involvement. Even as adults, church participation often continues as a family activity. At 21, Deidre lives with her parents and says "I like to go to church. Me and mom walk there." Once an adult leaves the family home, however, the practice of a personal faith may become more complicated.

Right to practice one's faith

The question must be asked, "Do adults with PWS have the opportunity to practice their faith and attend church functions of choice?" While every individual has the right to practice a personal faith, this is sometimes problematic in a residential setting other than the family home. For example, there can be issues with staff availability for supervision and transportation to church activities. When staff share a similar faith, the likelihood of participation seems greater. They will recognize the importance and make the effort to see that the individual gets to attend church. In a faith-based agency there is a greater commitment to support participation in church activities. For example, one man under the care of a faith-based agency attends church every Sunday and a church-sponsored friendship club every Tuesday evening. Also, where family and friends provide transportation there are seldom difficulties.

In a California study exploring church attendance of adults with developmental disabilities, the authors found that while the majority of the respondents lived in group homes, 48 percent attended church with a family member (McNair and Smith, 2000). In the present study, several adults with PWS, living outside of the family home, similarly attended church with a family member. One parent reported that her son didn't get to go to church because the caregivers didn't go themselves.

The guardian of one woman in the present study admitted that she hadn't considered the possibility of her sister participating in church activities as she herself did not. It was not that she was against participation in religion, rather the question had never come up before. She did, however, indicate that she would include the question in the next team meeting. Another woman, under the care of a faith-based agency, chose not to have church involvement. This was not an issue with the agency, which emphasized that transportation would be provided if she chose to participate. In the case of a young man under the care of his personal Friendship Society, formed from within his church community, it is a requirement for staff to accompany him to church and mid-week activities if they are on shift.

Meaningfulness of faith

A study examining the spiritual dimensions of Bar/Bat Mitsvah ceremonies for Jewish children with developmental disabilities showed that children can enjoy and benefit from religious education and rituals shared by others in their society (Vogel & Reiter, 2003). The authors asserted that overwhelming needs in other areas of a child's life often prevent participation in religious education and life-cycle rituals. Although this study dealt specifically with Jewish religious education and a Jewish rite of passage, the authors pointed out that the same implications exist for youngsters of all backgrounds.

As a young adult, John said that he wanted to be a preacher. He discussed his faith extensively on first meeting the writer. He sang several contemporary Christian songs a'capella, including one that he had written himself. He had done well in school academically, passing some regular grade 12 courses. As an adult he had begun a correspondence course in religion. He cried when talking about handicapped youth and faith. His faith was very important to him.

One couple described their son as having a "strong, simple faith." He knew what he believed and incorporated his understanding into his daily life. Another father described how his son prayed for forgiveness after consuming candies illicitly. He felt badly that he had done something wrong and felt better after confessing and asking for forgiveness.

For another young man, the meaningfulness of his faith is embodied in relationships. He likes it when the pastor takes him out for coffee, and he knows he can get counselling help if he needs it. It was the Pastor to whom he revealed details of an event that had traumatized him many years earlier, and which lived in constant memory.

For Joel, church is one of the most important things in his life. In addition to his faith practice, "he is very social and gets invited out a lot," says his father. Joel says, "Sunday is the best day of the week."

As mentioned at the beginning of this chapter, there are some who may be spiritual, but may not subscribe to a religion. One mother described her daughter's lifelong spirituality, acknowledging that "we didn't teach it." She said, "She always has a sense of what God wants". The strong sense of right and wrong is an important part of her life.

The understanding of right and wrong is implicit in all faiths. Assurance that one is doing what God wants can provide a personal strength and inner peace. In times of difficulty a faith community can provide an understanding, forgiving, and consistent context for dealing with problems. The personal and family support from within a faith community enhances the quality of life of those with PWS, and their parents.

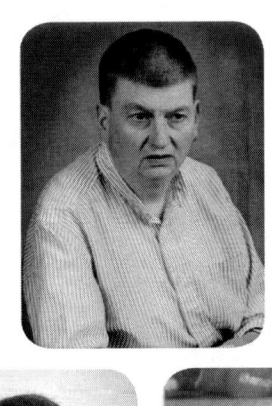

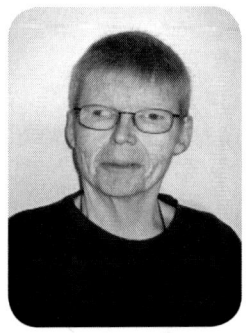
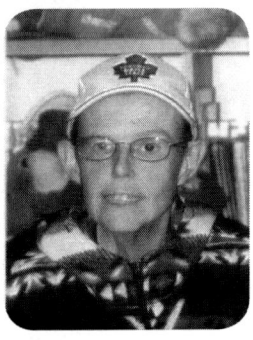

Men over 40 years of age

12

Government and
agency services

Provincial ministries of social services provide a philosophical
and regulatory framework for the provision of services to people
with disabilities. In Canada, these services have been influenced by
the concepts of normalization and community living. Current best
practice is guided by principles such as: protection of individual rights,
involvement of families, multi-disciplinary teaming, individualized
planning, empowerment of choice making, and meaningful community
inclusion and participation. Government and agencies are committed
to working respectfully, in an open and timely manner. Each will have
articulated operational principles which provide a bridge between their
mission statement and day-to-day activities. This chapter looks at the
experiences of PWS families with government and agency services
working within such frameworks.

Government services

As social services are a provincial responsibility, there may be
differences in eligibility requirements and resources available across
provinces to families with a PWS member.

Eligibility for child services

Establishing eligibility for services for children is easier than for adults.
Today, early identification leads to multi-disciplinary team involvement
and immediate services for infants. By the time a child reaches school

age, there is already a well-documented file history that can be used to justify eligibility for educational supports. Sometimes, however, parents must be encouraged to take advantage of available supports at a younger age. For example, some parents resist the need for formal respite, relying instead on the informal support of family and friends. From a government perspective, however, there is not a documented need as the family is coping just fine. If a real need does arise, there is no established history or paper trail. It is important to be aware of available services and to establish eligibility before a crisis presents itself.

Eligibility for adult services

Determining eligibility for adult services is not as easy as for children. Generally, eligibility requires assessment by appropriate professionals (e.g., medical specialists, registered or certified psychologists) and application. Usually there is sufficient formal assessment data on file if the school has been working in transition with government social services agencies. Eligibility for funding support is determined by the degree of individual need and not by diagnostic label. A label of PWS does not guarantee services, as some families have found out.

Eligibility criteria vary by province, although the intent is similar. For example, to be eligible in Alberta under the Persons with Developmental Disabilities Program (PDD) requires one to: be 18 years of age or older, have significantly below average intellectual capacity with onset prior to age 18, and have related limitations in adaptive skills (deficits in two or more of the following areas: communication, home living, community use, health and safety, self-care, social skills, self direction, functional academics, work, and leisure) (PDD, 2007). To be eligible under Community Living BC (CLBC, 2006) the person must have: a developmental disability, meaning significantly impaired intellectual functioning that manifests before the age of 18 and that exists concurrently with impaired adaptive functioning. A registered or certified psychologist must apply the diagnostic criteria as specified in the *DSM-IV* (Diagnostic and Statistical Manual of Mental Disorders, Revision IV). Most recently the government introduced an IQ below 70 as part of the definition of developmental disability.

Even after having received infant, child, and adolescent services, a family may be left without needed adult supports because the individual does not meet eligibility requirements. A high functioning young man in B.C., having an IQ of 90, for example, did not qualify for adult services after leaving high school. There was no transition planning. He was simply on his own like any other graduate. In reality, his parents were left to manage his future with no support. This is an example of someone with very special needs falling through the cracks. Apart from leisure activities with Special Olympics, he has had few successes to date. He has been re-assessed and has made the rounds of employment assistance programs, to no avail. He has no work and no prospects of being able to move into a more independent lifestyle unless something changes. Meanwhile, his mother, who recently retired, now finds herself preoccupied with the daily management of her son at an age when she thought that he would be leaving home and going to work, and when she and her husband could be enjoying a more relaxed lifestyle.

It should be noted that eligibility does not necessarily mean service. Given the economics of the day there may be waiting lists or a lack of appropriate services. This is a very important point for parents to consider, particularly in the two-year period before their child leaves the secondary school system. It is best to be working in transition with the appropriate social services agencies – otherwise there may be no services when they are needed. It is not just at the stage of school leaving that waiting lists occur. If moving from one community to another a similar situation can happen. In the case of a woman in her early thirties who moved to the Victoria area with her family, it took two years before she was able to get into a workshop program.

Individualized service dollars

In some jurisdictions, individualized funding offers people with developmental disabilities, and/or families/guardians, or support circles, the opportunity to directly manage the supports and services that an individual with PWS requires. In so doing, they assume full responsibility for staffing and programming as well as administration of regulatory requirements. In B.C., Vela Microboards can be formed to support individuals; in Manitoba a similar concept is run under a program called In Company of Friends; in Alberta it is known as Family Managed Supports.

In describing her son's experience with the In Company of Friends program, Gloria wrote:

> At 24 our son is living in the home of his choosing.... with the support of a network of his choice, he directs his own program, hires his own staff and is involved in all decisions. He is calm and proud.

She described his situation as "an enhanced quality of life" and illustrated by saying that "he doesn't HAVE to wait until 9 a.m. to go for coffee because that is what the log says." At the same time this model affects the parents' quality of life. While still involved in support, Gloria says "at least the time that would have been spent meeting with an agency and spinning wheels is now spent progressively." And she adds, "there never has to be a negative comment about my son at any meeting because the program is focussed on him and how to support him."

Along with the right to control programs and services, this approach necessarily means taking on significant responsibility and inherent problems. In times of low unemployment, for example, it can be hard to find and retain staff and individuals not used to private enterprise may have difficulty with the scope of requirements as an employer.

Some parents chose individualized funding because of their unhappiness with the traditional approach where agencies are contracted to provide services to groups of people with disabilities. Unfortunately, parent stories have a common theme - the squeaky wheel gets the oil! In most instances, parents received individualized funding because they were actively advocating for a better option for their child.

Parents as case managers

Individualized service dollars allow parents to remain integrally involved, often in the role of case manager. This satisfies some parents, knowing that they retain some influence over what is happening to their child. When parents function as case managers they are usually providing additional supports beyond what would be provided by an agency worker or social worker acting in the same capacity. For example, they may be personally helping with menu planning and shopping, monitoring independent living, transporting and accompanying to leisure and recreation activities, and assisting with job search and applications. In some cases, they would prefer to have others to do some of these tasks. The problem is finding the personnel, then training and supervising them. Sometimes it is just easier to do things oneself.

When an individual with PWS is not eligible for services, parents *must* act as case managers. It is difficult to abdicate this responsibility when there is no one else to take the role. Parents of adults who do not meet the eligibility criteria for services to people with disabilities are at risk for burn-out from an excessive load of caring and advocacy.

There may be no prospect for help until another ministry of government becomes involved, for example, the mental health or judicial systems. If the individual becomes a danger to self or others, or commits a crime, there may be an avenue for services. For parents thrust into this role, there is great frustration and little quality of life.

A mother, struggling with single parenting, working at two jobs, and needing to find residential accommodation and a day program for her 25-year-old son, in a market where there were waiting lists, angrily explained that the only other option was to give up her involvement in her son's life and relinquish his care to the province. Refusing to make this decision she has struggled on as case manager, giving up one of her jobs and relying on the help of friends and family. She has been forced into a situation where she has accepted a diminished quality of life for herself in order to try to ensure a better quality of life for her son.

Lack of resources

Being eligible for service does not necessarily mean that service will be provided. After five months, the mother described in the previous paragraph, was still unable to find an agency to provide residential care or a day program for her son.

One Calgary mother explained that her daughter had no day program since her worker had quit four months earlier. In the same city, one of the older participants in this study was featured in the newspaper for the same reason (Cryderman, 2008). After a support worker had left to work at a national chain supermaket for $1.50 more per hour, the agency was unable to find a suitable replacement. The sister and brother-in-law of the woman with PWS, who were both working full-time, were left to provide support to her independent living situation.

In some communities there is also a lack of program options. While most jurisdictions would like to have a range of options this may not always be possible. What is needed in the eyes of the parents may not actually exist. As suggested earlier, this encourages some parents to pursue the individualized funding option so that they can create what is needed. Sometimes parents need to band together in order to create the options. The establishment of PWS-specific group homes, for example, has only come about as a result of parent advocacy.

Administrative services

Social workers are the front-line bureaucratic representatives in working with families. Parents have strong emotions attached to social worker responsiveness to their needs. Kinash (2007c) identified social workers amongst human service workers, "persons who are paid to procure supports to minors and adults with PWS." Like some others within this sector, they were identified as "perpetrators of disabling attitudes." To be fair, social workers have been both criticized and praised.

There may also be a question of competence. As one B.C. mother put it, "things were fine up until graduation." Thereafter, dealing with adult services, she had frustrations with the government ministry staff. She related that a social worker telephoned to let her know that the respite worker had quit and a meeting was set for two weeks hence to discuss future service. When she arrived for the meeting she found that the social worker had been transferred out of town and that nobody was available to meet with her or to answer questions. When she asked for a copy of a letter from her daughter's file it could not be found. Her daughter was living at home at the time and the mother was getting one night of respite per month. Weeks later, without request, her daughter was offered a full-time residential placement. After the mother went through the adjustment to the idea with her daughter, a social worker realized that the young lady wasn't even on the waiting list and therefore was not eligible for the placement. It took another eight months before eligibility was established for the vacant bed.

Another B.C. mother explained how she successfully obtained a Declaration of Incompetence for her son and had Power of Attorney over his finances. Cheques from the Ministry of Children and Family (MC&F) were then made out to her. However, her son twice went to the MC&F office and convinced staff to give him the monthly cheques, which he then cashed at the bank, despite the fact that they were made out in his mother's name.

On the other hand, a couple from Manitoba could not provide enough praise for their social worker. She "moved heaven and earth for us," they said. They described her as "having a heart that understands." They related that she went to the OPWSA conference "on her own nickel." And when she was transferred from adult to child services she retained their daughter's adult file in order to continue service. They recognized that "she is exceptional," while others were just "a revolving door."

Promotion of independence

One important criticism, voiced with frustration, and in some cases with anger, must be recognized. While the principle of independence is generally accepted for people with disabilities, parents of adults with

PWS may feel betrayed by social services ministries which promote independence without any seeming concern for the welfare of the individual with PWS. One B.C. mother of a young woman who died in her own apartment at age 24, said categorically "if Social Services had never been involved she would have been far better off." After a period of hospitalization of the daughter, the parents had been asked if they would take her home with them, despite the fact that she had been living independently in the community with some supports prior to her hospital stay. The issue of rights, reinforced by social workers, had previously created conflicts in the parents' home. For example, while the parents maintained a "non-smoking" home, their daughter smoked and would not respect the parents' wishes for her to not smoke indoors. So smoking, which occurred multiple times daily, became a point of contention leading to conflict. Their daughter was high functioning, understood her rights and seemed to have the support of the social workers.

Another mother in the same province was angered that her 27-year-old daughter, who was in a stable and effective supported living environment, received a letter from the social services ministry promoting independent living. The mother felt it was highly inappropriate. As she stated, her daughter "would agree to anything" and "independent living is not an option."

Institutional services

While governments no longer operate large institutions for people with mental handicaps, they do still operate provincial institutions for other purposes, for example: youth custody centres, forensic assessment centres, and jails. On occasion individuals with PWS end up in these facilities. Here the complaints are usually associated with very strong emotion. One father sadly described how his daughter entered a juvenile institution at 113 pounds and left four years later at exactly double the weight. In another province, two adults were discharged from provincial institutions, after years of residency, both with morbid obesity.

The story of Trevor, the young man who went into an institution voluntarily for a forensic assessment is disturbing. The food restrictions were removed because of "his rights," and medications were removed and denied when requested in order to better assess him. He suffered humiliation, excessive weight gain, and shortly after his discharge he died. With multi-disciplinary professional involvements in institutional care, why should this happen?   The assumption that the professionals know what they are doing with PWS can be faulty. Even with health specialists such as nurses, doctors, and dieticians/ nutritionists, individuals with PWS can fall through the cracks. Parents must be vigilant when institutions are involved.

From the stories told, there are two important issues: social services versus judicial responsibility, and client rights versus responsibility to care. Should persons with developmental disabilities be incarcerated? Or should their "crimes" be dealt with through social services? And if they are admitted to a government facility, should individual rights outweigh the responsibility to care?   As Trevor's mother laments, an institution would not give alcohol to an alcoholic or deny insulin to someone with diabetes, so why would it give unlimited food to someone with PWS or deny prescribed medications?

Cooperation between parents and government services

Parents have the expectation that government services will support them in their parenting role. Unfortunately, not all employees are familiar with PWS. In their ignorance, they may make decisions that make things worse, much to the annoyance of the parents. For example, the parents of a runaway complained that police gave their son squares and chocolate milk while in their custody.   And one mother told the story of being called when her 14-year-old son was apprehended for shoplifting, expressing disappointment in what she felt was a lack of cooperation with those in authority:

> I received a call at work telling me that my son was being taken to the police station, and asking me to come and get him right away. My reaction was that a period of uncertainty at the police station would be good for him. I indicated this to the police representative and said I would come for him a little later. They told me that if I didn't come immediately they would take him to Social Services. I provided the name of his social worker (who was very familiar with the situation and my concerns), and suggested they might like to call him directly. I expected he would explain to the police, on a professional level, that a period in the station might be of some benefit. Instead the police, never took our son to the police station at all – but took him to Social Services immediately in the police car (an interesting ride for him

as social connotations weren't a factor), took him directly to the worker (who was in a meeting and interrupted). The worker had a meeting with him (dropping whatever was on his agenda) and then drove him back to school (where he was supposed to be in the first place). This appeared to be quite a pleasant experience for our son!

In this case the mother wanted her son to learn a lesson as a consequence of shoplifting. The actions of the police, however, did not support the parent's expectations. The teachable moment seemed to transform into a pleasant social outing.

What is viewed as a lack of cooperation may, in some cases, be adherence to inflexible policies and procedures. For example, the inability to obtain funding for services that parents feel they need, but for which there is not a sufficient paper trail. Parents may see this as a lack of cooperation, while the social worker feels bound to follow established policy and process. Thus bureaucratic procedures may contribute to unmet expectations.

Looking for efficiencies

Government is always looking for efficiencies, ways to provide services for less money. To service recipients this often looks like budget cutting. Parents, care providers, and agencies all complain about the lack of dollars available to do the job that is necessary. Everybody would like more money.

Despite a philosophical commitment to individualized programming, the reality is that it is more expensive to deliver. Thus, while parents argue for the need for one-on-one support of an educational assistant, the system will want to look at grouping options. Optimal individual programming may be sacrificed for the collective needs of everyone. Residential care may be more economically provided when accommodation is shared. One of the difficulties with employment opportunities has to do with the lack of individual support workers to accompany a worker on the job. In a workshop setting, on the other hand, one support worker can assist several workers.

After graduation from high school some young adults have been unable to get into appropriate programs. Waiting lists are a reality in adult services in some areas. As a consequence parents must take the initiative to provide programming, sometimes at considerable hardship to themselves. Parents have complained about having a young adult at home for a year or two while waiting for a program placement. Their frustration may not be the imposition on their personal quality of life so much as it is witnessing the demoralization of the young adult.

As governments look for efficiencies any proposals that show potential cost-savings will likely be entertained favourably. The problem is the lack of flexibility in the annual budget or the lead time necessary to get a proposal into the next budget. Parents need to understand the annual budget cycle when advocating for new programs and services.

A PWS question

Adults with PWS share many of the the concerns and frustrations of their parents in working with government services. Shortly before his death at age 42, John wrote "If the government has money to fund crisis situations why can they not prevent situations from becoming a crisis?" Recognizing his own needs, he went on to say "I need full support NOW before I get into a crisis situation."

Agency services

Families living in larger centres are likely to have more choices when seeking an agency to provide services. Those in smaller, more rural areas may have no choices. Parents are encouraged to do their homework before making a commitment with an agency. Not all agencies are equal. There are major considerations, for example: for-profit versus not-for-profit, faith versus non-faith-based, experienced versus inexperienced, and union versus non-union.

For-profit versus not-for-profit agencies

Agencies may be for-profit, that is to say an entrepreneurial endeavour where there is a profit motive for the owner, or they may be not-for-profit, that is to say an organization with registered charitable status. Either may receive government funds for the provision of services.

One of the drawbacks with for-profit agencies or private contractors is the matter of profit margin. These agencies may be reluctant to take on an individual with high supervision needs, recognizing that it may be more difficult to make a profit. A not-for-profit agency, on the other hand, is less likely to have this concern.

Families have been left to find alternatives when an agency has opted to discontinue service. In two residential examples, the young adults with PWS were considered to be too difficult to handle. In one case there was an escalating history of difficulties, in the other there was an almost immediate awareness of the care level being too difficult.

Another area of concern with for-profit agencies and private contractors has to do with continuity of service. Particularly when the agency is operated by an individual or a couple, there is a concern for the longevity of service. Will the operators still be in business five years from now? Do they have a long-standing commitment to this field of service, or will they change occupations when something more lucrative arises? The non-profit organization, on the other hand, is run by a board of directors. As any one member retires or otherwise discontinues service, he or she will be replaced, thus ensuring continuity of the organization. The question of continuity is particularly important to aging parents as they try to plan for their child's needs after their own passing.

Faith versus non-faith-based agencies

There is a long history of faith-based agencies providing social services in Canada. Some of the organizations are national in scope, others are regional, provincial, or even local.

As with secular agencies, faith-based agencies can receive government funding to provide services. Because they have a faith constituency which is vitally concerned about the provision of services, they also benefit from a level of philanthropic support which may or may not be available to the other agencies. Services are understood as a "ministry" provided to those in need. One does not usually have to be of the same faith in order to receive service. Staff, however, are expected to respect the common statement of faith of the agency.

Within many communities there are faith-based and secular agencies, offering families a choice. The Canadian Association for Community Living (CACL) operates 400 local associations across the country for the benefit of people with intellectual disabilities (CACL, 2008). The Association for Community Living (ACL) is an example of a non-faith-based agency. A number of PWS families included in this book are receiving services from their local ACL. Within each province there are also families receiving services from faith-based agencies, most of which operate on a local or regional level.

Secular and faith-based organizations were founded by people with similar concerns for the provision of services for children or adults with developmental handicaps. What is there to choose between the two? People of faith are more likely to choose a faith-based agency because they share a like-mindedness. However, the same thing can be said of those choosing a secular organization. On the other hand, some families without religious commitment may choose a faith-based agency because of what they believe is a stronger values-based service and commitment of staff.

Experience with PWS

While a knowledge of, and experience with, PWS is desirable, it is not always possible. Larger agencies, with regional, provincial, or national scope, are more likely to have resource people within their organization with experience with PWS. At times, however, parents opt to go with an individual service provider because of direct experience with PWS, and in some cases specifically with their child. For example, several families have hired their child's educational assistant or day program worker to provide respite care. They know the character of the individual and have confidence in the quality of the service and relationship.

On the other hand, there are individuals and agencies lacking in any direct knowledge of, or experience with PWS, who immediately go the extra mile in order to acquire the needed knowledge. By attending workshops, reading the literature, visiting and observing, or consulting with experts, they show their willingness to learn.

Union versus non-union workforce

Unions exist for the protection of their membership. Collective agreements spell out the rights of workers and management, including the ways in which workers change assignments or positions. Generally, seniority is the governing factor, assuming that workers meet the minimum qualifications for the position.

Union workers generally earn better salaries than non-union workers. Union establishments get more applicants and it follows that they may have more choice of qualified workers. The high turn-over of staff in the human services field in largely non-union workplaces is often because workers are attracted to higher paying positions within union environments. From the parents' perspective, employment stability is appreciated, provided that the worker is a good match. However, if the worker is not a good match, there may be difficulties in a union workplace as the worker will have rights within a collective agreement. For example, it may be difficult to have a worker take a different assignment or to lobby for a preferred worker who doesn't have enough seniority.

Nowhere have union issues been more contentious than in the public education system in B.C. Parents have had to contend with multiple educational assistants assigned during the course of a year, changes of assistants without consultation with parents, and a lack of continuity of assistants from year to year. With the advocacy of parents, however, some districts have been successful in negotiating concessions which recognize the importance of stability and continuity for the child. As a result, some EAs have been able to retain the same assignment with their student for as long as five or six years.

While unions also operate within residential and day program services in some areas, there were no reports of parental advocacy and union concessions in adult services.

Funding issues

Twenty years ago, parents criticized a system which would pay caregivers a liveable wage to provide a home and supervision for a young adult with PWS and yet pay parents little or nothing to provide the same level of care in the family home. Today, there are more options for residential placements and systems have more flexibility to meet individual circumstances.

Agencies receive all, or almost all, of their funding from government. With an economy which is "labour hungry," agencies will have difficulty recruiting and retaining staff. An article in the *Calgary Herald* (Cryderman, 2008) describes how some agencies are being pressured into signing one-year government contracts, locking themselves into status quo funding that will result in service cuts because they won't be able to retain staff. Social services, like education and health, have escalating costs and consume a large share of the provincial budgets.

Some PWS parents have complained about a lack of funding; others appear to be satisfied. It is apparent that two individuals with comparable needs may get different levels of funding depending on a variety of factors (e.g., province of residence, regional budget, degree of advocacy, experience level of the advocate). Experienced caregivers, for example, know how to make the best case for the highest level of funding support. By emphasizing the chronic nature and severity of challenges to providing care, they hope to get a better rate. Parents and guardians need to remain vigilant to ensure that caregivers are not perpetuating dependency or minimizing opportunities for client growth.

It may take a while for parents and new care providers to learn how to get fair and equitable treatment from the system. Parents recommend networking with others in similar circumstances and seeking guidance from those with more experience in order to learn the intricacies of funding.

Client rights versus food controls

Parents are usually quite adamant about the need for food access controls. Some agencies, however, will not agree to any restrictive food procedures, arguing that clients have a right to food access which cannot be denied. Here they demonstrate little understanding of current best practices with PWS, and their own unwillingness to accept the challenge of working with the syndrome. The PWSA-USA (2004) produced a helpful document titled *Adults with Prader-Willi Syndrome and Decisions Regarding Least Restrictive Environments and the Right to Eat.* Is strict dietary management too restrictive and a denial of rights? Is restricting the access to money, to limit the ability to buy food, a violation of personal rights of adults with PWS? The document takes the position that "failure to restrict food access is tantamount to medical neglect." It concludes by saying:

> restricting food is not an abrogation of rights; it is the standard of care for a person with Prader-Willi syndrome. Failure to restrict food and allowing a person to eat themselves to death is, in fact, a removal of 'rights' to a protected environment.

Parents have even complained that nutritionists/dieticians, the professionals expected to be most knowledgeable, have insisted on a diet with too many calories and have been unwilling to reduce the caloric intake to the levels recommended in PWS literature.

Restrictive procedures

When a client's behaviour becomes a threat to self or others, or threatens damage to the property of others, intervention is required. It is always expected that positive behaviour supports will be used to address the behaviours before restrictive procedures are employed. Two of the most common procedures are the use of time-out and physical restraint. Agencies are required to have policies in place for the application of restrictive procedures in order to prevent abusive situations. When considering an agency, parents should always request a copy of the policies.

In some cases the family may recommend the use of a procedure, and get a poor reception from the agency. For example, while a family might send a teen to his bedroom for a period of time-out with the understanding that he can return when he has calmed down, an agency will be required to closely monitor a time-out situation, requiring the availability of a staff person. For one woman, a chronic skin picker, family recommended the use of gloves and duct tape. This was initially rejected by the agency as too restrictive, but in the absence of successful alternatives it was eventually accepted as a reasonable intervention.

In another situation, a woman with PWS was subjected to video monitoring in the hallways of her building and to inspection of her apartment for food. These procedures were not considered restrictive or invasive as they were employed for her safety and protection, and utilized with her consent.

From the viewpoint of the person with PWS, however, supervision can be an invasion of their personal space and be too restrictive. Finding the balance between a controlling presence and an unobtrusive presence can be difficult. Over-restrictiveness might occur, for example, as a result of: personality factors, previous experience, inexperience, lack of knowledge, competing job tasks, health or fatigue level, or simply ease and convenience. While restrictions are necessary, they must always be balanced against client rights.

Staffing issues

Having knowledgeable and reliable staff is important to PWS parents. Staffing seems to be more stable in unionized environments where staff receive better wages and benefits.

Staffing crises. During fieldwork for the present study there was a crisis in human services work in Alberta. With a robust economy workers could earn more at fast food outlets than in community support worker roles for which they had college training. Thus agencies were having difficulty attracting and retaining qualified staff. The Alberta provincial average turnover rate in the community disability services sector was more than 40 per cent for 2005 (ACDS, 2006). Ironically, while an economic boom increases the quality of life of most, it may negatively impact services for people with disabilities.

When agencies have difficulty recruiting staff the only options are to take inexperienced or under-qualified staff. This was evident in a group home in Alberta where immigrant staff, with questionable

English language skills and knowledge of human services practice, were hired to work. A resident with PWS was evicted from the home and dismissed from the agency because of difficulties with his management. Was this decision a by-product of Alberta's staffing crisis in the human services field? A similar report was received from Winnipeg. An agency using unqualified staff with poor English language skills similarly terminated services to a woman with PWS. In both cases, the agencies were private, for-profit agencies.

Staff training. Given a lack of experience with, and knowledge of, PWS, it is incumbent on agencies to provide staff in-service training. In the first example above, it was explained that reading material on PWS was available for staff to read. The question remains, did the staff have sufficient English language skills to read and understand the material, or did they even try? On the positive side, the agency did employ a short period of job shadowing and shift overlap, both appropriate practices to improve communication and the sharing of staff knowledge.

Other agencies, including school districts, have encouraged and paid for staff attendance at regional PWS conferences. In B.C., an annual conference for para-educators has on occasion provided workshops specifically focussing on PWS in the classroom, attracting EAs from several districts. One school district even sent support staff to the PWSA-USA national conference when it was held in a neighbouring state.

Safety of staff. All workers have a right to safety in their work environment in Canada. The safety of staff is an important consideration for any agency or employer. Adults with PWS have been suspended from day programs (e.g., for striking or biting program staff) and charged with assault in residential programs. In five cases described to the writer, forced compliance to staff expectations seemed to precipitate each of the incidents. That is to say that the "assault" and violence only occurred as a reaction to the manner in which the staff were doing their job. One is left to wonder whether these incidents would have happened with more experienced and knowledgeable staff. Given that behavioural issues can be expected in working with the PWS population and that workers in the human service field are trained in behavioural interventions, should these incidents really have been treated as issues of worker safety? It is noteworthy that there were no reports of assault toward peers in any residential or day program setting.

Competence. Having syndrome-specific knowledge is only one aspect of competence. Most critical is the application of the knowledge. A good example is the ability to follow the individualized service plan. One mother in Manitoba raised the issue of competence when a staff person failed to follow the plan determined by the multi-disciplinary team that supported her son. While funded for a one-to-one worker for the day program, the worker failed to follow through with the objective to swim three times per week. According to the physiotherapist this activity was important for physical rehabilitation from an injury. It was reported that the young man "chose" not to participate in this activity. Is this a case of client rights or staff incompetence? From the mother's perspective, the requirements to protect her son's health should have taken precedence over his right of choice.

In another example, residential night staff would not wake a young man in order for him to go to the washroom during the night. As a result, he regularly wet the bed and had a body rash. Were the staff working in the best interest of the young man or themselves? Could they be considered incompetent or negligent? In another province, a young man with PWS and diabetes was not given his injection by a group home respite worker as required. Was the worker not competent to give the injection or incompetent at following directions?

While education and training do not guarantee competence, they are likely the best insurance against incompetence. Programs exist in all provinces for the training of workers in the human services sector. It is not unreasonable to query where staff were trained and what experience they have had with PWS.

Age of staff. In a magazine interview (Young, 1993), Margaret Willott raised a perspective that others have shared as well. She began by saying that she couldn't complain about the services that her daughter had been receiving, but then went on to say that "any problems that we might have had have been due to workers not understanding the syndrome." She then explained that her daughter was 33 years old and had a much younger worker:

So when you get a young 22 year old coming and saying, 'you can't do that. You're not allowed to do that,' to a 33 year old, it just doesn't work. [She] is handicapped but she's not all that badly mentally handicapped and she's quite capable of speaking for herself. She won't stand for that; she gets into a panic. If the worker pushes at that stage she's likely to fly off the handle. So, the workers should be mature enough to know that they don't lose anything by stepping back a bit. Young or inexperienced workers who think that they have all the answers and can teach others how to behave may cause a problem.

As the population of people with PWS ages, it is likely that this scenario will be repeated. In another case, an older worker acknowledged that she was a "mother figure" in the absence of the birth mother's involvement. Here the age difference was a positive factor.

Agency – parent relations

From an agency perspective, the adult with the disability is clearly the client. Even though parents of adults with disabilities may not have any legal rights with respect to control over their child's life, they usually feel a parental need for continued involvement after a move out of the family home is made. One mother complained that group home staff told her that she was not to visit without permission. While this decision may have been made to best facilitate the son's adjustment to the new living situation, it hurt the mother who had been so intimately involved with his life previously. It came across as though it was directed at her personally. In another province a mother reported that she had been asked not to visit her son for a month after he had moved into a new living situation, but she clearly understood that it was in order to help him get settled.

In one situation, a woman with PWS did not enjoy certain activities in her day program. The mother, while aware of this concern, did nothing about it. When questioned, she said that she did not want to cause repercussions. She had enough uncertainties about the agency that she did not feel comfortable advocating for her daughter.

Parents have reported good relationships with agency workers, and not-so-good relationships. In many cases there is respect; in some cases, however, there is little or no respect. After a high school experience where parents have been integral members of the team, they generally have an expectation of a similar level of involvement with adult programs. To the degree that parents come across as being positive and supportive, they may continue to be consulted. If, on the other hand, they come across in an aggressive or oppositional manner they will likely receive little consideration. Sometimes parents must acquire a new set of skills to be able to work successfully with adult agency staff.

Independence goals

Many parents balk at the idea of independence goals in an individualized education or program plan. They argue that their son or daughter will always require supervision and they cannot foresee times of independent function. They must understand, however, that agencies follow government policies which empower individuals with developmental disabilities to be more independent. They must also recognize that agencies will resist the one-on-one staffing that is required to provide the level of supervision that they want for their child. They should also consider the possibility that their own attitude of protection may at times place limitations on their child's development.

It is hoped that there are sufficient examples in this book to underscore the range and variability within PWS. There are many individuals with PWS who are able to function with little or no supervision for at least part of their day. While fully independent living may not be realistic, participation in work or leisure activities without one-on-one supervision may be possible for some. There are examples of individuals who can ride public transportation, attend community events, and function socially with friends without supervision. It is not unreasonable, from an agency perspective, to develop goals that would support such independence. From the point of view of the individual with PWS, such goals would add to their quality of life.

PWS voice

One of the messages from many adults with PWS is that they want to be heard. They want others to listen to them. They see themselves as adults, and have increasing awareness of their rights. They want to be involved in personal decision making. While they are generally tolerant of the degree of supervision in their lives, they become rebellious when others make all of the decisions for them. They accept that supervision is required for food access control; this is part of living with PWS. They object, however, when they are not allowed to make decisions about their daily life, when all choice making is taken away. While government and agency services are supposed to empower individuals in the control of their own lives, many personal stories suggest that this is difficult to translate into practice.

Hearing the PWS voice

Higher functioning adults with PWS are capable of engaging in self-advocacy. They make two important points:

- I am an adult (therefore treat me as an adult, not as a child).

• I have rights (therefore allow me to make my own decisions). Certainly social services guidelines respect these positions. Sometimes there are difficulties, however, in day-to-day interactions. Transition meetings for children moving to adult services may be difficult, for example, when parents strongly expect their own voice to be heard. Social workers who have been used to listening to the parents must exercise skill to enable the young adult's voice to emerge.

When a new worker is introduced to a family assumptions can be made which are disrespectful to the individual with PWS. For example, appearance or behaviour might lead the worker to believe that the individual is not able to express wishes and opinions, resulting in worker-parent dialogue to the exclusion of the person with PWS. Parents, concerned that their own views will be heard, may not be good advocates for their child with PWS at this time.

Some adults with PWS are sensitive to the issue of PWS voice, and see it as a matter of respect. One woman complained that her voice was ignored because she was short. She felt that she was treated like a child. This complaint has been echoed by others, most often in response to treatment in public settings, when employees such as receptionists and sales clerks speak to a taller companion, regardless of age, rather than speaking directly to the adult with PWS. When this happens with professionals and workers who should know better, it is most irksome to the person with PWS. Government services and agency personnel working with people with disabilities should always be sensitive to the matter of client voice.

Informed choice

Agency staff are expected to operate on the basis of "informed choice," that is to say that the individual must understand the options available to them and the implications of a choice. This may mean that a staff member may need to take extraordinary time in order to support choice making. Given a shortage of staffing hours, changing staff schedules, and the immediacy of competing tasks, it may be difficult for staff to take the time to get to know an individual's decision making capabilities. Because decision making can be a slow process for some individuals, staff may avoid engaging in decision making situations. Hearing and respecting PWS voice can be time consuming.

Choice and risk

In his autobiography, John (James, 2010) stated "I want to have

CHOICE to decide what I want in my life" (p. 93). By capitalizing "choice" he placed extra emphasis on this point. But how does an agency balance the right to make choices, with inherent risks, and the need for protection? Certainly parents expect that an agency, regardless of the type of service provided, will always provide quality care. Often there is an expectation that staff will function in a pseudo-parental role, providing structure and even making decisions for the individual when necessary (i.e., perpetuation of paternalism). But this is in conflict with prevailing philosophies about empowering individuals through personal choice making.

To protect themselves, agencies will provide protocols which address the concerns around risk and safety. The collective wisdom of a multi-disciplinary team will have input into establishing the protocols. As with parents, agency staff will always wrestle with the tension between supporting choice making, which may involve risk, and providing essential protections. One young man was told that he could not ride public transit into town on his own to trade some CDs. While he was capable of reading bus schedules and understood money, he was restricted to the group home because there wasn't an available staff person to accompany him. In this situation, they could not risk letting him go on his own, for fear of what he might do along the way. Individual choice was heard but not supported. Angered, the young man slipped out later in the day and went to town on his own anyway. Then he was considered a discipline problem!

Agency reaction

Without an opportunity to make meaningful choices there is a lack of personal control, which will lead to behavioural issues. From an agency perspective, behavioural issues usually result in greater supervision and more restrictions. If behaviour becomes unmanageable with the available resources, agencies will typically seek a higher funding level in order to provide more coverage and individualized service. Depending on the individual's history, an agency may pursue a medical route in order to get medications to reduce the behaviour concerns. If such routes fail, and service is too difficult or costly to provide, the agency may terminate service.

Parents of adults with PWS who have been with multiple agencies are quick to identify their complaints and make comparisons. With an agency change it has often been reported that behaviours improve (minimally for the honeymoon period), less medication is required, program satisfaction increases, and everyone is happier. From the perspective of the adult with PWS, improvement is based on some very simple principles: "they listen to me," "they treat me like an adult," and "they respect me."

Quality of life and professionals

Professionals have a responsibility to perform their duties according to the ethical codes and standards of practice for their discipline. The pressures of caseloads, the immediacy of emergencies, or the demands of the bureaucracy can sometimes limit their availability. These, along with individual personalities and circumstances, sometimes contribute to what parents consider to be an inappropriate or inadequate response to their needs. All professionals have the ability to augment or inhibit the quality of life of the individuals with PWS and their parents.

Calibre of professionals

James and Brown (1992), noted that the quality of life of individuals with PWS will be affected by the calibre of the rehabilitation professionals providing support. They pointed out that practitioners must be skilled, flexible individuals with appropriate personality traits.

When Kinash (2007c) invited an open-ended response from Alberta families with a PWS member to the topic of "attitudes," two groups were named by just over half of the families as "perpetrators of disabling attitudes" - human services workers and medical professionals. She pointed out that these sources of disabling attitudes are disturbing because human services and medical personnel are professionals who have chosen their career fields and are paid to provide supports. Their actions set the standards as they serve as role models for the public at large.

In the present study, parents and individuals with PWS generally expressed strong feelings when discussing workers and doctors. They either loved them and couldn't say enough good about them, or they decried their lack of sensitivity and professional competence, and wanted to get rid of them.

Negative attitudes toward human services workers evolved when they did not listen to, or communicate with, parents. Some workers appeared to place little value on the parents' experiences and knowledge and seemed bent on "re-inventing the wheel." Major parent criticisms included a lack of respect for the son or daughter, and professional incompetence. A disappointed and angry mother described how her diabetic and overweight son was provided pizza and beer, and permitted to smoke, while not taking his medications and insulin. To make things worse, residential staff accompanied him to a strip bar where he was allowed to spend his Christmas money on drinks and lap dances. He was also allowed to pawn his CD collection to get more spending money. The mother only learned about these activities after the fact. The attitudes of the workers did not respect the health care needs of her son or promote constructive social activities.

Social workers, too, have received criticism, chiefly around access to services. To be fair, it may not be the individual social worker who is to blame. Typical complaints include: "Nobody tells us what is available," "There are always wait lists," and "I get tired of the hoop-jumping." While these comments may reflect systemic issues, it is the social worker who is front line in interpreting and applying government and agency policies. How this is done can make a big difference.

Medical doctors have been more often criticized by PWS parents than other professionals (James & Brown, 1992). Criticisms were mainly aimed at General Practitioners and centred on the pursuit of the diagnosis, the manner in which the diagnosis was given, and support to the family after diagnosis. Little has changed in the last 20 years. It was in the context of birth and diagnosis that parents were most disappointed with General Practitioners in the present study. They were described by some as "cold and indifferent" or as "making unfounded hopeless forecasts." Parents understand that PWS is rare and that family doctors may not have any experience with it. It is not the lack of knowledge, rather it is the manner of treatment that disappoints them.

One mother related taking her five-year-old son with PWS to get medical attention. The family GP was away, so they saw another doctor at the clinic. He looked at the file and said, "I've never seen one of these before," referring to her child with PWS. Upset by his introduction, the mother retorted "You haven't seen what – a child with an earache?" The mother admitted she was quite angry and upset that a relatively young and popular doctor could make such a callous remark.

A mother who gave birth in 2007 described receiving the diagnosis without her husband present, being encouraged to explore the Internet while waiting for her husband to arrive, and then leaving the doctor's office with only an understanding of "the worst case scenario." This was a traumatic experience that lacked sensitivity. To be fair, one mother who moved to a new city, found that the new GP knew nothing about PWS on her first visit, but "by the second visit she was on top of it."

Amongst specialists, endocrinologists are the most often criticized. The issue is centred on their reluctance to prescribe growth hormone, or the slowness of the process to get assessment and approval for growth hormone.

The most extensive list of complaints known to the author is reserved for educators. Like human services workers, they provide a direct service for a significant portion of the day. The complaints are most often directed at teachers. Para-professionals (i.e., teacher assistants) generally fare well in the eyes of the parents. However, it is not uncommon when working with a difficult school situation to hear the parent say that "the teacher just doesn't get it!" Despite the advocacy of the parents, the PWS educational materials provided, the cumulative file evidence from the previous years, the psychology reports, and the medical history, some teachers still do not make adjustments for the learning and behavioural needs of the child. They are frequently criticized by parents for their lack of planning, failure to accommodate, insufficient communication, lack of sensitivity, and intimidating behaviours. A teacher, perhaps more than any other professional, can have a major impact on the quality of life of a PWS family during the childhood years.

Prevailing professional viewpoint

A consensus document from an international group of PWS experts, sponsored by the International Prader-Willi Syndrome Organization. concluded that "because of its many physical and behavioural manifestations, PWS should be managed in a multidisciplinary setting that emphasizes comprehensive care" (Eiholzer & Lee, 2006, p. 484). It must be recognized, however, that acknowledged PWS experts are largely medical doctors. They are most accustomed to working in clinical and hospital settings within a medical model. They are concerned with optimal health and longevity of life. When such experts say that something "should" be done parents tend to listen. But what about the other options?

Social services in Canada have embraced the principle of normalization for many years (Wolfensberger, 1972). They attempt to maintain the personal behaviours and characteristics of clients as "culturally normative" as possible. That is to say, to have them live in typical neighbourhoods where they can enjoy access to vocational, social, recreational, and other regular daily life opportunities.

Most individuals with PWS in Canada live in family or group homes in regular communities. While it is true that some of these may be in crisis, the majority are not. Most individuals and families are simply going about the routines of daily living without medical intervention, multi-disciplinary teams, or affiliation with PWS parent groups. Many parents reject group affiliation because it doesn't meet their needs; they reject the prevailing professional viewpoint for the same reason. They argue that multidisciplinary teaming is too intrusive, that congregate facilities are not "normal," and that comprehensive care denies the rights of individuals to make their own choices. In short, the independence and quality of life that they value for their children is in conflict with the prevailing professional view.

The prevailing professional view of what "should" happen in order to provide the best care would similarly not be accepted by many adults with PWS. The high levels of satisfaction expressed by those in supported independent living in Canada suggests that this would be their preferred option. It is a model which places priority on individual quality of life concerns. The promotion of PWS-specific group homes, touted by some professionals as the "best" option, is attractive to some parents but to fewer adults with PWS. Supported independent living and PWS-specific group homes are both desirable for a continuum of residential options.

The reality is that there is no "best" option for all with PWS; nor is life with PWS an "either - or" proposition. It isn't just live at home under strict controls or in a comprehensive multidisciplinary setting. It isn't just strict calorie counting or the Red Yellow Green diet that most professionals recommend. Life with PWS may or may not follow the recommendations of professionals or resemble the content of professional articles. Indeed, many families go about the tasks of daily living with little professional in-put.

Partnership needed

Parents have found approaches to the management of PWS that work for their individual situations. They recognize that there is a range within the syndrome. Most know that they are the real experts. They also know, however, that a balance of parent and professional input is most helpful. Some parents have learned to challenge the status quo and ask "why not?" They have become "squeaky wheels" in order to get services. They have learned that the decisions of professionals within a

The quality of lives of individuals with PWS have been improved by the advocacy of parents who have had a vision for a different option, in cooperation with professionals who have been interested in a creative solution and willing to operate "outside of the box."

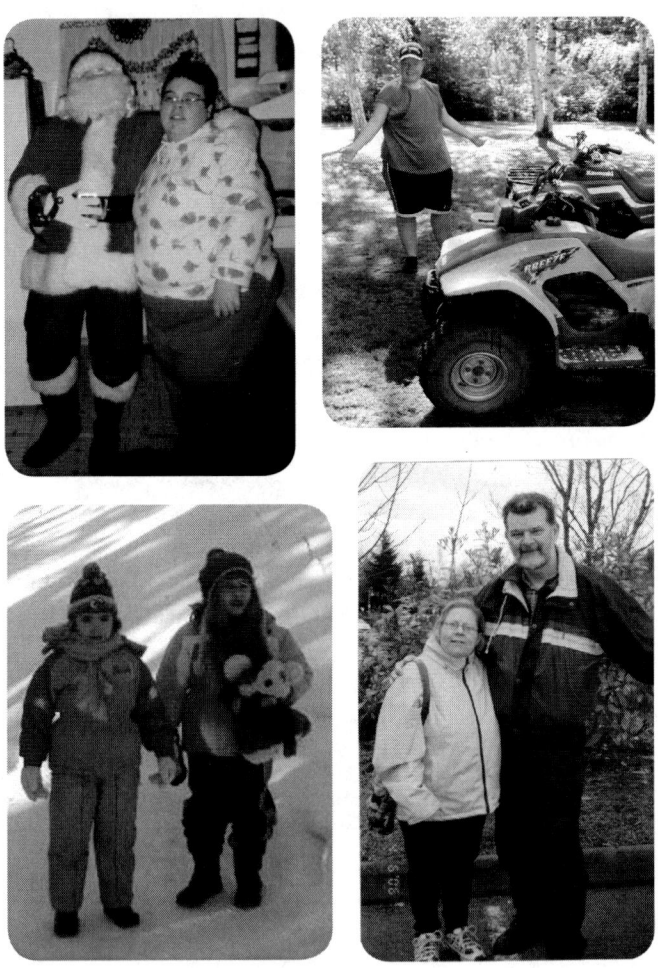

Happy times

13

Conclusion

Chapter 1 presented a philosophical framework for looking at quality of life. It asserted that any consideration of quality of life must focus on what is important to the individual. With this in mind, this book has attempted to consider those things which are important to individuals with PWS, at all ages, and to their parents or guardians. While the chapters are comprehensive in scope, they are not exhaustive. Their content was driven by structured and open-ended interviews, case histories, and published stories of more than 125 Canadian families with a PWS member.

Personal and family stories illustrate the range and variability within PWS. While there may be benefit in understanding the "behavioural phenotype," individual stories emphasize the uniqueness of each family circumstance. While there may be certain predispositions toward behaviours, the environment and how it is managed will have a large impact on the successful management of the syndrome. Readers should be encouraged by the positive experiences that have been related.

Clearly, the changes that have taken place in the last quarter century have changed the lives of parents of children with PWS. While the parenting issues are largely the same, the knowledge about PWS and the resources available have consistently improved, enhancing the quality of lives of parents. There is optimism for continued improvements in the future. While young adults experience the greatest stresses with weight management, residential placements, job opportunities, and social adjustments, older individuals with PWS have expressed considerable satisfaction with their quality of life.

Changes over time

While visiting PWS homes in the mid-1980s there was a lot of confusion about PWS. There were mothers who carried a burden of guilt for what they might have done during pregnancy, marriages which had split from inordinate stresses, and parents who were coping without any resources. The changes which have taken place in the last 25 years have lead to a greater understanding of PWS and better supports. These have included:

- *early diagnosis:* Pioneer parents struggled with knowing instinctively that there was something wrong, yet not being able to get a diagnosis. Today, parents are receiving a diagnosis in infancy. Starting with a diagnosis changes the direction of parents' energies; intervention becomes more focussed.

- *syndrome variability:* Whether one has a chromosome 15 deletion or disomy, or whether it is Type I or Type II, is contributing to a greater understanding of variability within the syndrome and holds hope for differentiated approaches to treatments.

- *multi-disciplinary teaming:* An early diagnosis brings with it a host of resources that did not exist for the pioneer parents. While there have always been general practitioners and pediatricians, today's parents have the involvement of: infant development workers; physio, occupational, and speech therapists; dieticians/ nutritionists; home nursing; clinics and research studies. The multi-disciplinary involvement, which begins in infancy with a medical focus, continues into childhood with an educational focus.

- *parent supports:* While many pioneer parents struggled to manage on their own, younger parents generally have: a multi-disciplinary team of professionals to provide support; a broader range of social services options; more formal and informal respite; and access to a regional, provincial, national, and international network of parents. There is also better community acceptance of people with disabilities today. With the support of PWS parent organizations, they can collectively lobby for improvements in services for their children.

- *individualized services:* The evolution from group funded services to individualized funding and service delivery, has changed all levels of the service system. While not all programs and services can be easily individualized, the impact for those who do benefit from this approach is encouraging. Individualized services allow for more creative ways to meet personal needs and desires, enriching quality of life for people with PWS.

- *inclusionary practices:* The progression from deinstitutionalization to integration, normalization, and community living has lead to greater public acceptance and inclusion for individuals with disabilities.
- *growth hormone treatment:* No single topic has received as much parent attention in the last decade as that of growth hormone treatment. While the process for determining eligibility is cumbersome and highly criticized, and the availability inequitable, the potential for increased growth velocity, decreased body fat and BMI, increased muscle development, improved physical abilities, improved respiratory function, and concomitant social acceptance ignite parent hopes and energies.
- *life expectancy:* It is clear that adults with PWS are living longer than was expected a generation ago. It is not unreasonable to assume that with early diagnosis and appropriate interventions, individuals with PWS will live into their "senior" years.

Social policy issues

Several of the changes noted in the previous section reflect changes in social policy directions. Pioneer families had to work through important social changes like institutionalization/deinstitutionalization and segregation/integration. Their generation helped to bring about educational inclusion, special education supports, respite, individualized funding, and community living opportunities. While these have been important improvements the fight is not over. There are several outstanding areas, particularly within the adult domain, that still require the advocacy of parents and the attention of policy makers:

- *eligibility for services:* Most jurisdictions use IQ 70 as a cut-off criterion for service for people with developmental disabilities. Individuals with PWS with IQs greater than 70 are often left to flounder without appropriate supports. Under the current system, until they become a mental health or judicial concern their needs are not likely to be addressed. Eligibility for support in educational and social services needs reform.
- *right to protection:* While individual right of choice should be highly valued, it is irresponsible, and may even be negligent, to uphold the individual right of choice knowing that the result may well lead to a worsening of the condition, even unto death.

Clarification of existing social services policy is needed.

- *opportunities for employment*: There is dignity in work. Many adults with PWS have skills that could contribute to the workforce if they were given a chance. Access to programs to assist job placement, job coaching, and entrepreneurship are needed.

- *need for qualified service providers*: In some jurisdictions, it is difficult to attract and retain qualified human services workers. Workers may be unqualified or under-qualified, with an insufficient knowledge of English to communicate or read and understand professional literature, program plans, and health protocols. Creative efforts are needed to train and retain workers in the human services field.

- *provision of respite*: While the provision of individualized service dollars creates more flexibility to address the need for respite, there needs to be greater availability and more equitable access in order to support the integrity of families. The focus needs to shift from crisis to more emphasis on prevention.

- *importance of leisure education*: The lack of employment options and the need to creatively address individualized day program hours suggests that there should be more emphasis on leisure activities, both individual and group type. The value of leisure skills training in developing self-concept and social skills is well understood. The in-home evidence of the value placed on fine arts, music, sports, and technology, suggests that more time should be spent in exposure to, and instruction in, life-time leisure and recreation activities.

- *need for clinical monitoring*: While children generally have the opportunity to be followed by a clinical team at a provincial children's hospital, the service is not always available for adults with PWS. In addition to monitoring health and development, clinics can disseminate the latest information, encourage best practices, and participate in research.

- *respect for PWS voice:* Some adults with PWS have become strong self-advocates and have taken on the cause of others with the syndrome. They desire a stronger PWS voice. They want to be heard. At the same time, if programs and services are to improve, there is a need for parents and professionals to listen to what they have to say. Creating opportunities for the PWS voice to be heard is a challenge, but from a quality of life perspective it is an absolute necessity.

The need for future research

The majority of PWS research is bio-medical in nature. From a quality of life perspective, however, there is a need for research from all of the disciplines involved with PWS, particularly those that are involved with direct service. The following topics are suggestive of areas that need exploration:

- *growth hormone*: While there is high interest among younger parents, not everyone is convinced of the need and benefits. There is a need for long-term studies which address the benefits and impact of short-term treatment; optimal age for, and length of treatment; long-term side effects of treatment; and adult mantenance requirements.
- *aging:* There is little available on this topic. Parents want to know about: the onset of dementia and Alzheimer's disease, long-term impact of obesity on mobility, non-dietary factors influencing longevity, syndrome management for seniors, and integrated opportunities within the seniors service sector.
- *diet and weight management:* Diet and weight management practices are of high interest. Weight management is dependent on much more than just diet. Further exploration is needed on its relationship to: significant others, residential changes, residential models, self-concept, traumatic events, day activities, and environmental controls. Family practices have evolved which need to be evaluated, for example: weekly weigh-ins; use of BMI targets; reliance on third-party or clinic monitoring; participation in independent living practices such as menu planning, grocery shopping, and food preparation; and the benefits of an organic diet.
- *allied and alternative health:* Some families want to explore beyond conventional western medical practices. Initially case studies need to be examined. What are the potential benefits from naturopathy, traditional Chinese medicine, chiropractic, massage therapy, and other body work practices?
- *residential models:* Of most interest are the comparative benefits of structured PWS group homes versus the benefits of the independent living model, and the various possibilities within this model.
- *inter-dependence/independence*: The teaching of independence is unrealistic as a goal for most students with PWS. On the other hand, teaching inter-dependence with a future goal of semi-independence in the community is more realistic, and consistent

with current best practice at the adult level in the Canadian experience. Curricula and instructional methods need exploration.

- *PWS siblings*: Sibling testimonies have described the best and worst of childhood memories. Adult sibling relationships are supportive and estranged. Research is needed to study sibling experiences, particularly in childhood.

- *psychological supports:* The reported high incidence of mental health concerns, particularly with UPD, suggests the need to study preventive measures, for example: best practices for "self" development; the nature and benefit of peer, family and other social supports; and the relationship of management practices to mental health issues.

- *peer supports:* Peers have been asked to assist in monitoring and supervising individuals with PWS without any training, minimal knowledge, and yet considerable adult expectations. Effective models and curricula need to be assessed.

- *entrepreneurial activities:* Given the lack of employment opportunities, entrepreneurship may offer a realistic alternative to employment. Models need to be studied, and case studies documented.

Life goes on

This project began in 2007. In the intervening time, the individuals and families in this study have been impacted by significant life events, such as: accidents and injuries, suspensions from school, loss of grandparents, participant death, parental death, diagnosis of terminal medical conditions, hospitalizations, changes in guardianship, changes of residence, resignations and retirement of support staff, termination of programs, loss of jobs, death of pets, changes to programs, interpersonal conflicts, loss of girl/boy friends, moving to new towns, and changing provinces. These events are not unique to individuals with PWS. They relate to health, aging, relationships, and economic circumstances. They underscore the normalcy of daily living.

Individuals with PWS demonstrate resiliency in the face of such life events. They adjust, as others do, with time. They grow through the experiences. While their satisfaction with life may be temporarily interrupted, their enjoyment returns. With supports provided by the home, school, and community, their quality of life improves.

Appendix A:

Prader-Willi syndrome organizations

The Foundation for Prader-Willi Research, Canada

19-130825 Yonge Street Suite #370
Richmond Hill, Ontario
L4E 0K2
Event website: www.onesmallstep.ca
Information website: www.fpwr.ca

A charitable organization comprised of parents, families, researchers, and others interested in addressing issues related to Prader-Willi syndrome (PWS) and childhood obesity. Founded in 2006 by parents of children with PWS, the mission of the Foundation for Prader-Willi Research Canada (FPWRC) is to eliminate the challenges of PWS through the advancement of research. Members of FPWRC believe that through research, treatments will be found that will lessen the restrictions placed on people with PWS. These advancements will provide those with the syndrome an opportunity to lead more independent lives. All proceeds support PWS research. Donations are payable to The Foundation for Prader-Willi Research, Canada.

In May of 2009 the FPWRC joined with the Canadian Prader-Willi Syndrome Association to become the national body representing PWS in Canada.

Canadian PWS provincial associations:

Alberta Prader-Willi Syndrome Association
c/o 9006-120 St.
Edmonton, AB T6G 1X7
Website: http://www.pwsaa.ca

British Columbia Prader-Willi Syndrome Association
c/o 2129 Lillooet Cr.
Kelowna, BC V1V 1W3
Website: http://www.bcpwsa.com

Ontario Prader-Willi Syndrome Association
2788 Bathurst St, Suite 303
Toronto, ON M6B 3A3
Website: www.opwsa.com
Email: opwsa@rogers.com
Tel: (416) 481-8657   Fax: (416) 481-6706

PWS Canada E-Group

http://health.groups.yahoo.com/group/PWScanada/

A parent/caregiver e-mail group offering support to anyone dealing with PWS.

Prader-Willi Syndrome Network

Website: http://www.pwsnetwork.ca/pws/

A network providing information and resources for service providers who work with individuals with PWS and their families. This site focusses on social service issues and not medical research or treatment.

Prader-Willi.ca

Website: www.prader-willi.ca
Email: terrance@prader-willi.ca

Prader-Willi.ca is a privately sponsored website that supports the quality of life of individuals with PWS and their families through the promotion of Canadian resources for non-medical aspects of PWS.

The Prader-Willi Syndrome Association (USA)

8588 Potter Park Drive, Suite 500
Sarasota, Florida 34238 USA
Website: www.pwsausa.org
Tel: (800) 926-4797
Tel: (941) 312-0400 Fax: (941) 312-0142

An organization of families and professionals working together to promote and fund research, provide education, and offer support to enhance the quality of life of those affected by Prader-Willi syndrome. Newsletter: *The Gathered View*.

International Prader-Willi Syndrome Association

Website: http://www.ipwso.org

A global organization of parents, friends, and professionals committed to enhancing the quality of life for people with PWS and their families. IPWSO has 81 member and associate member countries, representing some 25,000 families. Every three years the IPWSO sponsors an international ocnferrence hosted by different countries where professionals, scientists, and researchers enjoy a universal exchange or research, experience, and ideas. Newsetter: *Wavelength* (available free on-line).

Appendix B:
PWS timeline

1956   PWS first described by Drs. Prader, Labhart, and Willi

1968   Publication of the first Canadian paper on PWS, describing nine patients (Dr. D. Dunn, BC Children's Hospital)

1975   First issue of *The Gathered View* made the announcement of the organization of Prader-Willi Syndrome Parents and Friends

1977   The name of the organization changed to Prader-Willi Syndrome Association of the USA (PWSA-USA)

1979   First national PWSA-USA conference held in Minneapolis

1980   Formation of the Lower Mainland Prader-Willi Syndrome Association of British Columbia

1981   A small deletion on the upper part of the long arm of chromosome chromosome 15 first described

1982   Ontario Prader-Willi Syndrome Association (OPWSA) established

1983   A deletion on chromosome 15 donated by the father first described

1985   First scientific conference held in conjunction with the annual national PWSA-USA conference

1985   First Canadian PWS-specific group home attempted by the Lower Mainland Association of British Columbia

1986   Formation of the Alberta Prader-Willi Syndrome Association

1989   Alberta PWSA hosted the eleventh PWSA-USA annual conference in Calgary

        Maternal uniparental disomy (UPD) first described as an alternative causative mechanism for PWS

1991   DNA methylation analysis introduced for diagnosis

        Formation of the International Prader-Willi Syndrome Organization (IPWSO); The 1st International IPWSO Conference held in The Netherlands

        Central Canada Prader-Willi Syndrome Association, formed in the early 80s, ceased to exist as a legal entity, but continued as a support group. *PWSNews Canada* ends publication.

1992   First publication of *Wavelength*, the IPWSO newsletter for parents

1993   Consensus criteria for clinical diagnosis first published

1996   Lower Mainland PWSA changed name to the British Columbia Prader-Willi Syndrome Association (BCPWSA)

1998   Formation of the Canadian Prader-Willi Syndrome Association (CPWSA)

2000   FDA approval of growth hormone for PWS in the USA

2006   Foundation for Prader-Willi Research Canada formed

2009   The Foundation for Prader-Willi Research Canada joined with the Canadian Prader-Willi Syndrome Association to become the national body representing PWS in Canada

References

Akefeldt, A., Tomhaga, C. J., & Gilberg, C. (1999). A woman with Prader-Willi syndrome gives birth to a healthy baby girl. *Developmental Medicine and Child Neurology, 41*, 789-790.

Alberta Association for Community Living. (2009). PDD funding - You must choose a funding option by April 1, 2009. *AACL Information bulletin,* p. 4. Retrieved June 6, 2009, from http://aacl.org/Portals/O/InfoBulletinPDDfunding.pdf

Alberta Bone and Joint Institute. (2007, March 30). *News release: Alberta Bone and Joint Institute warns rising rates of obesity in children an alarming omen of early joint wear.* Retrieved May 18, 2010, from http://www.albertaboneandjoint.com/news_rel_Mar_07.asp

Alberta Council of Disability Services (ACDS). (October 27, 2006). *The cost of Alberta's economic wealth to citizens with developmental disabilities.* Calgary, AB: Author. Retrieved March 22, 2009, from http://www.mirafc.ca/website/documents/ACDS_Cost_of_Economic_Wealth.pdf

Alexander, R. C., & Greenswag, L. R. (1988). *Management of Prader-Willi syndrome.* New York: Springer-Verlag.

American Psychiatric Association. (2000). *Diagnostic and statistical manual of mental disorders* (4th ed.). Washington, DC: Author.

Antiochi, R., Stavrakaki, C., & Emery, P.C. (2003). Psychopharmacological treatments in persons with dual diagnosis or psychiatric disorders and developmental disabilities. *Postgraduate Medical Journal, 79*, 139-146.

Balko, K. (2005). *Red yellow green system for weight management.* Toronto, ON: Ontario Prader-Willi Syndrome Association.

Balko, K. (2006, October 20). *The ABCs of nutrition: Implementation of the Red Yellow Green System (RYG) of weight management.* Paper presented at the PWS Providers Day, Markham, ON.

Bavis, R. (2003, Winter). Letters to the editor. *The Star* [publication of the Developmental Disabilities Association, Richmond, BC], p. 3.

BBC News. (1998, January 10). Fat child's mother guilty of neglect. Retrieved January 11, 2009, from http://news.bbc/1/world/46077.stm

BBC News. (1998, February 27). Mother of obese teen escapes jail. Retrieved October 18, 2008, from http://news.bbc.co.uk/2/hi/americas/60819.stm

Beddoe, J. (2000, January). A message from the president. *Ontario Prader-Willi Syndrome Association Newsletter,* p. 1.

Berall, G. B., Allanson, J., & Desantadina, V. (2004). *Prader-Willi syndrome (January 2003 to December 2004) final report.* Canadian Paediatric Surveillance Registry 2004 Results. Ottawa, ON: Canadian Paediatric Society. Available on-line at http://www.cps.ca/English/Surveillance/CPSP/Studies/2004Results.pdf

Bertella, L., Girelli, L., Grugni, G., Marchi, S., Molinari, E., & Semenza, C. (2005). Mathematical skills in Prader-Willi syndrome. *Journal of Intellectual Disability Research, 49*(Pt. 2), 159-169.

Blackburn, L. (1992). Toddler's insatiable appetite could kill him; Victims of rare Prader-Willi Syndrome are in constant danger of eating themselves to death. *Whitehorse Star,* p. C8.

Boer, H., Holland, A., Whittington, J., Butler, J., Webb, T., & Clarke, D. (2002a). Psychotic illness in people with Prader-Willi syndrome due to chromosome 15 maternal uniparental disomy. *Lancet, 359,* 135.

Boer, H., Holland, A. J., Whittington, J.E., Butler, J.V., Webb, T., & Clarke, D.J. (2002b). Is psychotic illness inevitable in people with Prader-Willi syndrome due to chromosome 15 maternal uniparental disomy? *Lancet, 359,* 135-136.

Boyle, I. R. (2007, November/December). Dealing with a dual diagnosis of PWS and autism. *The Gathered View, 32*(6), 10.

Bradley, E., & Morris, S. (2001, October). Dual diagnosis: An overview. Paper presented to the Toronto/Peel Mental Health Task Force, Toronto, ON.

Bradley, L. (2009, April 01). Leaders honoured for helping children. *The Sudbury Star.* Retrieved February 20, 2010, from www.thesudburystar.com

Brown, I., & Brown, R. I. (2003). *Quality of life and disability.* New York: Jessica Kingsley.

Brown, R.I., & Hughson, A. (1993). Behavioural and social rehabilitation and training. Toronto: Captus Press.

Brown, R.I., Bayer, M.B., & MacFarlane, C. (1988). Quality of life amongst handicapped adults. In R.I. Brown (Ed.), *Quality of life for handicapped people* (pp. 111-140). New York: Croom Helm.

Butler, M .G. (2000). A 68 year old white female with Prader-Willi syndrome. *Clinical Dysmorphology, 9*(1), 65-67.

Butler, M.G., Bittel, D.C., Kibiryeva, N., Talebizadeh, Z., & Thompson, T. (2004). Behavioral differences among subjects with Prader-Willi syndrome and type I or type II deletion and maternal disomy. *Pediatrics, 113*(3), 565-573.

Butler, M.G., Hanchett, J.M., & Thompson, T. (2006). Clinical findings and natural history of Prader-Willi syndrome. In M.G. Butler, P.D.K. Lee, & B.Y. Whitman (Eds.), *Management of Prader-Willi syndrome* (3rd ed.) (pp. 3-48). New York: Springer.

Butler, M.G., & Meaney, J.F. (1991). Standards for selected anthropometric measurements in Prader-Willi syndrome. *Pediatrics, 88*(4), 853-860.

Canadian Association for Community Living (CACL). (2008). *All about CACL.* Retrieved December 8, 2008, from http://www.cacl.ca/english/aboutus/index_asp

Carpenter, P.K. (1994). Prader-Willi syndrome in old age. *Journal of Intellectual Disability Research, 38,* 529-531.

Carrel, A.L., Lee, P.D.K., & Mozul, H.R. (2006). Growth hormone and Prader-Willi syndrome. In M.G. Butler, P.D.K. Lee, & B.Y. Whitman (Eds.), *Management of Prader-Willi syndrome* (3rd ed.) (pp. 201-241). New York: Springer.

Carrel, A.L., Moerchen, V., Myers, S.E., Bekx, M.T., Whitman, B.Y., & Allen, D.B. (2004). Growth hormone improves mobility and body composition in infants and toddlers with Prader-Willi syndrome. *Journal of Pediatrics, 148*(6), 744-749.

Carter, T.O. (1991, September 9). An appetite for freedom. *British Columbia Report, 3*(2), 31.

Cassidy, S.B., Devi, A., & Mukaida, R.D. (1995). Aging in Prader-Willi Syndrome (Abstract 27). 2nd Prader-Willi Syndrome International Scientific Workshop and Conference Abstact Book, Somarka, Oslo, 15-18 June.

Chedd, N., Levine, K., & Wharton, R.H. (2006). Educational considerations for children with Prader-Willi syndrome. In M.G. Butler, P.D.K. Lee, & B.Y. Whitman (Eds.), *Management of Prader-Willi syndrome* (3rd ed.) (302-316). New York: Springer.

Christensen, C.S., & Hainline, B.E. (2001, September-October). PWS and obesity, and PWS look-alikes. *The Gathered View, 26*(5), 4-5.

Clarke, D. (1998). Prader-Willi syndrome and psychotic symptoms: 2. A preliminary study of prevalence using the psychopathology assessment schedule for adults with developmental disability checklist. *Journal of Intellectual Disability Research, 42*(Pt. 6), 451-454.

Clarke, D.J., Boer, H., Chung, M.C., Sturney, P., & Webb, T. (1996, April). Maladaptive behaviour in Prader-Willi syndrome. *Journal of Intellectual Disability Research, 40*(Pt. 2), 159-165.

Clarke, D., Boer, H., Webb, T., Scott, P., Fraser, S., Vogels, A., Borghgraef, M., & Curfs, L.M.G. (1998). Prader-Willi syndrome and psychotic symptoms: 1. Case descriptions and genetic studies. *Journal of Intellectual Disability Research, 42*(Pt 6), 440-450.

CLBC. (2006). *Eligibility for CLBC supports and services.* Retrieved March 15, 2009, from http://communitylivingbc.ca/policies_and_publications/policies

Community Living Research Project. (2008). *Residential alternatives in B.C.: An exploration of family members and self advocate experiences.* Vancouver, BC: UBC School of Social Work.

Criminal Code, R.S.C. 1985, c.C-46, s.265.

Crino, A., Schiaffini, R., Ciampalini, P., Spera, S., Beccaria, L., Benzi, F., et al. (2003). Hypogonadism and pubertal development in Prader-Willi syndrome. *European Journal of Pediatrics, 162,* 327-333.

Crisis Prevention Institute. (2006). Risks of restraints: Understanding restraint related positional asphyxia. Retrieved August 22, 2010 from http://www.crisisprevention.com

Crisis Prevention Institute (2010). About CPI. Retrieved August 22, 2010 from http://www.crisisprevention.com/About-CPI

Cryderman, K. (2008, March 12). Sister fears for future as home care falls short: New deal sought to retain staff for the disabled. *Calgary Herald.*

Department of Finance Canada. (2006. December 19). *Canada's new government establishes program eligibility for the children's fitness tax credit.* Retrieved from http://www.fin.gc.ca/news06/06-084e.html

Derogatis, L.R. (1983). *SCL-90-R: Administration, scoring and procedures manual-II* (2nd ed.). Towson, MD: Clinical Psychometric Research.

Dickson, L. (1987, February 23). Obsessive syndrome drives children to obesity. *The Ottawa Citizen,* p. D6.

Didden, R., Korzilius, H., & Curfs, L. (2007). Skin-picking in individuals with Prader-Willi syndrome: Prevalence, functional assessment, and its comorbidity with compulsive and self-injurious behaviours. *Journal of Applied Research in Intellectual Disabilities, 20,* 409–419.

Dimitropoulos, A., Feurer, I. D., Roof, E., Stone, W., Butler, M. G., Sutcliffe, J., & Thompson, T. (2000). Appetitive behavior, compulsivity, and neurochemistry in Prader-Willi syndrome. *Mental Retardation & Developmental Disabilities Research Reviews, 6*(2), 125-130.

Dorn, B., & Goff, B.J. (2003). *The student with Prader-Willi syndrome: Information for educators.* Sarasota, FL: PWSA(USA).

Drago, S. (2006). Vocational training for people with Prader-Willi syndrome. In M.G. Butler, P.D.K. Lee, & B.Y. Whitman (Eds), *Management of Prader-Willi syndrome* (3rd ed.) (pp. 370-380). New York: Springer.

Driscoll, D., & McCune, H. (1998, July-August). Recent advances in the research and treatment of obesity: How they relate to the Prader-Willi syndrome. *The Gathered View, XXIII*(4), 6-9.

Driscoll, D.J., & Butler, M.G. (2002, March-April). Beware of medical advice over the internet, *The Gathered View, 27*(2), 11.

Dykens, E. M. (2002). Are jigsaw puzzles 'spared' in persons with Prader-Willi syndrome? *Journal of Child Psychology and Psychiatry, 43*(3), 343-352.

Dykens, E.M. (2004, March). Maladaptive and compulsive behavior in Prader-Willi syndrome: New insights from older adults. *American Journal on Mental Retardation, 109*(2), 142-53.

Dykens, E.M., Cassidy, S.B., & King, B.H. (1999). Maladaptive behavior differences in Prader-Willi syndrome due to paternal deletion versus maternal uniparental disomy. *American Journal on Mental Retardation, 104*, 67-77.

Dykens, E.M., & Hodapp, R. (1995, April). Studies on behavioral and family issues in PWS: A progress report. *The Gathered View, XX* (2), 4-5.

Dykens, E.M., Hodapp, R.M., Walsh, K., & Nash, L. J. (1992). Profiles, correlates and trajectories of intelligence in Prader-Willi syndrome. *Journal of the American Academy of Child and Adolescent Psychiatry, 31*, 1125-1130.

Dykens, E.M., Leckman, J.F., & Cassidy, S.B. (1996). Obsessions and compulsions in Prader-Willi syndrome. *Journal of Child, Psychology and Psychiatry, 37*, 995-1002.

Dykens, E.M., & Shah, B. (2003). Psychiatric disorders in Prader-Willi syndrome: Epidemiology and management. *CNS Drugs, 17*(3) 167-178.

Eiholzer, U. (2005). Deaths in Children with Prader-Willi Syndrome. *Hormone Research, 63*, 33–39.

Eiholzer, U., Gisin, R., Weinmann, C., Kriemler, S., Steinert, H., Torresani, T., Zachmann, M., & Prader, A. (1998). Treatment with human growth hormone in patients with Prader-Labhart-Willi syndrome reduces body fat and increases muscle mass and physical performance. *European Journal of Pediatrics, 157*, 368-377.

Eiholzer, U., & Lee, P.D.K. (2006). Medical considerations in Prader-Willi syndrome. In M.G. Butler, P.D.K. Lee, & B.Y. Whitman (Eds.), *Management of Prader-Willi syndrome* (3rd ed.) (pp. 97-152). New York: Springer.

Eiholzer, U., & Lee, P.D.K. (2006). Appendix B: A comprehensive team approach to the management of Prader-Willi syndrome. In M.G. Butler, P.D.K. Lee, & B.Y. Whitman (Eds.), *Management of Prader-Willi syndrome* (3rd Ed.) (pp. 473-484). New York: Springer.

Eli Lilly. (2008, June). *Product monograph: Humatope* (Somatropin for injection). Toronto: Author. Retrieved November 21, 2008, from www.lilly.ca/searchable/pm/docs/16_HUMATROPE%20PM_9june08_MK.pdf

Ferenc, L. (2007, June 2). Campers light up at Shadow Lake. *The Star*. Retrieved March 22, 2009, from http://www.thestar.com/article/220693

Fidler, D.J., Hodapp, R.M., & Dykens, E.M. (2002). Behavioral phenotypes and special education: Parent report of educational issues for children with Down syndrome, Prader-Willi syndrome, and Williams syndrome. *Journal of Special Education, 36*(2), 80-96.

Fidler, D.J., Lawson, J.E., & Hodapp, R.M. (2003). What do parents want?: An analysis of education-related comments made by parents of children with different genetic syndromes. *Journal of Intellectual & Developmental Disability, 28*(2), 196-204.

Fieldstone, A., Zipf, W.B., Schwartz, H.C., & Berntson, G.G. (1997). Food preferences in Prader-Willi syndrome, normal weight and obese controls. *International Journal of Obesity and Related Metabolic Disorders, 21*(11), 1046-1052.

Fine, A. H. (1996). Leisure, living and quality of life. In R. Renwick, I. Brown, & M. Nagler (Eds.), *Quality of life in health promotion and rehabilitation* (342 – 355). Thousand Oaks, CA: SAGE.

Flacks, D. (August 22, 2009). From pain comes compassion. *The Star.* Retrieved February 8, 2010, from http://www.healthzone.ca/health/articlePrint/682640

FPWR Canada. (2009). Lauren's story. Retrieved February 08, 2010, from www.fpwr.ca/news-events/tributes/lauren-story

Fraser, A. (2008/09, Winter). Robbie. *RSCL Views* [Richmond Society for Community Living], p. 11.

Goff, B.J. (2006). Education and social issues for adolescents with PWS. In M.G. Butler, P.D.K. Lee, & B.Y. Whitman (Eds.), Management of Prader-Willi syndrome (3rd ed.) (pp. 344-355). New York: Springer.

Goldman, J.J. (1988). Prader-Willi syndrome in two institutionalized older adults. *Mental Retardation, 26*(2), 97-102.

Government of Canada. (1984). *The Charter of Rights and Freedoms: A guide for Canadians.* Ottawa: Publications Canada.

Grace. (1998, December). I lost over 100 pounds. *BC PWSA Newsletter*, pp. 3-4.

Grace, M. (1995, April). Future Prader-Willi options. *The Gathered View, XX*(2), 3.

Greaves, N., Prince, E., Evans, D.W., & Charman, T. (2006). Repetitive and ritualistic behaviour in children with Prader-Willi syndrome and children with autism. *Journal of Intellectual Disability Research, 50*(Pt 2), 92-100.

Greenswag, L.R. (1985, April). Residential needs. *The Gathered View,* *XX*(2), 3.

Greenswag, L.R. (1987). Adults with Prader-Willi syndrome: A survey of 232 cases. *Developmental Medicine and Child Neurology, 29,* 145-152.

Gunay-Aygun, M., Schwartz, S., Heeger, S., O'Riordan, M.A., & Cassidy, S.B. (2001). The changing purpose of Prader-Willi syndrome clinical diagnostic criteria and proposed revised criteria. *Pediatrics, 108*(5), 92-97.

Hain, B. (June 03, 2008). School mates walk for awareness. *Barrie Advance.* Retrieved February 05, 2010, from http://www.simcoe.com/article/106511

Halifax Daily News. (2001, July 30). *Boy with rare disorder chokes on marshmallow*, p.8.

Hall, B.D., & Smith, D.W. (1972). Prader-Willi syndrome: A resume of 32 cases including an instance of affected first cousins, one of whom is of normal stature and intelligence. *The Journal of Pediatrics, 81*(2), 286-293.

Harty, J.R., Hollowell, J.G., & Sieg, K.G. (1993, March). Tall stature: An atypical phenotype in Prader-Willi syndrome. *Clinical Pediatrics*, 179-180.

Heinemann, J. (2000, June/July)). For the love of grandparents. *The Gathered View, 25*(3), 4-5.

Heinemann, J. (2000, September/October). From kitchen to bedroom: Sexuality and Prader-Willi syndrome. *The Gathered View, 25*(4), 7,12.

Heinemann, J. (2000, November/December). Beyond the diet – For the professional: Issues in getting weight under control. *The Gathered View, 25*(5), 4-5.

Heinemann, J. (2003, May/June). Does a child with disabilities = A disabled marriage? *The Gathered View, 28*(3), 10.

Heinemann, J. (2008, October 25). Medical crisis prevention and intervention. Presentation at the BCPWSA Fall Conference, Vancouver, BC.

Heinemann, J., & McManus, B. (2005). Prader-Willi Syndrome (USA) database collection uncover areas of needed research. Retrieved from http://www.pwsausa.org/Scnceday/2005/databasecollections.htm

Heinemann, J., Wyatt, D.A., & Goff, B.J. (2006). Advocacy issues: Sexuality. In M.G. Butler, P.D.K. Lee, & B.Y. Whitman (Eds.), *Management of Prader-Willi syndrome* (3rd ed.) (pp. 457-464). New York: Springer.

Hinton, E.C., Holland, A.J., Gellatly, M.S., Soni, S., & Owen, A.M. (2006). An investigation into food preferences and the neural basis of food-related incentive motivation in Prader-Willi syndrome. *Journal of Intellectual Disability Research, 50*(Pt. 9), 633-642.

Hinton, E.C., Holland, A.J., Gellatly, M.S.N., Soni, S., Patterson, M., Ghatei, M.A., & Owen, A.M. (2006). Neural representations of hunger and satiety in Prader-Willi syndrome. *International Journal of Obesity, 30*, 313-321.

Hiraiwa, R., Maegaki, Y., Oka, A., & Ohno, K. (2007). Behavioural and psychiatric disorders in Prader-Willi syndrome: A population study in Japan. *Brain and Development, 29*, 535-542.

Hobbs, H. (1997). 'Structured' choice: Balancing the 'dignity of risk' against individual limitations. *The Gathered View, XXII*(2), p. 6.

Hodapp, R.M., Dykens, E.M., & Masino, L.L. (1997). Families of children with Prader-Willi syndrome: Stress support and relations to child characteristics. *Journal of Autism and Developmental Disorders, 27*(1), 11-24.

Hoefnagel, D., Costello, P. J., & Hatoum, K. (1967). Prader-Willi syndrome. *Journal of Mental Deficiency Research, 11*, 1-11.

Holland, A.J., Whittington, J.E., Butler, J., Webb, T., Boer, H., & Clarke, D. (2003). Behavioural phenotypes associated with specific genetic disorders: Evidence from a population-based study of people with Prader-Willi syndrome. *Psychological Medicine, 33*, 141-153.

Holm, V.A., Cassidy, S.B., Butler, M.G., Hanchett, J.M., Greenswag, L.R., Whitman, B.Y., & Greenberg, F. (1993). Prader-Willi syndrome: Consensus diagnostic criteria. *Pediatrics, 91*(2), 398-402.

Hornsey, C. (1997, February 15). Helping: United Way agency helps David 'bloom.' *The Windsor Star*, p. A5.

Horvath, B. (2006, October). Prader-Willi syndrome survey of Central West Region Service Providers, March 20, 2006. Toronto, ON: PWS Network Steering Committee.

Hoybye, C. (2007). Five-years growth hormone (GH) treatment in adults with Prader-Willi syndrome. *Acta Paediatrica, 96*, 410-413.

Hoybye, C., Hilding, A., Jacobsson, H., & Thoren, M. (2003). Growth hormone treatment improves body composition in adults with Prader-Willi syndrome, *Clinical Endocrinology (Oxf), 58*(5) 653-61.

Hoybye, C., Thoren, M., & Bohm, B. (2005). Cognitive, emotional, physical and social effects of growth hormone treatment in adults with Prader-Willi syndrome. *Journal of Intellectual Disability Research, 49*(Pt. 4), 245-52.

Hughes, J. (1990). Assessment of social skills: Sociometric and behavioral approaches. In C.R. Reynolds, & R.W. Kamphaus (Eds.), *Handbook of psychological and educational assessment of children* (pp. 423-444). New York: Guildford Press.

Huston, D. (2006). Blossom. *Volunteer Resources Newsletter*. Innisfail, AB: Innisfail Health Centre.

James, T. (2006). *Real life stories: Stephen*. Retrieved March 22, 2009 from http://members.allstream.net/~opwsa/reallifestories.htm

James, T.N. (1987). Social and psychological aspects of Prader-Willi syndrome. Unpublished doctoral dissertation. The University of Calgary.

James, T.N. (1995). *Social competence and community tolerance of Prader-Willi syndrome.* Paper presented at the 2nd Prader-Willi Syndrome International Scientific Workshop and Conference, Sormarka, Oslo. Abstract Book, p. 24.

James, T.N., & Brown, R.I. (1992). Prader-Willi syndrome: Home, school and community. London, UK: Chapman & Hall.

James, T.N. (2010). *Prader-Willi syndrome: Growing older.* Courtenay, BC: Poplar Publishing.

James, T.N., & Willott, G. (1989). *Residential options in western Canada.* Calgary, AB: Prader-Willi Syndrome Association of Alberta.

Jamin, T. (1990, May). Ray Ronald (1937-1990). *Under Prairie Skies* [L'Arche], 49, p. 2.

Johnson, R. (2004). *The way life is.* Victoria, BC: Trafford.

Joseph, B., Egli, M., Sutcliffe, J.S., & Thompson, T. (2001). Possible dosage effect of maternally expressed genes on visual recognition memory in Prader-Willi syndrome. *American Journal of Medical Genetics, 105*(1), 71-75.

Kazemi, F., & Hodapp, R.M. (2006). Transition from adolescence to young adult: The special case of Prader-Willi syndrome. In M.G. Butler, P.D.K. Lee, & B.Y. Whitman (Eds.), *Management of Prader-Willi syndrome* (3rd ed.)(pp. 356-369). New York: Springer.

Kellerman, T. (2002, January/February). Picky, picky, picky: A parent's perspective. *The Gathered View, 27*(1), 5.

Key, A.P.F., & Dykens, E.M. (2008). 'Hungry eyes': Visual processing of food images in adults with Prader-Willi syndrome, *Journal of Intellectual Disability Research, 52*(Pt. 6), 536-546.

Kinash, S. (2007a). *Dis-abling attitudes: Prader-Willi syndrome* [DVD]. Calgary, AB: University of Calgary.

Kinash, S. (2007b). *Prader-Willi syndrome through the lifespan* [DVD]. Calgary, AB: University of Calgary.

Kinash, S. (2007c). *A recipe for success*. Charlotte, NC: Information Age Publishing.

King, G. (1988). Help wanted: Relief for parents. *Entourage, 3*(2), 26-32.

Koenig, K., Klin, A., & Schultz, R. (2004). Deficits in social attribution ability in Prader-Willi syndrome [Abstract]. *Journal of Autism and Developmental Disorders, 34*(5), 573-582.

Laurnen, E.L. (1981). Scoliosis in Prader-Willi syndrome. In V.A. Holm, S.J. Sulzbacher, & P. Pipes (Eds.), *Prader-Willi syndrome* (293-298). Baltimore: University Park Press.

Ledbetter, D.H., Riccardi, V.M., Airhart, S.D., Strobel, R.J., Keenen, S.B., & Crawford, J.D. (1981). Deletion of chromosome 15 as a cause of the Prader-Willi syndrome. *New England Journal of Medicine, 304*, 325-329.

Lee, P.D.K. (1995). Endocrine and metabolic aspects of Prader-Willi syndrome. In L.R. Greenswag, & R.C. Alexander (Eds.), *Management of Prader-Willi syndrome* (2nd ed.)(pp. 32-57). New York: Springer-Verlag.

Levine, K., & Wharton, R.H. (1993). Children with Prader-Willi syndrome: Information for school staff. *Prader-Willi Perspectives: Prader-Willi Syndrome Information Series No. 1*. New York: Visible Ink .

Levine, K., Wharton, R., & Fragala, M. (1993). Educational considerations for children with Prader-Willi syndrome and their families. *Prader-Willi Perspectives, 1*(3), 3-9.

Lewis, B.A. (2006). Speech and language disorders with Prader-Willi syndrome. In M.G. Butler, P.D.K. Lee, & B.Y. Whitman (Eds.), *Management of Prader-Willi syndrome* (3rd ed.) (pp. 272-280). New York: Springer.

Lindgren, A.C., & Ritzen, E.M. (1999). Five years of growth hormone treatment in children with Prader-Willi syndrome. Swedish National Growth Hormone Advisory Group. *Acta Paediat Suppl, 88*(433), 109-111.

Lunman, K. (1990, June 20). Judge fines woman with food disorder. *Calgary Herald*, p. B1.

McLellan, W. (1998, January 9). Runaway eluded caregivers on incredible journey to U.S. *The Province*, p. A10.

McNair, J., & Smith, H.K. (2000). Church attendance of adults with developmental disabilities. *Education and Training in Mental Retardation and Developmental Disabilities, 35*(2), 222-225.

Mandel, V. (2003a, September 1). Binge eater freed from jail. Judge demands treatment for sufferer of rare disorder. *Windsor Star*. Retrieved September 01, 2003, from http://www.canada.com

Mandel, V. (2003b, September 5). Ontario to fund U.S. treatment program for teen-age sufferer of rare binge-eating disorder. Don Mills, ON: CanWest News. ProQuest document ID 403746801.

Mario, D. (2008, March 1). Giving: Telemiracle beneficiaries give back. *The Star-Phoenix,* p. A43.

Marlett, N. (1991). Voices of young adults who live with Prader-Willi syndrome: A beginning. *Journal of Practical Approaches to Developmental Handicap, 15*(10), 22-25.

Miller, J., Silverstein, J., Shuster, J., Driscoll, D.J., & Wagner, M. (2006). Short-term effects of growth hormone on sleep abnormalities in Prader-Willi syndrome. *Journal of Clinical Endocrinology Metabolism, 91*(2), 413-17.

Morris, S. (2003). Dual diagnosis. Retrieved May 18, 2010, from http://www.camh.net/Care_Treatment/Program_Descriptions/Mental_Health_Programs/Dual_Diagnosis/dual_diagnosis_morris_ppao2003.pdf

Myers, S.E., Whitman, B.Y., Carrel, A.L., Moerchen, V., Belcx, M.T., & Allen, D.B. (2006). Two years of growth hormone therapy in young children with Prader-Willi syndrome: Physical and neurodevelopmental benefits. *American Journal of Medical Genetics*, Part A 143A, 443-448.

Nagai, T., Obata, K., Ogata, T., Muralcami, N., Katada, Y., Yoshino, A., Sakazume, S., Tomita, Y., Sakuta, R., & Niikawa, N. (2006). Growth hormone therapy and scoliosis in patients with Prader-Willi syndrome. *American Journal of Medical Genetics*, Part A 140A, 1623-1627.

Nicholas, K. (1999). Conference benefits: Help & understanding for tough behaviors. *The Gathered View, 24*(2), 11.

Nicholls, R.D., Knoll, J.H.M., Butler, M.G., Karam, S., & Lalande, M. (1989). Genetic imprinting suggested by maternal heterodisomy in non-deletion Prader-Willi syndrome. *Nature (London), 342,* 281-285.

Nowak, A.J. (1995). Dental manifestations and management. In L. R. Greenswag, & R. C. Alexander (Eds.), *Management of Prader-Willi syndrome* (2nd ed.)(pp. 81-87). New York: Springer-Verlag.

Ontario Prader-Willi Syndrome Association (2006). *Red Yellow Green System for weight management.* Toronto, ON: Author.

PDD. (2007). *Persons with developmental disabilities.* Calgary, AB: South Alberta Community Board.

Poston, D.J., & Turnbull, A.P. (2004). Role of spirituality and religion in family quality of life for families of children with disabilities. *Education and Training in Developmental Disabilities, 39*(2), 95-108.

Pound, B. (December, 2002) . Therapeutic delight. *The Canadian Journal of Diagnosis*, 21.

Prader, A., Labhart, A., & Willi, H. (1956). Ein sydrom von adipositas, kleinwuchs, kryptorchismus, and oligophrenie nach myotonieartigem zustand im neugeborenenalter. (A syndrome of obesity, short stature, cryptochism, and oligoprenia, with amyotonia in the newborn period.) Schweizerische Medizinische Wochenschrift, *86*, 1260-1261.

Prader-Willi Syndrome Association (USA). (n.d.). Information for school staff. In *Pupils wanting success* [Educational package]. Sarasota, FL: Author.

Prader-Willi Syndrome Association of B. C. (n.d.). *Prader-Willi syndrome.* Vancouver: Author.

PWSA-USA. (2004). *Adults with Prader-Willi syndrome and decisions regarding least restrictive environment and the right to eat.* Retrieved March 15, 2009, from http:// www.pwsausa.org/postion/ps002.htm

PWSA-USA. (2007). Advisory for care providers exploring the dangers of positional asphyxia. Retrieved August 22, 2010, from www.pwsausa.org

Roof, E., Stone, W., Feurer, I.D., Thompson, T., & Butler, M.G. (2000). Intellectual characteristics of Prader-Willi syndrome: Comparison of genetic subtypes. *Journal of Intellectual Disability Research, 44*(Pt. 1), 25-30.

Rosner, B.A., Hodapp, R.M., Fidler, D.J., Sagun, J.N., & Dykens, E.M. (2004). Social competence in persons with Prader-Willi, Williams, and Down's syndromes. *Journal of Applied Research in Intellectual Disabilities, 17*, 209-217.

Schrander-Stumpel, C.T., Curfs, L.M., Sastrowijoto, P., Cassidy, S.B., Schrander, J.J., & Fryns, J.P. (2004). Prader-Willi syndrome: Causes of death in an international series of 27 cases. *American Journal of Medical Genetics, 124A*(4), 333-338.

Schultze, A. (2000, May). A woman with Prader-Willi syndrome gave birth to a girl with Angelman syndrome. *Wavelength, 9*(1), 17.

Sellinger, M.H., Hodapp, R.M., & Dykens, E.M. (2006). Leisure activities of individuals with Prader-Willi, Williams, and Down syndromes. *Journal of Developmental & Physical Disabilities, 18*(1), 59-71.

Smith, E. (2003/2004, Winter). Yes! Women with Prader-Willi syndrome can give birth. *Prader-Willi Alliance of New York, Inc. Newsletter, 13*(4), 14.

Special Olympics Canada. (2009). SOC official sports. Retrieved March 22, 2009, from http://www.specialolympics.ca/en/default.aspx?tabid-10000023

Stadler, D. (1995). Nutritional management. In L.R. Greenswag, & R.C. Alexander (Eds.), *Management of Prader-Willi syndrome* (2nd ed.) (pp. 88-114). New York: Springer-Verlag.

Steinhausen, H.C., Eiholzer, U., Hauffa, B.P., & Malin, Z. (2004). Behavioural and emotional disturbances in people with Prader–Willi syndrome. *Journal of Intellectual Disability Research, 48* (Pt. 1), 47-52.

Stevenson, D.A., Heinemann, J., Angulo, M., Butler, M.G., Loker, J., Ruupe, N., Kendall, P., Cassidy, S.B., & Scheimann, A. (2007). Gastric rupture and necrosis in Prader-Willi syndrome. *Journal of Pediatric Gastroenterolgie Nutr., 45*(2), 272-4.

Stewart, M. (1992, June 25). Toddler's disease produces appetite that threatens to cost him his life. *Vancouver Sun,* p. A3.

Symons, J. (1997, June).   Letters from Johnny.   *Wavelength & Scientific Newsletter,* 6(1), 12.

Symons, F.J., Butler, M.G., Sanders, M.D., Feurer, I.D., & Thompson, T. (1999). Self-injurious behavior and Prader-Willi syndrome: Behavioral forms and body locations. *American Journal on Mental Retardation, 104* (3), 260-269.

Thom, H. (1995, August). In loving memory of Trevor. *The Gathered View, XX.* (4), 11.

Thune, L.N. (1998, May-June). Osteoporosis, calcium, and PWS. *The Gathered View, XXIII*(3), 6-8.

Unterberger, D. (2003). Low-fat, low-sugar recipes for the Prader-Willi syndrome diet. Sarasota, FL: PWSA-USA.

VanHooren, R.H., Widdershoven, G.A.M., Van den Borne, H.W., & Curfs, L.M.G. (2002). Autonomy and intellectual disability: The case of prevention of obesity in Prader-Willi syndrome. *Journal of Intellectual Disability Research, 46*(7), 560-568.

Van Wageningen, E. (2004, March 30). Crown doesn't have appetite to proceed with charges against Prader-Willi teen. Don Mills, ON: CanWest News. ProQuest document ID 608621871.

Vela Microboard Association. (1997). Microboards [Brochure]. Surrey, BC: Author.

Villa Charities Newsletter. (2005). Prader-Willi home of success! Retrieved from http://www.villacharities.com/newsletter/archive/Summer2005/newsletter_main.asp?View=Vita2

Vogel, G., & Reiter, S. (2003). Spiritual dimensions of bar/bat mitzvah ceremonies for Jewish children with developmental disabilities. *Education and Training in Developmental Disabilities, 38*(3), 314-322.

Walley, R.M., & Donaldson, M.D.C. (2005). An investigation of executive function abilities in adults with Prader-Willi syndrome. *Journal of Intellectual Disability Research, 49*(Pt. 8), 613-625.

Waters, J., Jewson, N., Quinn, M., & Sharma, N. (2007). *Adults with Prader-Willi syndrome and their parents/carers: Report of a survey of members of PWSA(UK)*. Derby, UK: Prader-Willi Syndrome Association (UK).

Wett, M. (1989). *Proceedings of the 11th Annual National PWSA Conference*, Calgary, Alberta, Canada, p. 37.

Wharton, R. (2004, September-October). Stomach problems can signal serious illness. *The Gathered View, 29*(5), 6.

Whitman, B.Y. (1999, November). Using medications as a management strategy for persons with PWS. *Wavelength, 8*(12), 18-19.

Whitman, B.Y. (2006). Social work interventions: Advocacy and support for families. In M.G. Butler, P.D.K. Lee, & B.Y. Whitman (Eds.), *Management of Prader-Willi syndrome* (3rd ed.) (pp. 426-439). New York: Springer.

Whitman, B.Y., Myers, S., Carrel, A., & Allen, D. (2002). The behavioral impact of growth hormone treatment for children and adolescents with Prader-Willi syndrome: A 2-year, controlled study. *Pediatrics, 109*(2). Retrieved September 19, 2007, from http://www.pediatrics.org/cgi/content/full/109/2/e35

Whittington, J., Holland, A., Webb, T., Butler, J., Clarke, D., & Boer, H. (2004a). Cognitive abilities and genotype in a population-based sample of people with Prader-Willi syndrome. *Journal of Intellectual Disability Research, 48*(Pt. 2), 172-187.

Whittington, J., Holland, A., Webb, T., Butler, J., Clarke, D., & Boer, H. (2004b). Academic underachievement by people with Prader-Willi syndrome. *Journal of Intellectual Disability Research, 48*(Pt. 2), 188-2000.

Wigren, M., & Hansen, S. (2003). Rituals and compulsivity in Prader-Willi syndrome: Profile and stability. *Journal of Intellectual Disability Research, 47* (Pt. 6), 428-438.

Wigren, M., & Heimann, M. (2001). Excessive picking in Prader-Willi syndrome: A pilot study of phenomenological aspects and comorbid symptoms. *International Journal of Disability, Development and Education*, 48, 129-142.

Wolfensberger, W. (1972). The principle of normalization in human services. Toronto, ON: National Institute on Mental Retardation.

Wollmann, H.A., Schultz, U., Grauer, M.L., & Ranke, M.B. (1998). Reference values for height and weight in Prader-Willi syndrome based on 315 patients. *European Journal of Pediatrics, 157*, 634-642.

Yashinsky, D. (2008, January 8). Fishing not catching. *Toronto Globe & Mail*, p. L6.

Young, D. (1993). Prader-Willi syndrome. *Bridges, 2*(1), 6-9.

Young, J., Zarcone, J., Holsen, L., Anderson, M.C., Hall, S., Richman,D., Butler, M.G., &. Thompson, T. (2006). A measure of food seeking in individuals with Prader–Willi syndrome, *Journal of Intellectual Disability Research, 50*(Pt. 1), 18-24.

Ziccardi, M.K. (2006). Residential care for adults with Prader-Willi syndrome. In M.G. Butler, P.D.K. Lee, & B.Y. Whitman (Eds.), *Management of Prader-Willi syndrome* (3rd ed.)(pp. 381-394). New York: Springer.

Zellweger, H., & Schneider, H.J. (1968). Syndrome of hypotonia-hypomentia-hypogonadism-obesity (HHHO) or Prader-Willi syndrome. *American Journal of Diseases of Children, 115*, 588-598.

Index